To Dr

With my best regards

Aortitis

Clinical, Pathologic, and Radiographic Aspects

Aortitis
Clinical, Pathologic, and Radiographic Aspects

Editors

Adam Lande, M.D.

Clinical Associate Professor of Radiology
New York Medical College
Valhalla, New York
and
Attending Radiologist
Kingston Hospital
Kingston, New York

Yahya M. Berkmen, M.D.

Professor of Clinical Radiology
Cornell University Medical College
and
Chief, Pulmonary Radiology
The New York Hospital
New York, New York

Hugh A. McAllister, Jr., M.D.

Clinical Professor of Pathology
Baylor University College of Medicine
and
Chief, Cardiovascular Pathology
Texas Heart Institute
St. Luke's Episcopal Hospital
Houston, Texas

Raven Press ■ New York

Raven Press, 1140 Avenue of the Americas, New York, New York 10036

Made in the United States of America

Library of Congress Cataloging-in-Publication Data
Main entry under title:

Aortitis : clinical, pathologic, and radiographic
   aspects.

   Includes bibliographies and index.
   1. Aortitis. 2. Arteritis. I. Lande, Adam.
II. Berkmen, Yahya M. (Yahya Muhlis), 1929-
III. McAllister, Hugh A. [DNLM: 1. Aortitis—pathology.
2. Aortitis—radiography. WG 410 A6389]
RC694.5.A55A55 1986   616.1'38   85-20500
ISBN 0-88167-141-X

Preface

In the past few decades new forms of aortitis have been identified as separate clinical and pathological entities. At the same time, many systemic disorders have been shown to be associated with widespread arteritis. This is the first volume on aortitis to be published in this decade; it describes arteritis of the aorta and the large and medium sized elastic arteries, excluding arteritis of small muscular arteries. The volume is a compilation of information on various forms of aortitis heretofore scattered in the pages of numerous journals.

Aortitides of various etiologies frequently display similar clinical, pathological, and radiographic features. Because of the overlapping patterns, all factors have to be considered carefully in evaluating a particular type of aortitis. Many forms of aortitis are deceptive and misleading in their clinical presentation, and several have been named great imitators of medicine (syphilis, Takayasu's arteritis, giant cell arteritis). Symptomatology is varied, and patients are often treated for a variety of complaints without exploration of the underlying etiology. Some forms of aortitis have a peculiar affinity for favoring specific symptomatology with general systemic, cardiac, pulmonary, neurological, ophthalmological, dermatological, and other symptoms predominating. So, familiarity with the natural history of different types of aortitis, their clinical presentation, as well as their pathological and radiographic characteristics is essential if a correct diagnosis is to be made.

The purpose of this volume is to put into sharper focus various forms of aortitis, permitting their more accurate identification and differentiation. This volume provides new clinical information and new pathological and radiographic methods of aortitis diagnosis not found in any other publication. The section on radiology discusses the newest imaging modalities, including CAT and NMR; also, it presents the largest display of arteriography of aortitis in the literature. For the first time in the English literature, the surgical treatment of different types of aortitis is presented. The chapters on ophthalmology, neurology, and pediatrics are written by experts in their specific fields of interest.

Some types of aortitis thought to be rare or nonexistent in the United States have been shown to be relatively common. They are, however, notoriously missed in the daily clinical practice because of the lack of specific clinical and pathological criteria. This volume clarifies many misconceptions and fills an important clinical vacuum. It is a volume no clinician can afford to miss.

Adam Lande, M.D.

Contents

Contributors

John Baum   *Departments of Pediatrics and Medicine, University of Rochester School of Medicine and Dentistry, Rochester, New York 14620; and Arthritis and Clinical Immunology Unit, Monroe Community Hospital, Rochester, New York 14603*

Yahya M. Berkmen   *Department of Clinical Radiology, Cornell University Medical College, and Section of Pulmonary Radiology, New York Hospital, 525 East 68th Street, New York, New York 10021*

John C. M. Brust   *Department of Clinical Neurology, Columbia University College of Physicians and Surgeons, New York, New York 10027; and Department of Neurology, Harlem Hospital, New York, New York 10037*

Denton A. Cooley   *Division of Surgery, University of Texas Medical School of Houston, and Texas Heart Institute, St. Luke's Episcopal and Texas Children's Hospitals, Houston, Texas 77025*

J. Michael Duncan   *Division of Surgery, University of Texas Medical School of Houston, and Texas Heart Institute, St. Luke's Episcopal and Texas Children's Hospitals, Houston, Texas 77025*

Murk-Hein Heinemann   *Department of Ophthalmology, Cornell University Medical College, and New York Hospital, New York, New York 10021*

Gene G. Hunder   *Department of Medicine, Mayo Medical School, Rochester, Minnesota 55905*

Leslie D. Kerr   *Department of Medicine, Division of Rheumatology, Mount Sinai School of Medicine and Mount Sinai Hospital, New York, New York 10299*

Adam Lande   *Department of Radiology, New York Medical College, Valhalla, New York; and Department of Radiology, Kingston Hospital, 396 Broadway, Kingston, New York 12401*

Eulo Lupi Herrera   *National Institute of Cardiology of Mexico, "Ignacio Chávez," Mexico City, Mexico*

Hugh A. McAllister, Jr.   *Department of Cardiovascular Pathology, Texas Heart Institute, St. Luke's Episcopal Hospital, 6720 Bertner Street, Houston, Texas 77030; and Department of Pathology, Baylor University College of Medicine, Houston, Texas 77025*

Mario Seoane　*National Institute of Cardiology of Mexico, "Ignacio Chávez," Mexico City, Mexico*

Jesse Sigelman　*Department of Ophthalmology, Cornell University Medical College, and New York Hospital, New York, New York 10021*

Harry Spiera　*Department of Medicine, Division of Rheumatology, Mount Sinai School of Medicine and Mount Sinai Hospital, New York, New York 10029*

Renu Virmani　*Department of Cardiovascular Pathology, Armed Forces Institute of Pathology, Washington, D.C. 20306; and Department of Pathology, Vanderbilt University, Nashville, Tennessee 37232*

Aortitis: Clinical, Pathologic, and Radiographic Aspects, edited by A. Lande, Y. M. Berkmen, and H. A. McAllister. Raven Press, New York © 1986.

Historical Background of Aortitis

Yahya M. Berkmen

Department of Clinical Radiology, Cornell University Medical College, and Section of Pulmonary Radiology, New York Hospital, New York, New York 10021

When we speak of "history" we are usually thinking of the collective experience of the human race; but the individual experience that each one of us gathers in a single lifetime is history, just as truely.

Arnold J. Toynbee, *Change and Habit*

Recognition of aortitis as an entity dates back to the late sixteenth century when Ambroise Paré first associated aortic aneurysm with syphilis. Syphilis was then a widespread disease and remained so until the early part of the twentieth century, dominating the entire field of medicine as no other disease has ever done. This dominance found its expression in Sir William Osler's proverbial words: "Know syphilis in all its manifestations and relations, and all other things clinical will be added unto you." During this long period, syphilis was first the sole, and then the most prevalent, cause of aortitis. It may be said that the history of aortitis is the history of a rise and fall of the "empire" of syphilis.

Opinions differ regarding the geographic and chronologic origins of syphilis. It is well known, however, that an epidemic of unprecedented proportions swept Europe shortly after Columbus' return from the New World. It all seems to have started with the invasion of Italy in 1494 by Charles VIII of France. His army was mainly composed of missionaries from other countries including many Spaniards from Columbus' crew.

Originally the disease ran very acutely with high fever, severe headache, generalized pain, marked prostration, and a rapidly fatal outcome. This virulent course subsided within 50 years and took the more chronic and slowly progressive form that has been known since.

The disease created panic everywhere, and it was considered to be due to celestial vengeance against man's vices and sins. This ailment with no name and seemingly theretofore unknown in Europe dispersed with great devastation to the other parts of the world in an exceedingly short time. It made its appearance in Switzerland, Germany, and France in 1495, Holland and Greece in 1496, England and Scotland in 1497, Hungary and Russia in 1499. It reached India in 1498, China in 1505, and Japan in 1569.

Each nation blamed the other for spreading the disease: The Spanish called it Española disease, Italians called it Spanish disease, French called it Italian disease, Turks and English called it French disease. It was Turkish disease to the Persians, Polish disease to the Russians, and Portuguese disease in India and Japan.

Whether syphilis existed in Europe before Columbus' return from the New World is an unresolved issue. Disciples of both schools claim to have proof for their assertion.

The disease got its name from Girolamo Fracastoro's poem "Syphilis sive Morbul Gallicus" written in 1530. It was also called *lues venera* by Fernel in 1546.

Until the end of the nineteenth century, a great body of clinical information was collected about syphilis, and its treatment first with mercury and then with arsenic was introduced. Men like Paracelsus, Ambroise Paré, Jean Astruc, Morgagni, and Philippe Ricord among many others contributed to this knowledge. Finally in 1905 *Spirocheta pallida* was identified by Schaudinn and Hoffman as the organism of syphilis. In 1906–1907, Wasserman, Neisser, and Bruck developed a serologic test known as the Wasserman test, and in 1911 Noguchi introduced culture medium for Spirochetae. Discovery of penicillin at the end of the first half of this century marked man's victory over the disease which brought so much suffering and misery to an untold number of people for 400 years.

Syphilis was recognized as a cause of cardiovascular disease and aortic aneurysm by Ambroise Paré and later by Lancici, who died in 1720. However, it was in 1875 that Francis Welch furnished unequivocal evidence of a cause-and-effect relationship between syphilis and aortic aneurysms. It was also during the nineteenth century that the detailed morbid anatomy and histology of syphilitic aortitis were studied in detail. The grossly wrinkled intima of the aorta was described as having a "tree-bark" appearance and was considered typical of syphilitic aortitis. These gross features were accepted as pathognomonic for syphilis, and it was considered sufficient to make a specific diagnosis on the basis of the macroscopic appearance alone.

During the early part of the twentieth century, the association of aortitis with systemic diseases began to gain recognition. According to Pappenheimer and Von Glahn, in 1912 Rabe and Klotz independently gave the first descriptions of the histology of aortitis caused by rheumatic fever (27). This was followed by the publications of Pappenheimer and Von Glahn in 1924 and 1927 (27,28) on the same subject. In 1936 Mallory presented two similar cases of aortitis occurring in young males with "arthritis" and prophesied that "some of these as yet unclassified processes may produce lesions indistinguishable from those of syphilis" (24). Later, other observers confirmed the nonspecificity of tree-barking and, on the basis of macro- and microscopic similarities of various aortitides, concluded that it was frequently impossible to distinguish one form of aortitis from another apparently because of limited ways of response of the aorta to different insults (9,35).

In 1937 Sproul and Hawthorne (37) described a different type of nonspecific aortitis with giant cells and called it "chronic diffuse mesoaortitis," which in 1941 was renamed "giant cell chronic arteritis" by Gilmour (12). In a few years, clinical and histologic overlaps between giant cell arteritis and temporal arteritis of Horton and Magath (1932) (18), polymyalgia rheumatica of Barber (1957) (3), and polymyalgia arteritica of Hamrin et al. (1965) (15) became obvious. These entities have now been grouped together under the name giant cell arteritis and are considered to be part of a large spectrum of the same disease.

Meanwhile other systemic diseases associated with aortitis were described in rapid sequence: ankylosing spondylitis (5), scleroderma (33), relapsing polychondritis (29), Behçet's syndrome (17), Reiter's syndrome (13), systemic lupus erythematosus, Crohn's disease, psoriasis, etc.

Although syphilis was still the major cause of aortitis during the nineteenth century, in the second half of the century aortitis due to other inflammations came to be observed with increasing frequency. In 1847 Virchow and in 1853 Tufnell described suppurative aortitis with aneurysm formation. Osler in 1885 used the term of "mycotic" in reference to aortitis associated with subacute bacterial endocarditis. The period was marked by rampant infections of all varieties. Rheumatic fever and aortic and/or mitral valvular diseases as its sequelae were very common. These damaged leaflets, highly susceptible to superimposed infection, were frequently the seat of bacterial vegetations. Thus bacterial endocarditis remained as the single most common cause of mycotic aneurysms until the clinical application of antibiotics. To indicate this causal relationship, Eppinger introduced the term of "embolomycotic" in 1887.

It was not too long, however, before it was appreciated that infectious aortitis could occur without intravascular infection. Rappaport in 1926 referred to these cases as "primary mycotic aortitis" (30) and Crane in 1937 as "primary mycotic aneurysm" (8). The term "secondary" was reserved for the majority of mycotic aneurysms caused by bacterial endocarditis.

In 1945 antibiotics entered the medical scene and revolutionized the field of infectious diseases. The incidence of rheumatic fever diminished to a negligible minimum. The balance between secondary and primary mycotic aneurysm changed in favor of the primary variety. Blum and Keefer in 1962 proposed to substitute the term "cryptogenic" for "primary" and applied it to those mycotic aneurysms arising in the absence of endocarditis or other local systemic infections (7). Parallel to these changes, bacteria responsible for aortitis during the preantibiotic era, e.g., pneumococci, streptococci, and *Hemophilus influenzae*, have been mainly replaced by *Salmonella* and *Staphylococcus*.

Antibiotics favorably affected the incidence of syphilis, as has been mentioned. As syphilitic aortitis became a rarity, so did syphilitic aneurysms. Studies now suggest that syphilis is no longer a significant factor in the overall formation of aortic aneurysms (6). With this decline in the frequency of cardiovascular complications of syphilis, atherosclerosis became a predominant cause of aortic aneurysms. It seems almost as if nature has taken revenge and secondary infections have become a significant complication of atherosclerotic aortic aneurysms, known as infected aneurysms. *Salmonella*, again, has been the most commonly blamed culprit in these infections.

Since the end of World War II, intravenous drug abuse has spread throughout the United States in epidemic proportions (21). There has been a dramatic rise in the incidence of septic emboli, acute bacterial endocarditis, and mycotic aneurysms of the aorta. Coincidental with this, iatrogenic intravenous infections associated with intravenous catheters, angiography, cutdowns, and arterial access procedures has been utilized with increasing frequency, and their complications, especially those due to infection, have risen proportionally.

Technical advances in vascular surgery resulted in the performance of large numbers of bypass and graft procedures. Infections of these lifesaving interventions have become common. Infection in 1 to 3% of all grafts, with mortality rates approaching 50%, are being reported (39).

Among inflammatory aortitides and mycotic aneurysms, tuberculosis has always occupied a minor role. Weigert is credited with the description of tuberculous aortitis for the first time in 1882.

In 1856 Savory introduced a totally different type of arteritis (34). His patient was a young woman with obliteration of her vessels to both upper extremities and the left common carotid artery. This report apparently remained in oblivion for several decades, and when Takayasu, a Japanese ophthalmologist, reported ischemic retinopathy in a young woman (38) he was probably neither aware of Savory's article nor cognizant of the fact that he was describing a new disease, a form of aortitis that was to be known as Takayasu's arteritis.

Diverse clinical manifestations of Takayasu's arteritis have been responsible for much confusion which lasted until recently. In the earlier part of this century, different aspects of Takayasu's arteritis with its broad spectrum of sequelae have been individually described under various names as separate entities. Terms such as pulseless disease, brachiocephalic arteritis (41), aortic arch syndrome (32), brachiocephalic ischemia (26), brachial arteritis (10), aortic arch arteritis (4,23), sclerosing aortitis (16), aortitis syndrome (40), nonsyphilitic aortitis (31), the middle aortic syndrome (36), etc. testify to the erroneous application of terms to localized forms of Takayasu's arteritis (14).

Gradually, however, a unifying concept emerged as it became evident that all these cases described under different names were part of a larger and more complex disease, Takayasu's arteritis. The name suggested by Judge et al. (22) has been accepted and is used by the majority of authors today.

Among the numerous investigators who contributed to this realization, only a few can be mentioned here. Shimizu and Sano gave detailed clinical features of the disease in 1948. Frövig and Löken in 1951 (11) and Ask-Upmark in 1954 (1) reported the first groups of patients outside Japan. Ask-Upmark and Frajers in 1956 first noted that the disease was not necessarily confined to the aortic arch and its branches but could affect the entire aorta and all of its branches (2). Kimoto in 1960, Inada et al. in 1962 (19,20), Nako et al. in 1967 (25), and Sen in 1968 (35) have shown that Takayasu's arteritis and atypical coarctation of the aorta are one and the same disease.

The saga of aortitis is not complete. The mysteries of its immunologic and genetic aspects are now being probed, and its history is still in the making. It is hoped that this short overview of the history of aortitis will provide the reader with a perspective into the entity as a whole and pay tribute to those physicians who contributed to our understanding and knowledge of aortitis.

REFERENCES

1. Ask-Upmark, E. (1954): On the "pulseless disease" outside of Japan. *Acta Med. Scand.*, 149:161–178.
2. Ask-Upmark, E., and Frajers, C.-M. (1956): Further observations on Takayasu's syndrome. *Acta Med. Scand.*, 155:275–291.
3. Barber, H. S. (1957): Myalgic syndrome with constitutional effects—polymyalgia rheumatica. *Ann. Rheum. Dis.*, 16:230–237.
4. Barker, N. W. and Edwards, J. E. (1955): Primary arteritis of the aortic arch. *Circulation*, 11:486–492.
5. Bauer, W., Clark, W. S., and Kulka, J. P. (1951): Aortitis and aortic endocarditis—an unrecognized manifestation of rheumatoid arthritis. *Ann. Rheum. Dis.*, 10:470–471.
6. Bickerstaff, L. K., Pairolero, P. C., Hollier, L. H., et al. (1982): Thoracic aortic aneurysms—a population-based study. *Surgery*, 92:1103–1108.
7. Blum, L., and Keefer, E. B. C. (1962): Cryptogenic mycotic aneurysms. *Ann. Surg.*, 155:398–405.
8. Crane, A. R. (1937): Primary multiocular mycotic aneurysms of the aorta. *Arch. Pathol.*, 24:634–641.
9. De Takas, G. (1959): Arterial injuries and arterial inflammation. In: *Vascular Surgery*, p. 130. Saunders, Philadelphia.
10. Edling, N. P. G., Nystrom, B., and Seldinger, S. I. (1961): Brachial arteritis in the aortic arch syndrome. A roentgen and differential diagnostic study. *Acta Radiol.*, 55:417–432.
11. Frövig, G. A., and Löken, C. A. (1951): Syndrome of obliteration of arterial branches of aortic arch due to arteritis. *Acta Psychiatr. Neurol. Scand.*, 26:313–317.
12. Gilmour, J. R. (1941): Giant-cell chronic arteritis. *J. Pathol. Bacteriol.*, 53:263–277.
13. Good, A. E. (1974): Reiter's disease—a review with special attention to cardiovascular and neurologic sequelae. *Semin. Arthritis Rheum.*, 3:253–286.
14. Hachiya, J. (1970): Current concepts of Takayasu's arteritis. *Semin. Roentgenol.*, 5:245–259.
15. Hamrin, B., Jonsson, N., and Landberg, T. (1965): Involvement of large vessels in polymyalgia rheumatica. *Lancet*, 1:1193–1196.
16. Harrell, J., and Manion, W. C. (1970): Sclerosing aortitis and arteritis. *Semin. Roentgenol.*, 5:260–266.
17. Hills, E. (1967): Behçet's syndrome with aortic aneurysms. *Br. Med. J.*, 4:152–154.
18. Horton, B. T., and Magath, T. B. (1932): An undescribed form of arteritis of the temporal vessels. *Proc. Staff Meet. Mayo Clin.*, 7:700–707.
19. Inada, K., Shimizu, H., Kobayashi, I., et al. (1962): Pulseless disease and atypical coarctation of the aorta. *Arch. Surg.*, 84:306–311.
20. Inada, K., Shimizu, H., and Yokoyama, T. (1962): Pulseless disease and atypical coarctation of aorta with special reference to their genesis. *Surgery*, 52:433–443.
21. Jaffe, R. B., and Koschmann, E. B. (1970): Intravenous drug abuse—pulmonary, cardiac, and vascular complications. *Am. J. Roentgenol*, 109:107–120.
22. Judge, R. D., Currier, R. D., Gracie, W. A., and Figley, M. M. (1962): Takayasu's arteritis and the aortic arch syndrome. *Am. J. Med.*, 32:379–392.
23. Koszewski, B. J. (1958): Branchial arteritis or aortic arch arteritis: A new inflammatory arterial disease (pulseless disease). *Angiology*, 9:180–186.
24. Mallory, T. B. (1936): Case records of the Massachusetts General Hospital: Case #221411. *N. Engl. J. Med.*, 214:690–698.
25. Nako, K., Ikada, M., Kimata, S., et al. (1967): Takayasu's arteritis. *Circulation*, 35:1141–1155.
26. Ochsner, J. L., and Hewitt, R. L. (1967): Aortic arch syndrome (brachiocephalic ischemia). *Dis. Chest*, 52:69–82.
27. Pappenheimer, A. M., and Von Glahn, W. C. (1924): Lesions of the aorta associated with acute rheumatic fever, and with chronic cardiac disease of rheumatic origin. *J. Med. Res.*, 44:489–505.
28. Pappenheimer, A. M., and Von Glahn, W. C. (1927): Studies in the pathology of rheumatic fever—two cases presenting unusual cardiovascular lesions. *Am. J. Pathol.*, 3:583–594.
29. Pearson, C. M., Kroening, R., Verity, M. A., and Getzen, J. H. (1967): Aortic insufficiency and aortic aneurysm in relapsing polychondritis. *Trans. Assoc. Am. Physicians*, 80:71–90.
30. Rappaport, B. Z. (1926): Primary acute aortitis. *Arch. Pathol. Lab. Med.*, 2:653–658.
31. Restrepo, C., Tejeda, C., and Correa, P. (1969): Nonsyphilitic aortitis. *Arch. Pathol.*, 87:1–12.

32. Ross, R. S., and McKusick, V. A. (1963): Aortic arch syndromes: Diminished or absent pulses in arteries arising from arch of aorta. *Arch. Intern. Med.*, 92:701–740.

33. Roth, L. M., and Kissane, J. M. (1964): Panaortitis and aortic valvulitis in progressive systemic sclerosis (scleroderma)—report of a case with perforation of an aortic cusp. *Am. J. Clin. Pathol.*, 41:287–296.

34. Savory, W. S. (1856): Case of a young woman in whom the main arteries of both upper extremities of the left side of the neck were throughout completely obliterated. *Med. Chir. Trans. Lond.*, 39:205.

35. Sen, P. K. (1968): Obstructive disease of the aorta and its branches. *Indian J. Surg.*, 30:289–327.

36. Sen, P. K., Kinare, S. G., Engineer, S. D., et al. (1963): The middle aortic syndrome. *Br. Heart J.*, 25:610–618.

37. Sproul, E. E., and Hawthorne, J. J. (1937): Chronic diffuse mesoaortitis. *Am. J. Pathol.*, 13:311–323.

38. Takayasu, H. (1908): A case with peculiar changes of the central retinal arteries. *Acta Soc. Ophthalmol. Jpn.*, 12:554.

39. Thompson, J. E., and Garrett, W. V. (1980): Peripheral arterial surgery. *N. Engl. J. Med.*, 302:491–503.

40. Ueda, H., Morooka, S., Ito, I., et al. (1969): Clinical observations on 52 cases of aortic arch syndrome. *Jpn. Heart J.*, 10:277–288.

41. Wickbom, I. (1957): Arteriography in brachiocephalic arteritis (pulseless disease or Takayasu's syndrome). *Acta Radiol.*, 48:321–329.

Aortitis: Clinical, Pathologic, and Radiographic Aspects, edited by A. Lande, Y. M. Berkmen, and H. A. McAllister. Raven Press, New York © 1986.

Pathology of the Aorta and Major Arteries

Renu Virmani and *Hugh A. McAllister, Jr.

*Department of Cardiovascular Pathology, Armed Forces Institute of Pathology, Washington, D.C., 20306; and Department of Pathology, Vanderbilt University, Nashville, Tennessee 37232; *Department of Cardiovascular Pathology, Texas Heart Institute, St. Luke's Episcopal Hospital, Houston, Texas 77030; and Department of Pathology, Baylor University College of Medicine, Houston, Texas 77025*

NORMAL AORTA

The aorta is the main trunk of the systemic arteries and carries oxygenated blood to all the body organs and tissues. It is an elastic artery composed of three layers: a thin tunica intima, a thick tunica media composed of numerous longitudinally oriented elastic laminae, and a thin outer collagenous layer, the adventitia. The media with its spirally arranged elastic lamellae provides tensile strength and elasticity. The aorta consists of thoracic and abdominal portions. The thoracic aorta is composed of the ascending aorta, arch, and descending aorta. The ascending aorta is about 3 cm wide in an adult and extends from the aortic valve to 5 to 6 cm cephalad to join the arch. The arch of the aorta gives rise to all brachiocephalic vessels, lying almost anteroposterior within the superior mediastinum and closely related to left phrenic and vagus nerves. The descending thoracic aorta is the continuation of the arch and lies in the posterior mediastinum to the left of the vertebral column; it then comes to lie in front of the vertebral column and passes through the diaphragm at the level of the 12th thoracic vertebra.

Tunica Intima

The intima at birth is lined by a single layer of flattened endothelial cells and is limited toward the media by the internal elastic lamina. As age advances, a narrow connective tissue layer is interposed between the endothelial layer and the elastic laminae (91). The intima gradually thickens over the years. Soon after birth or by a few months, connective tissue appears which is induced by the migration of smooth muscle cells from the media, through the orifices in the internal elastic lamina. The smooth muscle cells then produce the fibrous connective tissue (48–50).

The fully developed intima consists of three distinct layers. The first to form is the musculoelastic layer, which lies adjacent to the internal elastic lamina (50). It

The opinions or assertions contained herein are the private views of the authors and are not to be construed as official or as reflecting the views of the Department of the Army or the Department of Defense.

is composed of smooth muscle cells which lie parallel to the longitudinal axis of the vessel. The other component comprises the elastic lamellae, which are closely associated with the smooth muscle cells and are either produced by the smooth muscle cells or are the product of the splitting of the internal elastic lamina. The musculoelastic layer is loosely arranged in the collagen and acid mucopolysaccharide ground substance (50). This musculoelastic layer gets fully developed toward the latter half of the first decade of life (38,91).

The second layer to develop is the elastic hyperplastic layer consisting of elastic fibers running at first parallel to the longitudinal axis of the vessel; as their numbers increase they become circumferential (91). The elastic fibers are embedded in a background of acid mucopolysaccharide with a few collagen fibers and smooth muscle cells (49). This layer is well developed by the second decade, but it continues to grow and may not be easily separated from the elastic hyperplastic layer (49,91).

The third layer, which is closest to the internal elastic lamina, consists of connective tissue intermingled with occasional elastic tissue fibrils within a background of acid mucopolysaccharide. This layer is the most inconsistent (91), but with increasing age the collagen becomes hyalinized and there is a decrease in mucopolysaccharides. The intima is thicker in the abdominal aorta than the thoracic aorta in adults. The three individual layers may be difficult to identify (91) in older individuals.

Tunica Media

The media consists of numerous layers of longitudinally oriented elastic laminae. The space between elastic lamellae contains smooth muscle cells and collagen fibrils in mucopolysaccharide ground substance. Varying numbers of branches extend from the elastic lamellae and intermix with smooth muscle cells and connective tissue. The spaces between elastic lamellae increase with age, and there is a decrease in medial elastic elements and partial replacement with collagen (91). This decrease in elasticity ultimately leads to dilatation of the aorta during old age. Collagen bundles are more numerous in the thoracic aorta, but the amount varies with different levels. In the ascending aorta, arch, and upper thoracic aorta the collagen is mainly aggregated in the inner media, whereas in the middle and lower thoracic aorta it occurs mainly in the outer media (14). Collagen bundles are uncommon in the media of the abdominal aorta.

The outer one-third to one-half of the media in the thoracic aorta is penetrated by adventitial vasa vasorum and lymphatics. It has been shown that vasa vasorum in mammalian elastic arteries are dependent on the number of units of elastic lamellae in the media, and only arteries with more than 28 such units have medial vasa vasorum. In humans only in the thoracic aorta which has more than 29 units are vasa vasorum found within the media (91). The number of elastic lamellae are maximum in the ascending aorta (approximately 56) and are most tightly opposed in the innermost part, i.e., close to the tunica intima. The arch is somewhat thinner than the ascending aorta, and continuous elastic lamellae are seen only in the outer two-thirds of the media. The media is further reduced in width in the upper descending thoracic aorta, with elastic laminae being closely opposed in the inner-most part of the media but spaced further apart in the outer half (14). The thoracic aorta just above the diaphragm has elastic lamellae which are regularly spaced, smoother, and less branched (14), whereas in the abdominal aorta the adventitia is almost as thick as the media and there is an increase in the number of elastic fibers in the outer media and the adventitia. The elastic laminae number approximately 28; they gradually decrease in number and are quite thin in the inner media compared to the outer media. However, the internal elastic lamina is well marked in the abdominal aorta (135,136) (Fig. 1).

Adventitia

The collagenous adventitia is the outermost layer and is not separated from the media by a distinct external elastic lamina; instead there is a dense network of medium-sized, short elastic lamellae interspersed in collagen. The thoracic aorta from its origin to the diaphragm has a thin adventia with few elastic fibers, whereas the abdominal aorta has a thick adventitia with an increase in elastic fibers. Within the adventitia are blood vessels (vasa vasorum), lymphatics, and nerves in loosely arranged collagen and elastic fibers. In the paramedial zone the collagen fibers are plump and appear hyalinized with a few smooth muscle cells longitudinally arranged (91).

AGING AORTA

The elastic fibers fragment with advancing age, and the smooth muscle cells decrease in number. The smooth muscle cells that remain may lose certain organ-elles, including nuclei. Collagen fibers apear to incrcasc with aging, and the amount of acid mucopolysaccharide also increases. Unless the increase in collagen is unusually marked, these changes cause the aorta to weaken, so that its lumen enlarges with age. This generalized dilatation, which is both a transverse and a longitudinal enlargement, has been described by Cooley (22) as "annuloaortic ectasia." Dilatation of the aorta during old age is not limited to the tubular portion but may extend into the sinus of Valsalva and cause aneurysms which have also been observed in syphilitic aortitis (51,122), Marfan's syndrome, and Ehlers-Danlos syndrome (108,123,126). The degenerative changes of the aorta seen with age involve focal or diffuse fragmentation of the elastic lamellae, and this is accom-panied by focal collections of acid mucopolysaccharide ground substance (5), what Erdheim in 1930 (34) described as "cystic medial necrosis." This focal weakness in the aortic root dilatation may cause displacement of the commissural attachments and result or aggravate aortic incompetence. This weakness with cystic medial change, especially in the setting of systemic hypertension, can cause aortic dissec-tions. Marfan's syndrome, which is an inherited connective tissue disorder, also has a high incidence of dissection and pathologically is associated with extensive degeneration of elastic fibers and accumulation of large amounts of acid mucopo-lysaccharide (5,109).

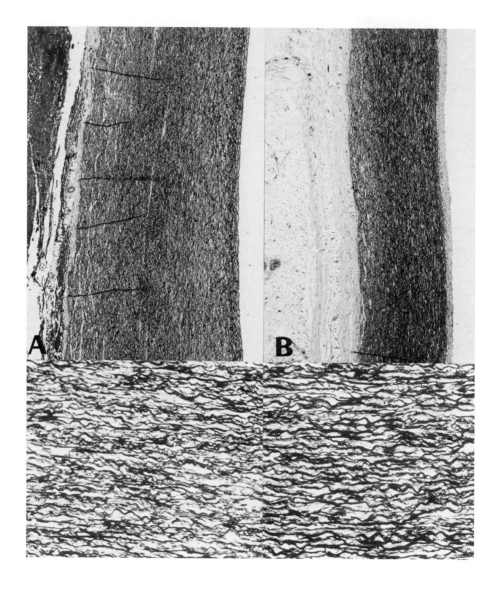

Another change in the aorta with age is the accumulation of amyloid. Amyloid has been uniformly noted to be present in all aortas in individuals beyond the age of 55 (23,116). All aortic amyloid is resistant to potassium permanganate reaction. Tryptophan is present in all amyloid deposits. Aortic amyloid does not react with antisera to amyloid fibril protein ASc, or human prealbumin proteins previously demonstrated in generalized senile cardiac amyloid (23). This amyloid, as seen by electron microscopy, occurs as irregular, tight lumps and consists of fine fibrils less than 100 Å in diameter lying in complete disorder (23).

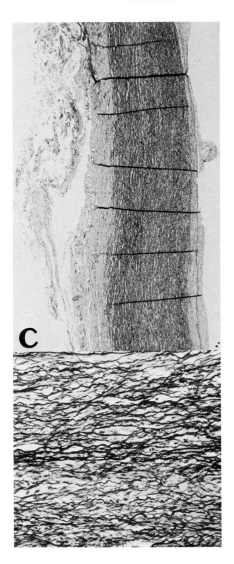

FIG. 1. Sections of the ascending aorta **(A)**, thoracic aorta **(B)**, and abdominal aorta **(C)** from a 22-year-old man who died in a motor vehicle accident. Note the thickness of the media in the ascending aorta compared to that of the thoracic and abdominal aorta and the presence of vasa vasorum in the ascending and thoracic aorta but its absence in the abdominal aorta. Also, the adventitia is thin in the portion of aorta above the diaphragm compared to that below the diaphragm. The adventitia in abdominal aorta is thickened, and there is an increase in collagenous tissue with hyalinization and a few smooth muscle cells. (Movat stain, × 20.) The lower panel is a high-power view of the media. (Movat stain, × 125.)

PATHOLOGY COMMON TO ALL TYPES OF AORTITIS

Because the aorta is a mesenchymal organ, any injury to the aorta, whether mechanical toxic, infectious, immunologic, or due to other causes, may produce a similar morphologic pattern, during either the acute or the healing phase (71). In most types of aortitis the inflammation is limited to the media and adventitia without involvement of the intima. An exception to this rule is aortitis secondary to rheumatic fever in which there is fibrinoid necrosis and inflammatory reaction of the intima and/or media and adventitia. In the healing or chronic phase of aortitis, the cellular infiltrate resolves and the damaged tissue is replaced with collagen. Maturation and subsequent retraction of the collagen results in wrinkling and a "tree-bark" texture. This appearance of the internal surface of the aorta is characteristic for most forms of aortitis, irrespective of the etiology (68). The intimal irregularity may be due to scar formation and retraction as part of the spectrum of intimal inflammation, or it may be secondary to scar retraction of the media and adventitia in the absence of prior intimitis. In advanced aortitis the characteristic appearance of the aortic intima is frequently altered by secondary dystrophic calcification and atherosclerosis. An injured intima with focal loss of endothelial integrity predisposes to accelerated atherosclerosis (71). Occasionally the atherosclerotic changes are so severe as to totally obscure the preceding aortitis. The distinguishing features of the spectrum of aortitis range from the active, florid, inflammatory stage to the "burned-out, scarred tombstone" stage and are usually identified by means of careful microscopic analysis (71,78).

Although microscopically nonspecific inflammatory changes may occur in any form of aortitis and atherosclerosis, severe atherosclerosis is invariably accompanied by medial destruction and a chronic inflammatory infiltrate composed of lymphocytes and plasma cells, thereby simulating aortitis. However, certain types of aortitis do exhibit predilection for certain sites of the aorta and specific gross and/or microscopic findings, e.g., rheumatoid, rheumatic, ankylosing spondylitis, tuberculous lesions, syphilitic aortitis, and mycotic aneurysms (especially when bacteria or fungi are cultured or demonstrated histochemically) which help to distinguish the various aortitides. Also, during the acute phase of aortitis of any etiology, a few giant cells may be present; in giant cell aortitis these cells are abundant and usually dominate the histologic picture (71). It is of utmost importance that the pathologist, before examining the histologic section, has a detailed clinical history, findings of the physical examination, laboratory results, and the results of any specific investigation that may have been performed, e.g., aortogram, computed tomography (CT) scan, echocardiographic findings in the heart, etc. It is well known that certain aortitides have common histologic findings, but the clinical setting in which these occur may help to distinguish one form of aortitis from another.

Syphilitic Aortitis

During the 1960s the majority of inflammatory lesions of the aorta were secondary to syphilis (56). The various pathologic features seen in syphilis are well recognized. Because of the multitude of clinical presentations involving multiple organs, tertiary syphilis has therefore been described as one of the great imitators of medicine (71). The incidence of syphilitic aortitis at autopsy used to be approximately 1% during the 1950s and 1960s; however, today only an occasional case of syphilis is seen at the autopsy table (51). This decrease in the incidence of syphilis coincided with the discovery of penicillin (71) and the institution of rigorous public health measures.

Syphilitic heart disease may be clinically and pathologically divided into five categories (53): (a) aortitic, syphilitic; (b) syphilitic aortic aneurysm; (c) syphilitic aortic valvulitis or aortic root dilatation with regurgitation; (d) syphilitic coronary ostial stenosis; and (e) gamma formation within the aortic wall or myocardium. The first four are the common manifestations and involve the aorta and the closely related structures.

Of the 126 patients examined by Heggtveit (52,53), 42 were considered to have only syphilitic aortitis, i.e., without complications, and 84 had one or more of the three major complications, i.e., aneurysm, aortic regurgitation, coronary ostial stenosis. Clinically the diagnosis of syphilis was made in only 20% of cases, and this was when an aneurysm involved the proximal segment of the aorta or there was aortic regurgitation in the presence of positive serology.

Aortitic, Syphilitic Aortitis

Characteristically, in syphilitic aortitis the proximal aorta is affected, probably because of rich vascular and lymphatic circulation. The process usually does not extend beyond the renal arteries. On gross examination the aortic intima has a "tree-bark" appearance, and depressed scars may be seen from which radiate wavy lines "spider" scars. These are covered by thickened plaques which are white and shiny (56). In late stages the characteristic lesions may be obscured by atheroscle-

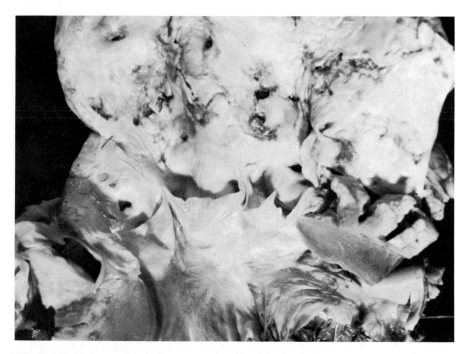

FIG. 2. Ascending aorta, aortic valve, and left ventricular outflow tract in a 58-year-old man with a positive VDRL. Note the presence of wrinkling focally, but the characteristic appearance has been obscured by the atherosclerotic change. Also the disease process does not extend below the sinotubular junction.

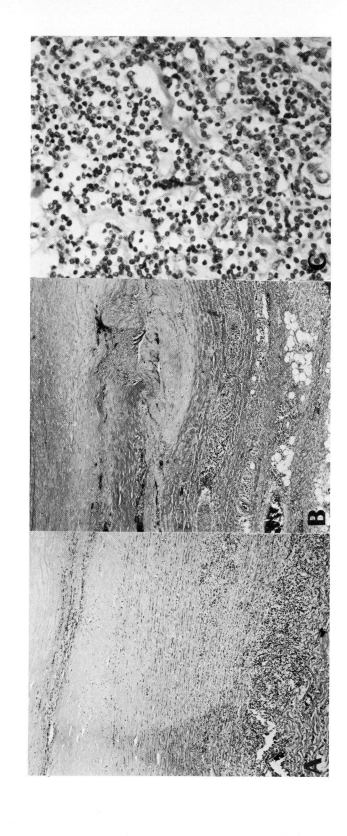

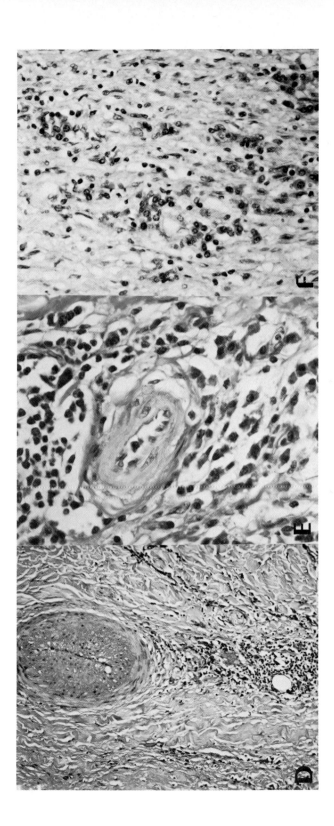

FIG. 3. Histologic sections of the ascending aorta showing perivascular lymphocytic and plasma cell infiltration in the adventitia and thickening of the vasa vasorum (**A,B**). Photomicrographs of the media demonstrating perivascular cuffing by chronic inflammatory cells consisting of lymphocytes and plasma cells (**C**) with endarteritis obliterans (**D,E**). The vessels within the media (**E**) also show inflammatory cell infiltrate accompanying vessels. (H&E; **A** ×30, **B** ×40, **C** ×300, **D** ×115, **E** ×450, **F** ×300.)

rosis (Fig. 2). The aortic wall is thickened with maximum thickening of the adventitia and intima. With time, dilatation and calcification occur which may be seen on roentgenograms. It is said that if the dilatation of the ascending aorta exceeds 3.8 cm in diameter, syphilis, not senile change, is the most likely diagnosis. However, Marfan's disease and aortic insufficiency must be excluded in the differential diagnosis. The aorta also elongates and becomes more tortuous in syphilis. However, elongation of the aorta in syphilis is limited to the thoracic aorta and is not as marked as in senile ectasia (71).

Microscopic examination shows a perivascular inflammatory infiltrate consisting of lymphocytes and plasma cells around vasa vasorum of the adventitia, and this inflammation extends into the media accompanying the vessels (Fig. 3). This inflammation causes destruction of the elastic tissue and smooth muscle cells, leading to wrinkling and scarring of the intima. The vasa vasorum are severely stenotic due to severe endarteritis obliterans with marked intimal proliferation (52–54,56). The inflammatory infiltrate in the adventitia and media resolves, leaving marked fibrosis interrupting the elastic and smooth muscle cell continuity. Lesions of microgummas may be seen in the aorta (Fig. 4) or the myocardium. These consist of caseous necrosis with surrounding diffuse infiltration with mononuclear cells—mainly lymphocytes and plasma cells and occasional giant cells and polymorphonuclear leukocytes. Gummas are seen in the media in 20% of cases; they are rarest in the myocardium (56). Rarely spirochetes may be recognized in the microgummas in the heart and aorta.

Syphilitic Aortic Aneurysms

With syphilitic aortic aneurysms the multiple foci of inflammation in the adventitia and media of the aorta result in destruction and weakening of the aortic wall such that dilatation and eventual aneurysm formation may occur. Aneurysms are usually located in the ascending aorta and the aortic arch (Fig. 5) and rarely may occur in the proximal branches of the arch vessels; that is, aneurysms usually occur

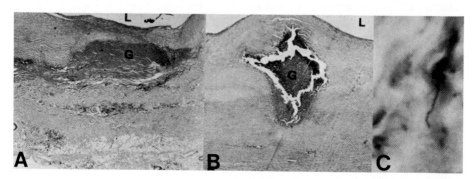

FIG. 4. A,B: Histologic sections of the ascending aorta showing gumma-like necrosis *(G)* with surrounding fibrosis and chronic inflammation in the perivascular regions in the adventitia. (H&E, ×10.) **C:** Spirochete. (Warthin-Starry stain, ×700.)

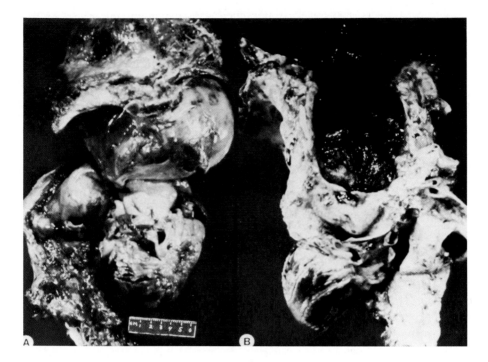

FIG. 5. Anterior and posterior views of the heart, the arch, and the ascending, descending, and thoracic aorta. The ascending aorta and the arch contain a large aneurysm. At the arch the aneurysm is ruptured posteriorly.

above the diaphragm. Aneurysms below the renal arteries in syphilis are extremely rare (71). Syphilitic aneurysms may be saccular or fusiform, and according to Kampmeier (65) the frequency at various sites is as follows: sinus of Valsalva, less than 1%; ascending aorta, 36%; transverse arch, 24%; descending arch, 5%; descending thoracic aorta, 5%; and multiple sites, 4%. Large aneurysms of the ascending aorta may cause compression and/or obstruction of the superior vena cava producing superior vena cava syndrome. Rupture of an aneurysm usually occurs 6 to 8 months after the symptoms appear, and it may rupture into various sites: left pleural cavity, esophagus, mediastinum, pericardium, superior vena cava, pulmonary veins, and retroperitoneal tissues (51). Bony erosion into vertebral bodies, sternum, and ribs is caused by aneurysm pressure and pulsation. Dissection of the aorta involved by syphilis is rare because the media is disrupted and replaced by scar tissue (108). Once an aneurysm has appeared and produced symptoms, death usually occurs within 2 years.

Aneurysms of the sinus of Valsalva have been categorized into two groups by Merten et al. (86): In the first the aneurysm is associated with fusiform dilatation of the ascending aorta, and in the second the aneurysm is localized in the sinus of Valsalva. These syphilitic sinus aneurysms dilate and attain a large size, are unpredictable, and are asymmetrical with a tendency to rupture outside the heart. The congenital aneurysms of the sinus of Valsalva are small and affect the right coronary sinus, less frequently the noncoronary sinus, and rarely the left coronary sinus. At one time, syphilis accounted for the majority of aneurysms of the thoracic aorta, but today atherosclerosis and cystic medial necrosis predominate.

Syphilitic Aortic Valvulitis with Dilatation

Heggtveit (51) reported aortic insufficiency in 29 of 100 cases of syphilitic aortitis. The cause of aortic insufficiency includes dilatation of the aortic ring especially when syphilis involves the sinus of Valsalva or thickening and widening of the valve commissures which may or may not be accompanied by valvular sclerosis, foreshortening, and rolling of the free margins of the cusps. In a few cases the aortic cusps are uninvolved; but the dilatation of the aortic ring causes functional insufficiency.

Syphilitic Coronary Artery Ostial Stenosis

Ostial stenosis is usually secondary to intimal thickening caused by aortitis, and this partially or completely obstructs the take-off of the coronary arteries; superimposed atherosclerosis may further aggravate the stenosis. Heggtveit (51) reported stenosis of one or both coronary ostia in 26 of 100 cases of syphilitic aortitis. The right was stenosed in 5 cases, the left in 6, and both right and left in 15. The extent of stenosis was considered to be severe in 15 and moderate in 11. The combination of ostial stenosis and aortic incompetence may lead to angina pectoris and myocardial infarction. Among Heggtveit's 26 patients, 24 had recent or healed infarcts. However, in 17 cases associated coronary atherosclerosis was present.

A definite diagnosis of syphilitic aortitis is difficult to establish in persons over 50 years of age, as blood serology may be negative or positive with a low titer, and a history of primary syphilis is absent. Also, the coexistence of atherosclerosis and hypertension may overshadow or mask the underlying syphilitic aortitis (53).

Although syphilis once accounted for as much as 5 to 10% of all cardiovascular deaths, syphilitic disease of the heart and aorta today is relatively rare. However, the resurgence of syphilis during the last 20 years may in the future cause an increase in the number of cases with syphilitic involvement of the cardiovascular system.

We have studied 77 patients with various aortitides varying in age from 19 to 87 years (mean 49 years) who were diagnosed histologically to have aortitis of the ascending aorta and aortic arch. Syphilitic aortitis was diagnosed in 27 patients, their ages ranged from 30 to 81 years; all but two were men. Eighteen had evidence of aortic regurgitation, 21 had congestive heart failure, and 10 had a history of anginal and/or acute myocardial infarction. In 18 patients the VDRL had been positive. Morphologic examination revealed the presence of aortic aneurysms in 20 (Fig. 5), 17 had thickening of aortic valve, and 18 had ostial stenosis involving one or both ostia (of these, 9 had superimposed severe coronary atherosclerosis).

Histologic examination revealed thickening of vasa vasorum with marked inflammatory cuffing by lymphocytes and plasma cells in the adventitia (Fig. 3) with extension into the media causing disruption of elastic fibers and varying degrees of inflammation and occasional giant cell reaction. Gummas were occasionally seen in the aorta, and rarely spirochetes were demonstrated on special stains (Fig. 4).

Rheumatic Fever

Vascular lesions in rheumatic fever are not prominent but have been well described. Aortic lesions were first recognized by Romberg in 1894 (57), and subsequently aortitis has been described as either limited to the intima or extending deeper to involve both media and adventitia. When all three layers of the aortic wall are involved, rheumatic aortitis is considered to be a true panaortitis (53,69). Baggenstoss and Titus (3) stated that the ascending and thoracic aorta contain the most numerous lesions. However, Fassbender (35) noted that the abdominal aorta is more frequently affected. Lande and Berkman (71) stated that aortitis in rheumatic fever may be segmental or that the entire aorta may be affected, from the aortic valves to the bifurcation. Grossly, the lesions as described by Klotz (70) are nodular, fibrous thickenings; Von Glahn and Pappenheimer (128) described them as elevated, transparent plaques and ridges of brown color; and Moore noted them to be yellow, elevated, nodular, and streaked (89). In chronic rheumatoid disease there is a great loss of elasticity of the entire aorta, and the vessel wall is thicker (70). Histologically, the adventitial vessels are congested with edema and cellular infiltration by lymphocytes and plasma cells. There are foci of fibrinoid necrosis seen perivascularly with various stages of granulomatous reaction consisting of the characteristic basophilic cells within or at the border of fibrinoid necrosis; giant cells and lymphocytes accompany this reaction. However, classic Aschoff bodies do not form. With time, the adventitia thickens by laying of collagenous tissue, and the vessel walls of the vasa vasorum may also thicken. In acute stages the arterioles partially penetrate the media accompanied by lymphocytes, plasma cells, and occasionally basophils. The intimal lesions are similar to those seen in the atrial subendocardium, with bands of fibrinoid necrosis surrounded by basophilic cells, multinucleated giant cells, and polymorphonuclear leukocytes. Verrucae may be rarely seen, and these heal into a scar. The aortic wall is usually thickened, and the aorta is often dilated occasionally with a fusiform aneurysm (70). Typical rheumatic involvement of the mitral and aortic valves is usually present.

The incidence of rheumatic heart disease has markedly decreased because of awareness of the association of group A beta-hemolytic streptococcal pharyngeal infections with rheumatic fever and aggressive treatment with penicillin.

Rheumatoid Arthritis

The association of rheumatoid joint disease and heart disease has been recognized for centuries. However, most of the cardiac lesions that were described were consistent with rheumatic carditis. It is only in 1950 that Bywaters (15) distinguished the lesion of rheumatoid arthritis from rheumatic heart disease. This overlap of rheumatic heart disease with rheumatoid arthritis occurred because rheumatic heart disease was more common at autopsy in patients with rheumatoid arthritis than in the general population (113). In 1958 Cruickshank (24) pointed out that rheumatoid heart disease occurred in patients over 40 years of age who had the disease more than 5 years with widespread joint involvement; mitral and aortic valve were most frequently involved, and the classic rheumatoid granulomas could be seen microscopically. Rheumatoid nodules may occur in the pericardium, myocardium, valves, and aorta as described by Sokoloff (121) and Ellman et al. (32); however, the most common site is the pericardium leading to fibrous adhesions.

On gross examination the rheumatoid nodules are firm, varying in size from a few millimeters to several centimeters (8). On cut surface they are grayish and show areas of yellowish necrosis which may be cystic. Microscopically, the central areas of necrosis are surrounded by palisading, closely packed mesenchymal cells, mostly fibroblasts, macrophages, and occasional giant cells; outside this is an inflammatory zone of lymphocytes and plasma cells of varying intensity. Early lesions of rheumatoid arthritis may have an acute inflammatory infiltrate. Rare cases of myocarditis with rheumatoid arthritis occur which do not exhibit the classic morphologic findings described above. Histologically, the lesions may be focal or generalized infiltrations of lymphocytes, plasma cells, palisading histiocytes, and fibroblasts.

Patients with rheumatoid arthritis may develop rheumatoid granulomas in the aorta (24,71) or may have a morphologically nonspecific panaortitis that mimics syphilitic aortitis (53). Usually the aorta is affected only in the first 2 to 5 cm; occasionally its entire length is involved, either continuously or with clearly demarcated skip areas (133).

We have (111) reported clinical and morphologic findings in 38 patients aged 34 to 79 (mean 60 years) with severe rheumatoid arthritis; 28 were males and 10 were females. The duration of disease varied from 6 months to 40 years with a mean of 11 years. Clinical cardiac manifestations included chronic congestive heart failure in 16 patients, precardial murmurs of mitral and/or aortic origin in 8 patients, pericardial friction rub in 3 patients, cardiac tamponade in 1 patient, and chest pain in 3 patients. Electrocardiographic changes ranged from complete heart block and/or bundle branch block (8 patients) to nonspecific ST–T wave changes (5 patients). At autopsy the heart weight was increased in 19 patients. Rheumatoid nodules were present in the heart in 18 patients (47%), and the myocardium of the left ventricle was the most frequent site (13 patients). Valvular rheumatoid nodules were less frequent (5 patients), and they occurred with equal frequency in the aortic and mitral valves. Pericardial rheumatoid nodules were seen in 13 patients, but scarring was present in 16 patients. Epicardial coronary arteries were involved with rheumatoid nodes in 5 patients and the aorta in 3 patients. All 3 patients with aortic involvement had medial and adventitial involvement, and 1 patient had intimal involvement as well. All had central areas of necrosis surrounded by palisading fibroblasts and occasional giant cells with adjoining lymphocytic and plasma cell infiltrates (Fig. 6). In all 3 of these patients the lesions occurred in the ascending aorta.

Ankylosing Spondylitis

Ankylosing spondylitis is an idiopathic inflammatory disorder characterized by progressive bilateral sacroilitis. The inflammation usually involves the vertebrae, peripheral joints, and eye (29). Prior to the 1950s the cardiac lesions were often confused with those of rheumatic heart disease and syphilitic aortitis. However, by the late 1950s several reports documented the aortic involvement peculiar to ankylosing spondylitis: dilatation of the aortic valve ring; fibrous thickening; scarring and focal inflammatory infiltrate in the aortic valves which sag into the ventricular cavity; and dilatation of the sinus of Valsalva with destruction of the elastic and muscle fibers of the aortic media with patchy inflammation (1,29,45). The aortic valve cusps are shortened and thickened at the basal attachments and distal margins, and a subaortic fibrous ridge or "bump" is present (13,125) (Fig. 7). Ankylosing spondylitis primarily affects the wall of the aorta behind the sinus of Valsalva with extension into the tubular portion of the aorta for a few centimeters only. The fibrosis may involve the adventitia, media, or intima and progress to calcification. In the active phase of aortitis there is endarteritis obliterans and perivascular infiltration by lymphocytes and plasma cells (13,67). The coronary ostia may be narrowed by this fibrotic process (107). Also, the aortitis with mononuclear inflammation consisting predominantly of lymphocytes and plasma cells, and thickened vasa vasorum (Fig. 8) extends below the aortic valves into the membranous portion of the septum, into the muscular septum, and down the anterior mitral leaflet causing it to thicken (Fig. 7). This extension below the aortic valve causes conduction disturbances because of close proximity to the atrioventricular bundle (11). Clinically, patients with long-standing ankylosing spondylitis usually have aortic regurgitation, but mitral regurgitation is infrequent. Heart block and conduction defects have also been described. The incidence of aortic involvement in ankylosing spondylitis varies from 1 to 10% and appears to be related to the duration of the disease (45).

The lesions of the myocardium are nonspecific, consisting of fibrosis, perivascular lymphocytic infiltrate, and an increase in mucinous ground substance. Fibrinous obliteration of the pericardial cavity has been seen at autopsy, but pericarditis is not a feature of ankylosing spondylitis.

Although the precise etiology of ankylosing spondylitis remains uncertain, the presence of unusually high frequency of the imperative antigen HLA-B27 in up to 95% of affected patients (and in 50% of their first-degree relatives) provides overwhelming evidence of genetic linkage (11,12). The frequent associations between ankylosing spondylitis and such seemingly unrelated disorders as ulcerative colitis, regional enteritis, Reiter's syndrome, and psoriasis have until recently been unexplained. It now appears that among patients with these underlying disorders those with the B27 antigen are most likely to develop ankylosing spondylitis (16,81).

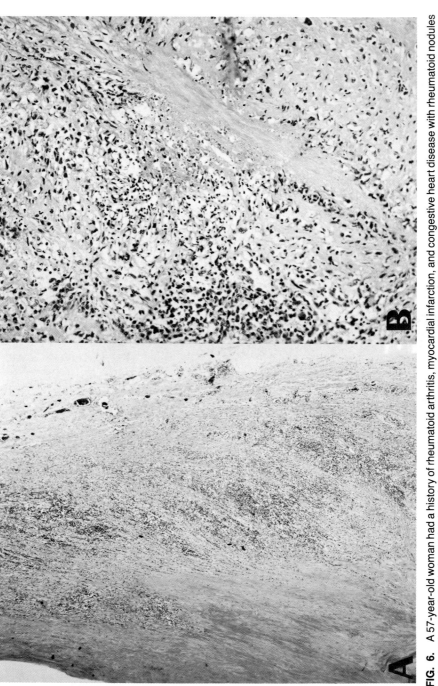

FIG. 6. A 57-year-old woman had a history of rheumatoid arthritis, myocardial infarction, and congestive heart disease with rheumatoid nodules in the aortic, mitral, and tricuspid valves, left ventricle, coronary arteries, and aorta. **A,B:** Photomicrographs demonstrated aortic and coronary artery involvement with a classic rheumatoid granuloma in the media and adventitia of the aorta. (H&E; **A** ×25, **B** ×160.) (*Continued*).

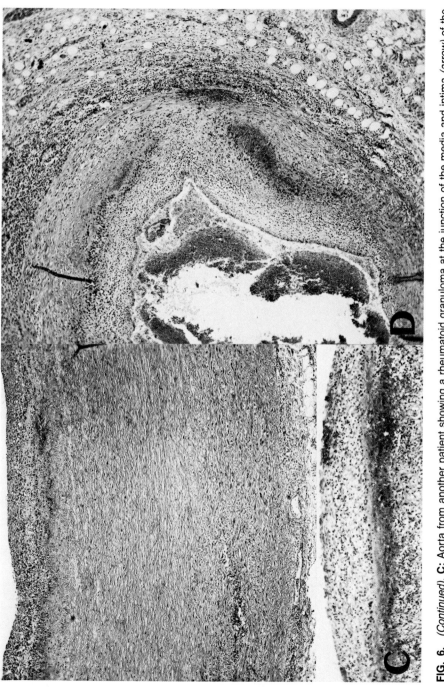

FIG. 6. *(Continued).* **C:** Aorta from another patient showing a rheumatoid granuloma at the junction of the media and intima *(arrow)* of the ascending aorta in a patient dying with advanced rheumatoid arthritis. (H&E; **C** ×60.) **D:** Section of the coronary artery showing rheumatoid nodules within the wall of the artery.

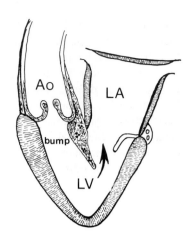

FIG. 7.   Classic involvement of the heart in ankylosing spondylitis. The ascending aorta for only a few centimeters and the aorta behind the sinus of Valsalva are involved by chronic inflammatory cell infiltrate and fibrosis. The inflammation and fibrosis extends into the aortic valve, producing shortening and thickening and into the anterior leaflet of the mitral valve producing a bump. *AO*, aorta; *LA*, left atrium; *LV*, left ventricle.

Ankylosing spondylitis must be differentiated from syphilitic aortitis. The former primarily affects the wall of the aorta behind the sinus of Valsalva and extends for only a short distance into the tubular portion of the aorta. Syphilis tends to spare the aortic valves, whereas ankylosing spondylitis extends into the aortic valve cusp at least in the basal portions and causes thickening. Also, the adventitial process, i.e., thickening, extends into the membranous and muscular portion of the ventricular septum and into the anterior mitral leaflet (13).

Reiter's Syndrome

Reiter's syndrome is characterized by the well-recognized triad of nongonococcal urethritis, conjunctivitis, and polyarthritis with sacroiliac disease especially in young men (134). Cardiac involvement in Reiter's syndrome is considered uncommon. The symptoms of cardiovascular disease may appear as early as 17 months or as late as 23 years after the onset of Reiter's syndrome (71,90). The cardiac manifestations consist of aortitis with dilatation (present in 2 to 5% of patients), aortic regurgitation, pericarditis, myocarditis, and various conduction delays (10, 25,93,101,131,137). First-degree heart block is the most common electrocardiographic abnormality (25,26) and is usually transient. Sobin and Hagstrom (120) noted dilatation of the aortic ring with microscopic evidence of fibrosis of the conduction tissue and a lymphocytic and plasma cell infiltrate. The cardiac involvement in Reiter's syndrome is remarkably similar to ankylosing spondylitis with predominant involvement of the ascending aorta, disruption of elastic tissue, and infiltration by inflammatory cells (102). Rare cases of distal aortitis in Reiter's syndrome have also been reported, and the histology is again nonspecific (40,90).

Behçet's Syndrome

Behçet in 1937 described a clinical syndrome of relapsing iridocyclitis and ulcers of the mouth and genitalia (6). It is now known that there is systemic small-vessel arteritis causing multiple organ system involvement and affecting the skin and mucous membranes, joints, eyes, and central nervous system. Other organ systems that are less frequently involved are the gastrointestinal tract, pancreas, kidney, and heart. Vascular involvement of peripheral veins with phlebitis and spontaneous thrombosis of deep veins has been reported (19,33,94,106). Manifestations of involvement of the heart are less frequent, but when they do occur they include pericarditis, myocarditis, acute myocardial infarction, acute aortic regurgitation, right heart endocardial fibrosis, right ventricular mural thrombosis with pulmonary emboli, ruptured aneurysm of the sinus of Valsalva into the left ventricular cavity, and active endocarditis of the mitral and aortic valves (16,21,33,63,64,67,73,75).

Relapsing Polychondritis

Relapsing polychondritis is an uncommon disorder but clinically a distinct systemic disease characterized by intermittent inflammation of cartilagenous structures of the ear, nose, joints, larynx, and trachea (104). It usually occurs during the third to sixth decades and is often fatal within several years. Pearson et al. (103) recognized aortic disease as a complication of this disorder. Aortic aneurysms have been reported to occur in 10% of cases (103), and fatal rupture has been reported (58).

Relapsing polychondritis is morphologically characterized by a focal lesion of the aorta with loss of glycosaminoglycans. There is destruction of the media with increased vascularization, perivascular infiltration of mononuclear cells, and increase in collagen, and a decrease of elastic tissue and sulfated acid mucopolysaccharides. These lesions in the aorta are distinct from those of Erdheim's cystic medial necrosis. Marfan's syndrome, syphilitic aortitis, and giant cell aortitis. The loss of glycosaminoglycans and the inflammatory reaction in the aorta have been considered secondary to the release of lysosomal enzymes from damaged cells (103). Although the majority of patients have aortic insufficiency, a few with mitral insufficiency have been reported with dilatation of the mitral annulus. The cusps may be thickened and inflamed, and papillary muscles may show chronic inflammation (98). Aortic dissections have been reported (46,117) and suggest similarities with Marfan's syndrome.

Mycotic Aneurysms

Mycotic aneurysms result from destruction of the vessel wall by a suppurative or granulomatous infection. Osler (96) used the term "mycotic" to denote aneurysms that were infectious in origin. The term "mycotic" aneurysm does not imply fungal infection. In recent years the term "mycotic" has been largely replaced with "infective," although syphilitic aneurysms are usually excluded from this designation (53,92).

The source of infection has been suggested by Mendelowitz et al. (85) to be:

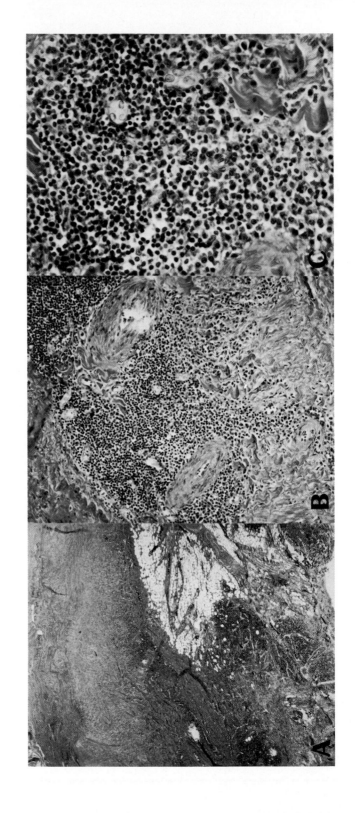

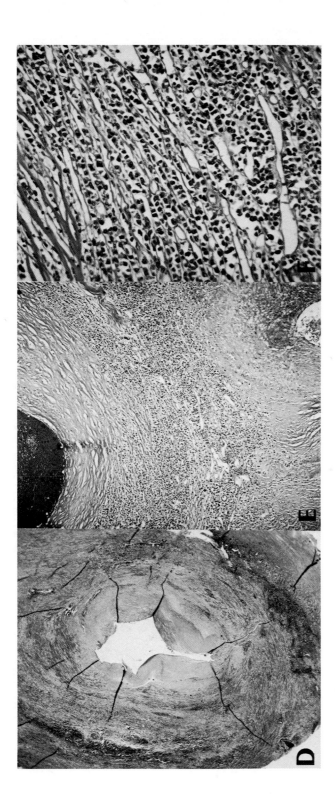

FIG. 8. A 58-year-old man had ankylosing spondylitis and a history of myocardial infarction, intractable congestive heart failure, and mitral and aortic regurgitation. At autopsy he had thickened ascending aorta (**A**) with marked fibrosis and chronic inflammatory cell infiltration by predominantly plasma cells and lymphocytes (**B,C**). The inflammation and fibrosis extended to involve the coronary arteries (**D–F**) and aortic and mitral valves. (H&E; **A** ×20, **B** ×115, **C** ×300, **D** ×10, **E** ×45, **F** ×180.)

1. Embolic (e.g., from infective endocarditis)
2. Bacterial with (a) normal artery, (b) previous atherosclerosis, (c) previous syphilis, or (d) a congenital arterial anomaly
3. Contiguous infection secondary to (a) osteomyelitis, (b) abscesses, cellulitis, or lymphadenitis
4. Arterial trauma including aortectomy or other aortic surgery (53,85)

An aorta previously affected by a congenital or acquired lesion is more likely to be a site of infection than an undamaged vessel. If infection comes from the lumen, the intimal and internal elastic lamella are destroyed and there may be inflammation in the media and around the vessel; if the vessel wall is attacked from outside by being involved in an area of inflammation or by infection of the vasa vasorum, a saccular aneurysm may result through the area of weakened wall. The more pyogenic organisms such as *Staphylococcus* evoke a neutrophilic response; less virulent organisms cause more chronic reaction with lymphocytes and plasma cells. Almost any artery may be involved: the aorta, coronary arteries, and the cerebral and mesenteric arteries. Not all mycotic infections of the aorta result in aneurysm formation; in fact, some, though rarely, cause only suppurative aortitis (4) (Fig. 9). Since the advent of antibiotics there has been a striking decrease in the incidence of primary mycotic aneurysms and an increase in secondary infections in preexisting aneurysms (7). During the preantibiotic era, most mycotic aneurysms were associated with streptococcal, staphylococcal, and pneumonococcal infections (4). More recently, such lesions have been associated with 50% of cases, and *Salmonella* group has emerged as the most common etiologic agent (4,7,30,85,119). *Salmonella* organisms are ingested frequently by man and commonly produce bacteremia. Therefore patients with atherosclerosis of the aorta are susceptible to *Salmonella* colonization of a plaque, producing aortitis and aneurysm formation.

Tuberculous Aortitis

Tuberculous aortitis involves the thoracic and abdominal aorta with equal frequency and usually results from contiguous spread of the tuberculous process from a tuberculoma (Fig. 10) in the lungs or a periaortic lymph node or from adjacent empyema or osteomyelitis (79). Hematogenous spread of tuberculosis to the aorta is less frequent. If the aorta is sufficiently weakened, an aneurysm may result. Such aneurysm may be either true or false (118,127). Dissecting aneurysms secondary to tuberculosis or suppurative infection have been occasionally reported (83,100).

Sarcoid Aortitis

Sarcoidosis is a systemic granulomatous disease of undetermined etiology with most frequent involvement of the lymph nodes and lung. Cardiac involvement has been well recognized with the majority of patients dying suddenly (88,110). Considerable attention has been paid to vascular involvement seen in sarcoidosis. It

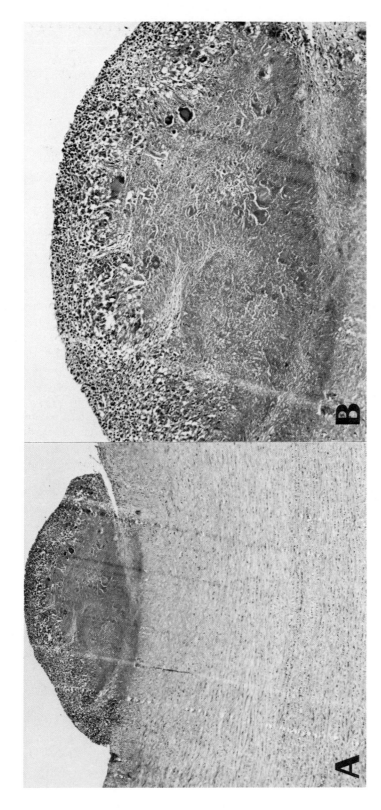

FIG. 9. Mycotic infection of the aorta with a mushroom-like growth on the intimal surface of the aorta in a compromised host. Note the central area of necrosis surrounded by granulomatous inflammation including giant cells. The area of necrosis on Gomori silver methamine stain contained fungal forms consistent with *Aspergillus*. There was no invasion of the wall of the aorta. (H&E; **A** ×40, **B** ×100.)

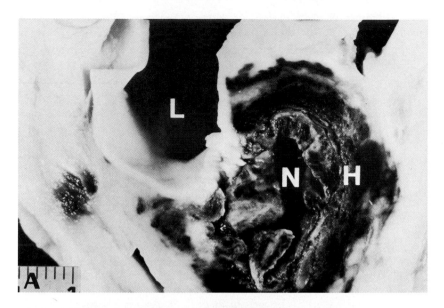

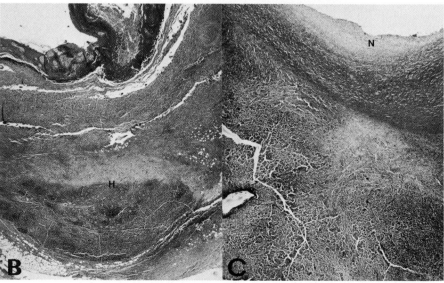

FIG. 10. An 11-year-old white male from a middle-class family presented with fever and arthritic pain in the ankles. On investigation he was found to have nodular densities in both lung fields. He died suddenly and unexpectedly. At autopsy the ascending aorta was ruptured **(A)**, and on histologic sectioning extensive areas of necrosis were seen in the adjoining hilar nodes which appeared to rupture into the wall of the aorta **(B,C)**. Acid-fast stains demonstrated occasional acid-fast bacilli, and the lungs showed extensive replacement by caseating granulomas (a rare presentation and occurrence). *H*, hilar lymph node; *L*, lumen of aorta; *N*, necrosis. (H&E, **B,C** ×15.)

occurs predominantly in small and medium-sized arteries of the lung, and rarely lesions have been reported in the vessels of the eye and brain. To our knowledge only four patients with aortic involvement by sarcoid have been reported. Sarcoid lesions in the aorta were found predominantly in the adventitia. The abdominal and descending thoracic aorta and the pulmonary, subclavian, and iliac arteries have been reported to be involved by noncaseating, well-formed granulomas with even aneurysms in the involved segments of the aorta (82,124). We have seen a case of sarcoid-like granulomas in the adventitia of the aorta (Fig. 11) in a patient with aortic incompetence and pericarditis.

DISEASES OF THE AORTA AND PERIPHERAL ARTERIES CONSIDERED IN THE DIFFERENTIAL DIAGNOSIS OF AORTITIS

Aortic Atherosclerosis

The surgical pathology of aortic atherosclerosis is the direct result of advanced lesions and their complications: progressive luminal narrowing, aneurysms, and distal embolization. By definition, an aneurysm is a localized dilatation of any segment of the aorta (50). True aneurysms of the aorta are of two types: fusiform and saccular (50,108). In fusiform aneurysms the entire circumference of the aortic wall is dilated, such that the diameter of the aorta at the level of the aneurysm is markedly increased. This is the most common type of aortic aneurysm, and with rare exceptions all aneurysms affecting the abdominal aorta are of the fusiform variety (50,108).

Although atherosclerosis occurs primarily in the intima, secondary atrophy of the media beneath the atheroma results in fibrous replacement and loss of musculoelastic units; this loss makes the aorta vulnerable to dilatation and ultimately to the formation of an aneurysm. Most abdominal aneurysms begin inferior to the origin of the renal arteries and terminate at the iliac bifurcation of the aorta (42). It is not entirely understood why the abdominal aorta is the site of predilection for aneurysm formation in atherosclerosis, but it may reflect severe involvement by atherosclerosis in this area rather than in the thoracic aorta. Erect posture of man has been proposed to account for the increased susceptibility of the abdominal aorta to atherosclerosis (50). Others believe that the standing pulse-wave reflected from the bifurcation is an important factor in the localization of aneurysms in the abdominal aorta (9,44). Most aneurysms are present anteriorly or anterolaterally and to the left of the midline; this probably is the result of lumbar spinal curvature (43). Thrombus may be present within the aneurysm, and the aortic lumen usually remains patent. Therefore such aneurysms are not accompanied by signs of aortic occlusion.

Data indicate that of all patients with abdominal aneurysms approximately 25% are entirely asymptomatic (50). The major complication of abdominal aortic aneurysm is rupture. In the past correlations between the size of the aneurysm and the incidence of rupture were stressed. Reportedly no ruptures occurred when the

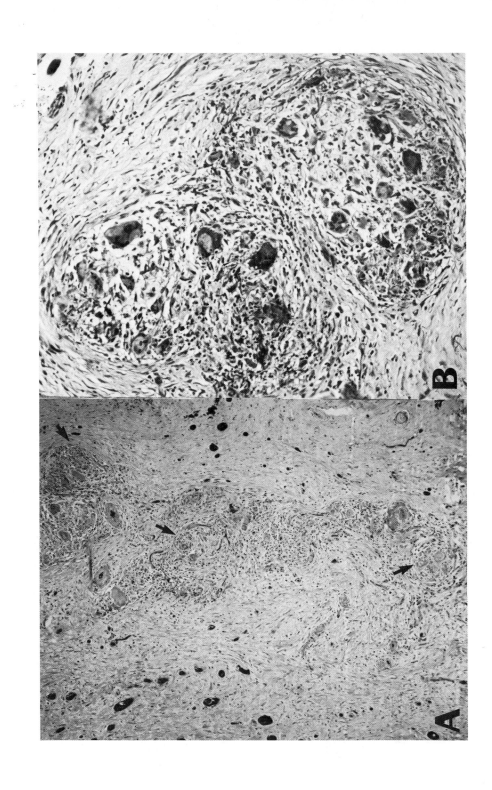

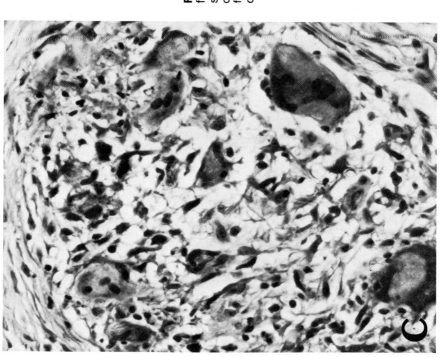

FIG. 11. A: Histologic section of adventitia of the ascending aorta showing marked fibrosis and chronic inflammation with focal noncaseating granulomas (*arrow*) consistent with sarcoidosis. **B,C:** Higher magnifications of the area containing noncaseating granulomas with extensive giant cell formation. Special stains were negative for organisms. The patient had focal nodular densities in both lung fields and mediastinal enlargement on chest x-ray. (H&E; **A** ×60, **B** ×160, **C** ×400.)

aneurysm was less than 4 cm; the incidence of rupture is 5% when lesion is less than 5 cm, 16% when the aneurysm is less than 6 cm, and 76% when it is larger than 7 cm (27,50,79). However, smaller aneurysms occasionally undergo rupture secondary to superimposed infection. Therefore all resected abdominal aortic aneurysms should be cultured and stained for bacteria, especially if the aneurysm is less than 7 cm in diameter (79). Infection usually occurs in the ulcerated intimal surface of an atherosclerotic abdominal aneurysm and does not occur in normal aorta.

Treatment is surgical resection of the infected abdominal aortic aneurysm with graft replacement (2). Therapy with antibiotics is difficult because of limited access to bacteria.

Embolization until recently was considered rare because it was believed that the masses of laminated thrombi in abdominal atherosclerotic aneurysms rarely gave rise to distant emboli. In 1966 Edwards et al. (31) reported on 82 consecutive patients with proved embolization; 94% of the emboli arose from intracardiac thrombi, and in only three patients were the emboli derived from ulcerated atherosclerotic lesions of the aorta. Darling et al. (28) in 426 instances of arterial emboli found that only 1.5% originated in abdominal aorta or iliac aneurysms. However, Wagner and Martin (129) reviewed the English language literature on peripheral arterial embolization, and of the 85 atheroemboli they found 45% were derived from aneurysms and 43% were unexplained. In another 4-year prospective study (1968–1972), emboli to the lower extremities arose from thrombi within asymptomatic aortic atherosclerotic aneurysms in 39 patients (76). These authors recommended that in all cases of peripheral arterial occlusive disease the presence of abdominal aortic aneurysms must be ruled out.

Inflammatory Aneurysms of the Abdominal Aorta

Inflammatory aneurysm was first described as a distinct entity by Walker et al. (130). It has been considered an unusual variant of atherosclerotic aneurysm, but the etiology and pathogenesis of inflammatory aneurysm is uncertain (112). The site of these aneurysms is similar to that of most atherosclerotic aneurysms, i.e., infrarenal, with frequent iliac involvement. The male/female ratio is 9:1, as it is for atherosclerotic abdominal aneurysms (39,130).

The inflammatory aneurysm is recognized at surgery as a thick-walled aneurysm caused by the presence of extensive periaortic inflammation and fibrosis (about 1 cm). The inflammatory–fibroblastic process extends from the aorta into the retroperitoneum, where it may displace and obstruct the ureters. The fibroblastic proliferation may involve the duodenum, mesentery, small intestine, sigmoid colon, renal artery and vein, and inferior vena cava (39,95,112,130). The inner surface of the wall consists of atherosclerotic plaque. The demarcation between plaque, attenuated media, adventitia, and periadventitial fibrous tissue are lost (Fig. 12).

Microscopically, the aortic wall consists of complex atherosclerotic plaque with the media underneath attenuated, fragmented, or totally replaced by fibrous tissue

(Fig. 12). The atherosclerotic plaque consists of fibrocalcific plaque with red blood cells, lymphocytes, histiocytes, lipid, cholesterol clefts, and fibrin. The adventitia no longer consists of loose connective tissue; instead, there is dense connective tissue in direct continuity with the atherosclerotic component. The connective tissue extends beyond the aortic adventitia and entraps fat (Fig. 12), nerves, ganglia, and lymph nodes. Within the fibrous tissue there is either focal or diffuse heavy lymphocytic and plasma cell infiltration. Some patients may have phlebitis with occlusion of small periaortic veins (36).

There is no morphologic or microbiologic evidence to suggest either primary infection or secondary infection of an atherosclerotic aneurysm as a basis for inflammatory aneurysm (36). Because of the lack of hemosiderin pigment in the aneurysmal wall, slow blood leakage leading to periaortic inflammation and fibrosis is not considered a cause of inflammatory aneurysm (112). The preponderance of this disease in elderly men and the absence of aortic arch involvement makes Takayasu's disease unlikely. Nevertheless, a precursor lesion of aortitis cannot be completely excluded (36,130). Serologic tests for syphilis have been negative in patients with inflammatory aneurysms, and no association with rheumatoid disease has been reported. Histologic changes in the retroperitoneum of patients with idiopathic retroperitoneal fibrosis may be identical to those found in inflammatory aneurysms (130). Although retroperitoneal fibrosis appears to begin in the periaortic connective tissue, most patients do not have an associated aortic aneurysm (87).

Dissecting Aneurysms of the Aorta

Dissections of the aorta have been studied extensively (55,59,72), yet dissecting aortic aneurysms remain highly lethal and the etiopathogenesis is poorly understood. The mean age of patients with aortic dissection is 60 years, and these aneurysms are two or three times more common in men than women. At least 70% of patients with dissection have systemic hypertension (18,108), which probably accounts for the higher incidence among Blacks (59).

Aortic dissections are characterized by transverse intimomedial tear (no more than one-third to one-half the circumference) with longitudinal splitting of the media following a course that is parallel to the direction of blood flow. The most common location is the ascending aorta a few centimeters above the aortic valve. The second most common site is the distal arch or descending thoracic aorta. Dissections usually extend distally along the greater curvature of the aorta and usually do not involve the entire circumference. Dissections may extend to involve the arch vessels and distally the common iliacs or any of the abdominal branches producing regional ischemia. The aortic root dissections commonly affect the right coronary artery and may cause inferior myocardial infarction. The dissections are usually in the outer media at the junction of the middle and outer thirds and are characterized anatomically by hemorrhage.

The primary defect in the media of the aorta is considered by some to be responsible for the dissection (8,34,41). This process involves two basic defects

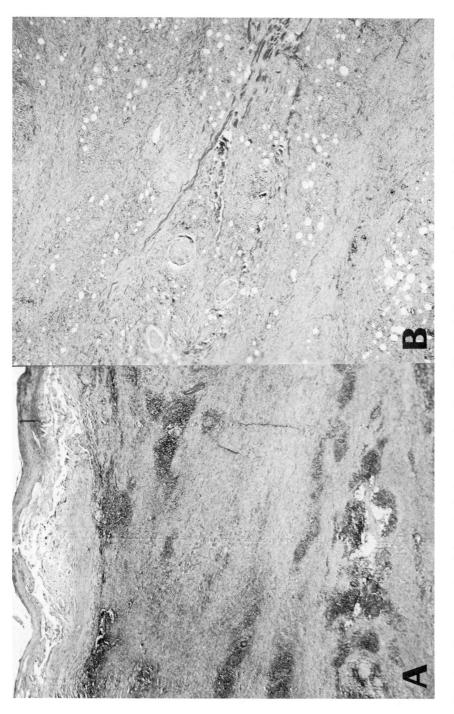

FIG. 12. Histologic section of the abdominal aneurysm in a 49-year-old male. **A:** Note extensive atherosclerosis involving the intima with almost complete loss of media and extensive adventitial fibrosis entrapping fat and nerves (**B**). (H&E; **A** ×15, **B** ×25.) (*Continued.*)

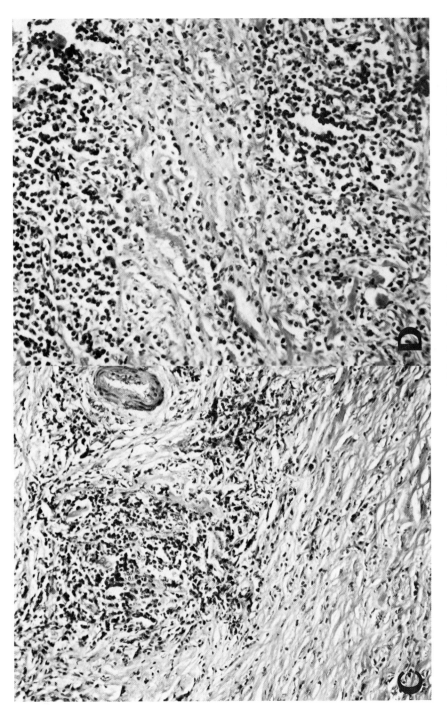

FIG. 12. *(Continued.)* **C,D:** Higher magnifications showing fibrosis and chronic inflammation. (H&E; **C** ×160, **D** ×250.)

that are observed in varying proportions: (a) focal loss and disruption of elastic lamellae of the media; and (b) loss of medial smooth muscle cells. These defects, which are caused by loss and disruption of elastic lamellae and loss of smooth muscle cells, are filled by increased amounts of acid mucopolysaccharides (hence the term cystic medial necrosis). However, because these changes occur to some degree as a consequence of aging, the patient's age must be taken into account. However, not all accept the concept of cystic medial necrosis as the cause for aortic dissection. Schlatmann and Becker (115), in a study of 100 normal aortas, found a good correlation of change with aging and concluded that changes in the aorta of cystic medial necrosis represented a form of injury caused by hemodynamic events and not as specific changes responsible for dissection. Rare medial disorders associated with dissection are granulomatous aortitis and bacterial aortitis. In contrast to granulomatous aortitis, cystic medial necrosis causes thinning rather than thickening of the aortic wall unless dissection has healed. Neither the adventitia nor the intima are thickened, and the vasa vasorum are not hypertrophied. In the most common form of cystic medial degeneration, which usually occurs after the age of 40 years, the predominant defect is focal smooth muscle cell loss (42). The less common form, which affects younger groups and is frequently associated with familial diseases such as Marfan's syndrome, Ehlers-Danlos syndrome, osteogenesis imperfecta, or cutis laxa, is characterized predominantly by defects in elastic tissue (37). Most patients have intermediate forms in which the two types of degeneration coexist. When dissection of the aorta has occurred, the presence of cystic medial degeneration may be overlooked unless the surgical pathologist examines the thin rim of normal aorta at the proximal and distal ends of the specimen (78).

External Blunt Trauma

Posttraumatic aneurysms usually occur in the upper descending thoracic aorta just distal to the ligamentum arteriosum and are discovered by chance, or because of continuous expansion late rupture may occur. Because the adventitia can withstand great mechanical forces and remain intact, when tearing of the inner layers of aorta occurs the adventitia helps prevent rupture and formation of an aneurysm. The inner margins of the traumatic aneurysm are formed by the edge of the original laceration. In time, the intimal surface may show atherosclerotic change and even calcification. When diagnosed early, surgical removal is recommended (80).

Diseases of the Peripheral Arteries

Atherosclerosis

Among the peripheral artery diseases that result in circulatory insufficiency of the extremities, atherosclerosis is by far the most frequent. The iliac, femoral, popliteal, and tibial arteries are usually affected. Intimal disease is most severe in the proximal arterial tree, and smaller, unnamed distal ramifications are relatively spared. Diseased arteries are thickened and tortuous, with irregularly narrowed

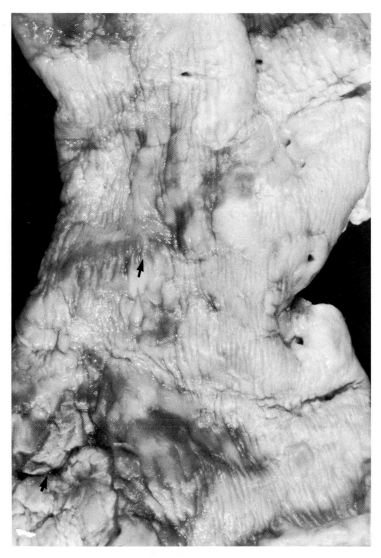

FIG. 13. Gross appearance of the aorta in a 74-year-old patient with giant cell aortitis. Note the wrinkling and focal atherosclerotic change *(arrow)*.

lumens that frequently contain both mural and occlusive thrombi of various ages. Histologically, intimal thickening represents advanced, complicated atherosclerotic plaque. The media of sclerotic peripheral arteries is often calcified, and many of these calcified arteries contain osseous foci (114).

Medial sclerosis is characterized by ring-like calcification within the media of small to medium muscular arteries. Although Monckeberg's medial sclerosis may occur together with atherosclerosis, these two disorders are totally distinct (42).

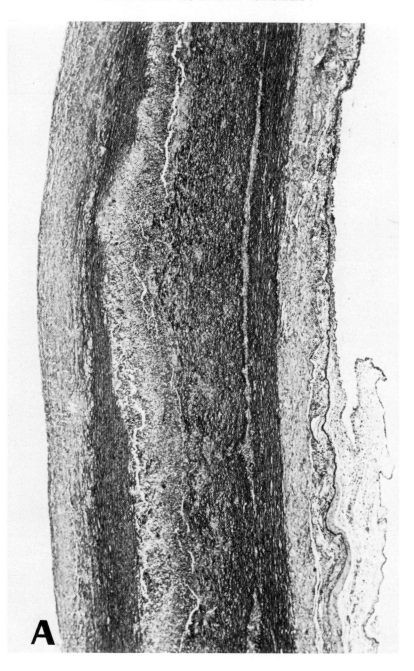

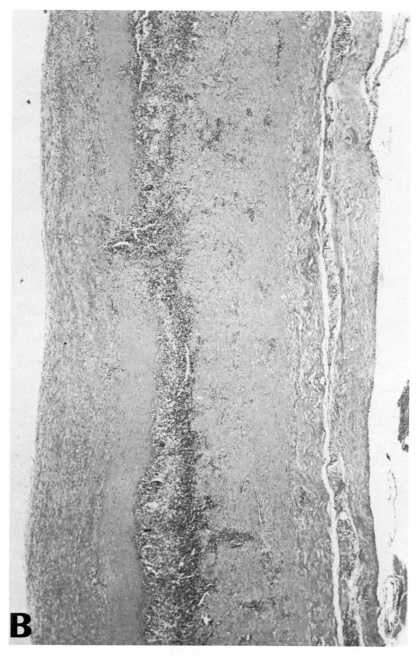

FIG. 14. Histologic section of the aorta showing extensive destruction of the media **(A)** and marked inflammation **(A,B)**. (**A:** Movat stain; ×15. **B:** H&E; ×15.) *(Continued.)*

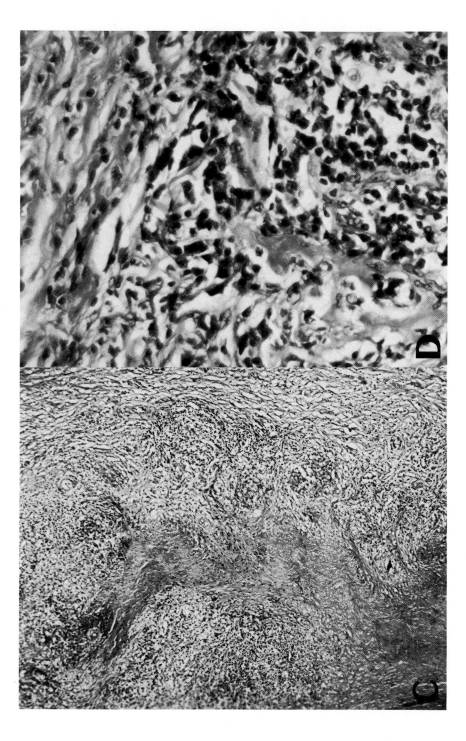

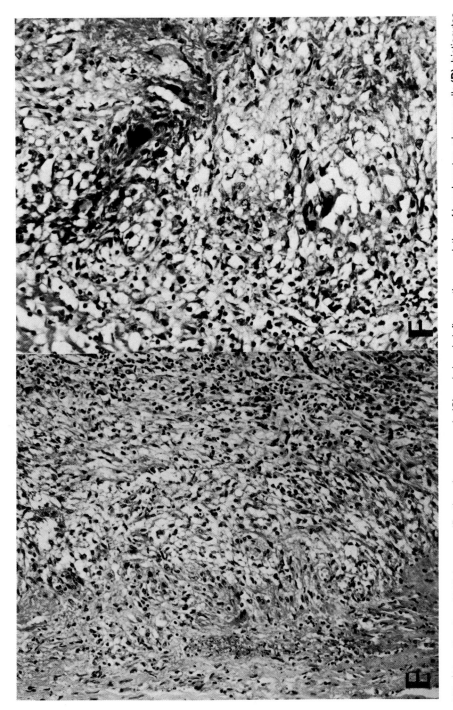

FIG. 14. *(Continued.)* Higher magnification shows necrosis (**C**) and chronic inflammation consisting of lymphocytes, plasma cells (**D**), histiocytes (**E**), and giant cells (**F**). (**C–F**: H&E; **C** ×25, **D** ×400, **E** ×160, **F** ×250.)

Monckeberg's sclerosis most severely affects the femoral, tibial, radial, and ulnar arteries and the arteries that supply the genital tract in both sexes. The calcification is not associated with any inflammatory reaction, and the intima and adventitia are largely unaffected. In the pure, uncomplicated form of Monckeberg's sclerosis, these medial lesions do not encroach on the vessel lumen (42). However, calcification of the internal elastic lamina and the adjacent media may also occur in hyperparathyroidism, vitamin D intoxication or hypersensitivity, pseudoxanthoma elasticum, and juvenile intimal sclerosis (idiopathic arterial calcification of infancy) with associated fibromuscular hyperplasia of the intima resulting in significant luminal compromise (77). These changes also may involve the coronary arteries (20). Intimal proliferation associated with medial calcification is particularly prominent in juvenile intimal sclerosis.

Fibromuscular Dysplasia

Fibromuscular dysplasia most commonly affects the renal arteries, although any of the muscular arteries and the branches of the aorta may be involved. The most commonly affected arteries include the cervical portion of the internal carotid artery and the celiac, superior mesenteric, inferior mesenteric, and iliac arteries. Less commonly, the vertebral artery and the branches of the external carotid artery are involved (133).

There are four morphologic types of fibromuscular dysplasia (47,105). The first type, medial fibroplasia, is generally referred to as fibromuscular hyperplasia, although true muscular hyperplasia is not present. In this variant, the internal elastic membrane is thinned and replicated, and destruction and thickening of the media are focally present. In the foci of medial thickening, much of the muscle is replaced by collagen. However, microaneurysms and small saccular aneurysms may appear in areas of muscular thinning. This is the most common type of fibromuscular dysplasia, and it is rarely complicated by dissection or rupture.

A second type of fibromuscular dysplasia consists of intimal fibroplasia, characterized by circumferential accumulation of collagen and intimal smooth muscle cells inside the internal elastic lamina. This type of dysplasia is particularly associated with dissecting aneurysms in the arterial wall; it occurs most commonly in children and young adults (47,105).

The third type of dysplasia involves true hyperplasia of smooth muscle and fibrous tissue in the media. It is sometimes associated with rupture of the external elastic lamina and medial dissection.

The fourth type, adventitial fibrosis, is characterized by a dense collagenous collar that produces external arterial stenosis. Varying lengths of the artery may be involved, and a considerable amount of the media is often replaced. The disease may be focal, or it can extend into the segmental renal arteries. It usually occurs in young women, most often in the arteries that lead to the right kidney (47,105).

Thromboangiitis Obliterans (Buerger's Disease)

Thromboangiitis obliterans (Buerger's disease) involves medium-sized and small arteries and veins of the extremities. It occurs predominantly in males who have a smoking history. These arterial occlusive lesions initially occur in distal, medium-sized, and small vessels such as the anterior tibial, posterior tibial, radial, ulnar, plantar, palmar, and digital arteries, rather than in the brachial or femoropopliteal arteries. At a later stage, the disease may extend proximally to major arteries (133).

Microscopically, highly cellular organizing and recanalizing thrombi fill the lumens of the diseased arteries; however, cellularity diminishes with the age of the lesion. There is no evidence of prior intimal or medial disease, and the internal lamina is intact. In the acute stage, the intima, media, and adventitia are diffusely infiltrated with polymorphonuclear leukocytes, but there is no evidence of vessel wall necrosis. This is invariably associated with thrombus formation with pockets of microabscesses. As the lesion progresses, increasing intimal and adventitial fibrosis occurs. Occasionally, a cellular organizing thrombus contains granulomatous foci and scattered giant cells of the Langhans type (79). In the subacute stage mononuclear cells predominate, and giant cells may be present in varying numbers. The inflammatory infiltrates of the acute lesions and the dense adventitial fibrosis of older lesions commonly involve the contiguous connective tissue and adjacent veins. Nerves in the neurovascular bundle frequently become enveloped in the dense fibrous tissue that surrounds the vessels. Because this disease involves relapses and remissions, it is possible to find lesions at different stages of development within the same artery or arteries (132). Superficial migratory thrombophlebitis, which is present during the early stage in many patients, may reappear during exacerbations of thromboangiitis obliterans.

Giant Cell Arteritis

Giant cell arteritis (temporal arteritis, cranial arteritis, granulomatous arteritis, polymyalgia arteritis) is a disease of the elderly with an average annual incidence of 74 per 100,000 population aged 50 and older (61,62). This disease reaches its peak in patients over 70 years of age. Giant cell arteritis has been mainly reported in patients of European ancestry, and 65% of patients are women. The onset of illness may be abrupt or insidious. There may be rapid onset of polymyalgia rheumatica defined as aching and stiffness in the neck, shoulder girdle, and/or hip girdle associated with an elevated erythrocyte sedimentation rate (60). These symptoms may be accompanied by headache, but more often the disease is insidious with nonspecific constitutional manifestations, e.g., malaise, fatigue, weight loss, and anorexia. Psychosis, mental depression, and confusion may occur also. A low-grade fever is frequently present. Visual manifestations are present in 25 to 50% of patients and consist of transient visual blurring, diplopia, ptosis, and partial or complete visual loss.

Giant cell arteritis is characterized by focal, granulomatous inflammation of small to medium-sized arteries principally affecting the cranial vessels, especially

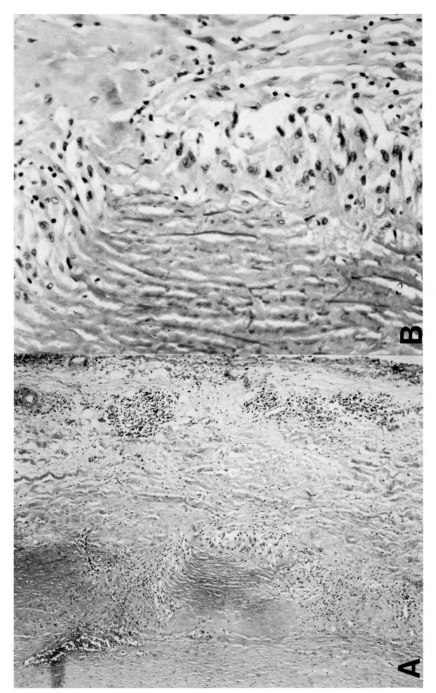

FIG. 15. Healing giant cell aortitis. Note the decreased inflammation and mild inflammation with histiocytic and lymphocytic infiltrate with only an occasional giant cell reaction. (H&E; **A** ×60, **B** ×250.)

the temporal arteries in older individuals. Other arteries that may be involved are the internal carotid, external carotid, central retinal, vertebral, ophthalmic, and posterior ciliary arteries.

However, large artery involvement is clinically detectable in approximately 10% of patients; this usually occurs in the severe form of the disease. The affected arteries develop nodular enlargement which can be palpated when the arteries are superficial, as in the temporal area. The most important aspect of this disease for the surgical pathologist is to remember the focal nature of this disease, the "skip" lesions. A biopsy specimen removed from a segment of artery adjacent to a sharply demarcated area of inflammation may be entirely normal. This has been documented in 28% of patients by serial sections of long segments of involved vessels (68). In some cases biopsy from one side may be normal, with the contralateral biopsy positive for disease. If on gross examination a portion of the vessel is abnormal, that segment must be biopsied first (61).

The characteristic histologic findings are a mononuclear inflammatory cell infiltrate throughout the vessel wall, disruption of the internal elastic lamina with fragmentation, and a giant cell reaction of the Langerhan's type in the region of the fragmented internal elastic lamina (62,66,68,74,99). These lesions vary in intensity within short segments of the artery, and their morphologic appearance depends on the degree of activity. The intima is grossly thickened by a mixed inflammatory cell infiltrate, edema early in the disease process, and dense fibrous tissue later on. The media is infiltrated early by a population of acute and chronic inflammatory cells and later by lymphocytes. The media is normally preserved, but focal necrosis of smooth muscle cells sometimes occurs. Involvement of the adventitia is variable, but cellular infiltration frequently occurs early in the disease process, and delicate adventitial fibrosis predominates in chronic lesions. Strikingly, the contiguous connective tissue is rarely involved, with either inflammatory cells or subsequent fibrosis. In healed lesions intimal fibrosis predominates, and minimal cellular reaction remains; however, elastic tissue stains demonstrate extensive disruption of the internal elastic lamina. Giant cells may be totally absent, but their presence or absence does not affect the diagnosis or the clinical course of the disease. The changes of healed temporal arteritis must be differentiated from normal aging changes of temporal arteries (97,99).

The changes in the aorta grossly are those common to all aortitides, i.e., longitudinal wrinkling and "tree-bark" appearance (Fig. 13). In the aorta the lesions are primarily confined to the media, with fragmentation of the elastic laminae (Fig. 14), smooth muscle loss, and medial scarring depending on the stage of the disease. Large numbers of giant cells interspersed with lymphocytes and plasma cells are seen in the acute phase (Fig. 14). However, the cellular infiltrate in the healing phase may be sparse with only occasional giant cells and chronic inflammatory cells seen (Fig. 15). There is increased medial vascularity with an accompanying perivascular mononuclear infiltrate. Focal areas of elastic tissue dropout are best appreciated by elastic stains. Because of extensive destruction of the media with little or no adventitial fibrosis, "giant cell aortitis," has frequently been associated with aneurysmal dilatation of the aorta and aortic insufficiency as well as rupture and dissection. In the healing stages in the aorta a wide variety of clinical conditions which have similar morphologic findings must be excluded. These are ankylosing spondylitis, rheumatoid arthritis, Takayasu's disease, Reiter's syndrome, and scleroderma. Because these diseases may have similar findings Marquis et al. (83) combined these clinical conditions under the heading "idiopathic medial aortopathy and arteriopathy." However, the clinical presentation can strongly suggest the etiology. Therefore the combination of clinical and histologic findings can point the pathologist and the clinician in the right direction (18).

Giant cell arteritis must be differentiated from Takayasu's disease, as histologically and clinically there is considerable overlap. They can be distinguished predominantly on the basis of age and epidemiologic differences. Takayasu's disease occurs in young females and mainly involves the large vessels, whereas giant cell arteritis occurs almost exclusively in persons over 50 years of age and involves extracranial vessels in the majority of cases. Headache and polymyalgia rheumatica are more characteristic of giant cell arteritis.

Giant cell arteritis is easily distinguished from polyarteritis. The histopathologic absence of fibrinoid necrosis and the clinical course are sufficiently different to enable distinction between them.

REFERENCES

1. Ansell, B. M., Bywaters, E. G. L., and Doniach, I. (1958): The aortic lesion of ankylosing spondylitis. *Br. Heart J.*, 20:507–515.
2. Austin, D. J., Thompson, J. E., Patman, R. D., and Rant, P. S. (1969): Infected arteriosclerotic aneurysm of the abdominal aorta. *Am. J. Surg.*, 118:950–952.
3. Baggenstoss, A. H., and Titus, J. L. (1968): Rheumatic and collagen disorders of the heart. In: *Pathology of the Heart and Blood Vessels*, 3rd Ed., edited by S. E. Gould, pp. 695–697. Charles C Thomas, Springfield, Illinois.
4. Bardin, J. A., Collins, G. M., Devin, J. B., and Halasz, N. A. (1981): Nonaneurysmal suppurative aortitis. *Arch. Surg.*, 116:954–956.
5. Becker, A. E. (1975): Medionecrosis aortae. *Pathol. Microbiol.*, 43:124–128.
6. Behçet, H. (1937): Uber rezidivierende, aphthose, durch ein Virus verursachte Geschwure am Mund, am Auge und an den. *Genital. Dermatol. Wochnschr.*, 105:1152–1157.
7. Bennett, D. E., and Cherry, J. K. (1967): Bacterial infection of aortic aneurysms: A clinicopathologic study. *Am. J. Surg.*, 113:321–326.
8. Bennett, G. A., Zeller, J. W., and Bauer, W. (1940): Subcutaneous nodules of rheumatoid arthritis and rheumatic fever. *Arch. Pathol.*, 30:70–89.
9. Blakemore, A. H., and Voorhees, A. B., Jr. (1954): Aneurysm of the aorta: A review of 365 cases. *Angiology*, 5:209–231.
10. Block, S. R. (1972): Reiter's syndrome and acute aortic insufficiency. *Arthritis Rheum.*, 15:218–220.
11. Bottinger, L. E., and Edhag, O. (1972): Heart block in ankylosing spondylitis and uropolyarthritis. *Br. Heart J.*, 34:487–492.
12. Brewerton, D. A., and James, D. C. (1975): This histocompatibility antigen (HL-A27) and disease. *Semin. Arthritis Rheum.*, 4:191–207.
13. Bulkley, B. H., and Roberts, W. C. (1973): Ankylosing spondylitis and aortic regurgitation: Description of the characteristic cardiovascular lesion from study of eight necropsy patients. *Circulation*, 48:1014–1027.
14. Bunce, D. F. M. (1974): *Atlas of Arterial Histology*. Warren H. Green, St. Louis.
15. Bywaters, E. G. L. (1950): The relation between heart and joint disease including "rheumatic heart disease" and "chronic post-rheumatic arthritis (type Jaccoub)." *Br. Heart J.*, 12:101–131.

16. Calin, A., and Fries, J. F. (1975): Striking prevalence of ankylosing spondylitis in healthy W 27-positive males and females. *N. Engl. J. Med.*, 293:835–839.
17. Carlson, R. G., Lillehei, C. W., and Edward, J. E. (1970): Cystic medial necrosis of the ascending aorta in relation to age and hypertension. *Am. J. Cardiol.*, 25:411–415.
18. Castleman, B., editor (1971): Case records of the Massachusetts General Hospital. *N. Engl. J. Med.*, 284:120–1210.
19. Chajek, T., and Fainara, J. (1975): Behçet's disease: Report of 41 cases and a review of the literature. *Medicine (Baltimore)*, 54:179–196.
20. Cheitlin, M. D., McAllister, H. A., Jr., and DeCastro, C. (1975): Myocardial infarction without atherosclerosis. *JAMA*, 231:951–959.
21. Comess, K. A., Zibelli, L. R., Gordon, D., and Fredrickson, S. R. (1983): Acute, severe, aortic regurgitation in Behçet's syndrome. *Ann. Intern. Med.*, 99:639–640.
22. Cooley, D. A. (1979): Annuloaortic ectasia. *Ann. Thorac. Surg.*, 28:303–304 (editorial).
23. Cornwell, G. G., Westermark, P., Murdock, W., and Pitkamen, P. (1982): Senile aortic amyloid. *Am. J. Pathol.*, 108:135–139.
24. Cruickshank, B. (1958): Heart lesions in rheumatoid disease. *J. Pathol. Bacteriol.*, 76:223–240.
25. Csonka, G. W., and Oates, J. K. (1957): Pericarditis and electrocardiographic changes in Reiter's syndrome. *Br. Med. J.*, 1:866–869.
26. Csonka, G. W., Litchfield, J. W., and Oates, J. K. (1961): Cardiac lesions in Reiter's disease. *Br. Med. J.*, 1:243–247.
27. Darling, R. C. (1970): Ruptured arteriosclerotic abdominal aortic aneurysm: A pathologic and clinical study. *Am. J. Surg.*, 119:397–401.
28. Darling, R. C., Austen, W. G., and Linton, R. R. (1967): Arterial embolism. *Surg. Gynecol. Obstet.*, 124:106–114.
29. Davidson, P., Baggenstoss, A. H., Slocumb, C. H., and Daugherty, G. W. (1963): Cardiac and aortic lesions in rheumatoid spondylitis. *Mayo Clin. Proc.*, 38:427–435.
30. Davies, O. G., Thornburn, J. D., and Powell, P. (1978): Cryptic mycotic abdominal aortic aneurysm: Diagnosis and management. *Am. J. Surg.*, 136:96–101.
31. Edwards, E. A., Tilney, N., and Lindquist, R. R. (1966): Causes of peripheral embolism and their significance. *JAMA*, 196:133–138.
32. Ellman, P., Cudkowicz, L., and Elwood, J. S. (1954): Widespread serous membrane involvement by rheumatoid arthritis. *J. Clin. Pathol.*, 7:239–244.
33. Enoch, B. A., Castillo-Olivares, J. I., Khoo, T. C., Grainger, R. G., and Henry, L. (1968): Major vascular complications in Behçet's syndrome. *Postgrad. Med. J.*, 44:153–159.
34. Erdheim, J. (1930): Medionecrosis aortae idiopathica cystica. *Virchows Arch. [Pathol. Anat.]*, 276:187–229.
35. Fassbender, H. A. (1975): *Pathology of Rheumatic Diseases.* pp. 57–62. Springer-Verlag, Berlin.
36. Feiner, H. D., Raghavendra, B. H., Phelps, R., and Rooney, L. (1984): Inflammatory abdominal aortic aneurysm: Report of six cases. *Hum. Pathol.*, 15:454–459.
37. Ferrans, V. J., and Boyce, S. W. (1983): Metabolic and familial diseases. In: *Cardiovascular Pathology*, edited by M. D. Silver, pp. 945–1004. Churchill Livingstone, New York.
38. Geer, J. C., and Haust, M. D. (1972): Smooth muscle cells in atherosclerosis. In: *Monograph on Atherosclerosis*, Vol. 2, edited by O. J. Pollak, H. S. Simms, and J. E. Kirk. Karger, New York.
39. Goldstone, J., Malone, J. W., and Moore, W. S. (1978): Inflammatory aneurysms of the abdominal aorta. *Surgery*, 83:425–430.
40. Good, A. E. (1974): Reiter's disease: A review with special attention to cardiovascular and neurologic sequelae. *Semin. Arthritis Rheum.*, 3:253–286.
41. Gore, I. (1952): Pathogenesis of dissecting aneurysm of the aorta. *Arch. Pathol.*, 53:142–153.
42. Gore, I. (1968): Diseases of non-coronary arteries. In: *Pathology of the Heart and Blood Vessels*, edited by S. E. Gould, pp. 953–1005. Charles C Thomas, Springfield, Illinois.
43. Gore, I., and Hirst, A. E., Jr. (1973): Arteriosclerotic aneurysms of the abdominal aorta: A review. *Progr. Cardiovasc. Dis.*, 16:113–150.
44. Gosling, R. G., Newman, D. L., Bowder, N. L. R., and Twinn, K. W. (1971): The area ratio of normal aortic junctions: Aortic configuration and pulse-wave reflection. *Br. J. Radiol.*, 44:850–853.
45. Graham, D. C., and Smythe, H. A. (1958): The carditis and aortitis of ankylosing spondylitis. *Bull. Rheum. Dis.*, 9:171–174.

46. Hainer, W. W., and Hamilton, G. W. (1969): Aortic abnormalities in relapsing polychondritis: Report of a case with dissecting aortic aneurysm. *N. Engl. J. Med.* 280:1166–1168.
47. Harrison, E. G., Jr., and McCormack, L. J. (1971): Pathological classification of renal arterial disease in renovascular hypertension. *Mayo Clin. Proc.*, 46:161–167.
48. Haust, M. D. (1977): Arterial endothelium and its potentials. In: *Atherosclerosis: Metabolic, Morphologic and Clinical Aspects*, edited by G. W. Manning and M. D. Haust. Plenum Press, New York.
49. Haust, M. D. (1978): Atherosclerosis in childhood. In: *Perspectives in Pediatric Pathology*, Vol. 4, edited by H. R. Rosenberg and R. P. Bolande. Year Book, Chicago.
50. Haust, M. D. (1983): *Atherosclerosis—Lesions and Sequelae.* Vol. 1, edited by M. D. Silver, pp. 195–207. Churchill Livingstone, New York.
51. Heggtveit, H. A. (1964): Syphilitic aortitis: A clinicopathologic autopsy study of 100 cases, 1950 to 1960. *Circulation*, 29:346–355.
52. Heggtveit, H. A. (1965): Syphilitic aortitis: Autopsy experience at the Ottawa General Hospital since 1950. *Can. Med. Assoc. J.*, 92:880–881.
53. Heggtveit, H. A. (1983): Nonatherosclerotic diseases of the aorta. In: *Cardiovascular Pathology*, Vol. 2, edited by M. D. Silver, pp. 710–713. Churchill Livingstone, New York.
54. Heggtveit, H. A., Hennigar, G. R., and Morrione, T. G. (1963): Panaortitis. *Am. J. Pathol.*, 42:151–172.
55. Hirst, A. E., Johns, V. T., and Kline, S. W. (1958): Dissecting aneurysm of the aorta: A review of 505 cases. *Medicine (Baltimore)*, 37:217–219.
56. Hudson, R. E. B., editor (1965): Cardiovascular syphilis. In: *Cardiovascular Pathology*, Vol. 1, pp. 1168–1190. Williams & Wilkins, Baltimore.
57. Hudson, R. E. B., editor (1965): Pathology of acute rheumatism. In: *Cardiovascular Pathology*, Vol. 1, pp. 939–941. William & Wilkins, Baltimore.
58. Hughes, R. A. C., Berry, C. L., Seifert, M., et al. (1972): Relapsing polychondritis: Three cases with a clinico-pathological study and literature review. *Q. J. Med.*, 163:363–380.
59. Hume, D. M., and Porter, R. R. (1963): Acute dissecting aortic aneurysms. *Surgery*, 53:122–154.
60. Hunder, G. G., and Allen, G. L. (1973): The relationship between polymyalgia rheumatica and temporal arteritis. *Geriatrics*, 28:134–140.
61. Huston, K. A., and Hunder, G. G. (1980): Giant cell (cranial) arteritis: A clinical review. *Am. Heart J.*, 100:99–107.
62. Huston, K. A., Hunder, G. G., Lie, J. T., Kennedy, R. H., and Elveback, L. R. (1978): Temporal arteritis: A 25 year epidemiologic, clinical and pathologic study. *Ann. Intern. Med.*, 88:162–167.
63. Huycke, E. C., Robinowitz, M., Cohen, I. S., Burton, N. A., Fall, S. M., Boling, E., and Hough, D. (1985): Rheumatoid granulomatous endocarditis with systemic embolism in Behçet's disease. *Ann. Intern. Med. (in press).*
64. James, D. G. (1979): Behçet's syndrome. *N. Engl. J. Med.*, 301:431–432.
65. Kampmeier, R. H. (1938): Saccular aneurysm of the thoracic aorta: A clinical study of 633 cases. *Ann. Intern. Med.*, 12:624–651.
66. Kimmelstiel, P., Gilmour, M. T., and Hodges, H. H. (1952): Degeneration of elastic fibers in granulomatous giant cell arteritis (temporal arteritis). *Arch. Pathol.*, 54:159–168.
67. Kinsella, T. D., Johnson, L. G., and Sutherland, R. I. (1974): Cardiovascular manifestations of ankylosing spondylitis. *Can. Med. Assoc. J.*, 3:1309–1311.
68. Klein, R. G., Campbell, R. J., Hunder, G. G., and Carney, J. A. (1976): Skip lesions in temporal arteritis. *Mayo Clin. Proc.*, 51:504–510.
69. Klinge, F. (1933): Die rheumatische Narbe. *Ergeb. Allg. Pathol.*, 20:106–132.
70. Klotz, O. (1912): Rheumatic fever and the arteries. *Trans. Assoc. Am. Physicians*, 27:181–188.
71. Lande, A., and Berkman, M. Y. (1976): Aortitis: Pathologic, clinical, and arteriographic review. *Radiol. Clin. North Am.*, 14:219–240.
72. Leonard, J. C., Hasleton, P. S., and Leonard, J. C. (1979): Dissecting aortic aneurysms: A clinical-pathologic study. *Q. J. Med.*, 189:55–63.
73. Lewis, P. D. (1964): Behçet's disease and carditis. *Br. Med. J.*, 1:1026–1027.
74. Lie, J. T., Brown, A. L., Jr., and Carter, E. T. (1970): Spectrum of aging changes in temporal arteritis. *Arch. Pathol.*, 90:278–285.
75. Little, A. G., and Zarins, C. K. (1982): Abdominal aortic aneurysm and Behçet's disease. *Surgery*, 91:359–362.

76. Lord, J. W., Jr., Rossi, G., Daliana, M., Drago, J. R., and Schwartz, A. M. (1973): Unsuspected abdominal aortic aneurysms as the cause of peripheral arterial occlusive disease. *Ann. Surg.*, 177:767–771.

77. McAllister, H. A., Jr. (1982): Endocrine heart disease. In: *Cardiovascular Pathology*, edited by M. D. Silver, pp. 1035–1057. Churchill Livingstone, New York.

78. McAllister, H. A. Jr., and Ferrans, V. J. (1982): The heart and blood vessels. In: *Principles and Practice of Surgical Pathology*, edited by S. G. Silverberg, pp. 615–652. Wiley, New York.

79. McAllister, H. A., Jr., and Ferrans, V. J. (1982): Granulomas of the heart and major blood vessels. In: *Pathology of Granulomas*, edited by H. L. Ioachim, pp. 75–123. Raven Press, New York.

80. McCollum, C. H., Graham, J. M., Noon, G. P., and DeBakey, M. E. (1979): Chronic traumatic aneurysms of the thoracic aorta: An analysis of 50 patients. *J. Trauma*, 19:248–452.

81. McEwen, C., DiTata, D., and Lingg, C. (1971): Ankylosing spondylitis and spondylitis accompanying ulcerative colitis, regional enteritis, psoriasis and Reiter's disease: A comparative study. *Arthritis Rheum.*, 14:291–318.

82. Maeda, S., Murao, S., Sugiyama, T., Utaka, I., and Okamoto, R. (1983): Generalized sarcoidosis with "sarcoid aortitis." *Acta Pathol. Jpn.*, 33:183–188.

83. Marquis, Y., Richardson, J. B., Ritchie, A. C., et al, (1968): Idiopathic medial aortopathy and arteriopathy. *Am. J. Med.*, 44:939–954.

84. Meeham, J. J., Pastor, B. H., and Torre, A. V. (1957): Dissecting aneurysm of the aorta secondary to tuberculous aortitis. *Circulation*, 16:615–620.

85. Mendelowitz, D. A., Ramstedt, R., Yao, J. S. T., and Bergan, J. J. (1979): Abdominal aortic salmonellosis. *Surgery*, 85:514–519.

86. Merten, C. W., Finby, N., and Steinberg, I. (1956): The antemortem diagnosis of syphilitic aneurysm of the aortic sinuses: Report of 9 cases. *Am. J. Med.*, 20:345–360.

87. Mitchinson, M. J. (1970): The pathology of idiopathic retroperitoneal fibrosis. *J. Clin. Pathol.*, 23:687–689.

88. Morales, A. R., Levy, S., Davis, J., and Fine, G. (1974): Sarcoidosis and the heart. *Pathol. Ann.*, 9:139–155.

89. Moore, R. A. (1976): Cellular mechanism of recovery after treatment with penicillin: Subacute bacterial endocarditis. *J. Lab. Clin. Med.*, 31:1279–1293.

90. Morgan, S. H., Asherson, R. A., and Hughes, G. R. V. (1984): Distal aortitis complicating Reiter's syndrome. *Br. Heart J.*, 52:115–116.

91. Movat, H. A., More, R. H., and Hause, M. D. (1958): The diffuse intimal thickening of the human aorta with aging. *Am. J. Pathol.*, 34:1023–1031.

92. Navarette-Reyna, A., Rosenstein, D. L., and Sonnenworth, A. C. (1965): Bacterial aortic aneurysm due to Listeria monocytogenes. *Am. J. Clin. Pathol.*, 43:438–444.

93. Neu, L. T., Reider, R. A., and Mack, R. E. (1960): Cardiac involvement in Reiter's disease: Report of a case with review of the literature. *Ann. Intern. Med.*, 53:215–220.

94. O'Duffy, J. D., Carney, J. A., and Deodhar, S. (1971): Behçet's disease—report of 10 cases, 3 with new manifestations. *Ann. Intern. Med.*, 75:561–570.

95. Olcott, C., IV, Holcroft, J. W., and Stoney, R. J. (1978): Unusual problems of abdominal aortic aneurysms. *Am. J. Surg.*, 135:426–431.

96. Osler, W. (1885): The Gulstonian lectures on malignant endocarditis. *Br. Med. J.*, 1:467–470.

97. Ostberg, G. (1973): An arteritis with special references to polymyalgia arteritica. *Acta Pathol. Microbiol. Scand. [A] [Suppl.]*, 237:1–59.

98. Pappas, and Johnson, M. (1972): Mitral and aortic valvular insufficiency in chronic relapsing polychondritis. *Arch. Surg.*, 104:712–714.

99. Parker, F., Healey, L. A., Wilske, K. R., and Odland, G. F. (1975): Light and electron microscopic studies on human temporal arteries with special reference to alterations related to senescence, atherosclerosis and giant cell arteritis. *Am. J. Pathol.*, 9:57–72.

100. Parkhurst, G. F., and Decker, J. P. (1955): Bacterial aortitis and mycotic aneurysm of the aorta: A report of twelve cases. *Am. J. Pathol.*, 31:821–835.

101. Paronen, I. (1948): Reiter's disease—a study of 344 cases observed in Finland. *Acta Med. Scand. [Suppl.]*, 212:1–114.

102. Paulus, H. E., Pearson, C. M., and Pitts, W., Jr. (1972): Aortic insufficiency in five patients with Reiter's syndrome: A detailed clinical and pathologic study. *Am. J. Med.*, 53:464–472.

103. Pearson, C. M., Droening, R., and Verity, M. A. (1967): Aortic insufficiency and aortic aneurysm in relapsing polychondritis. *Trans. Assoc. Am. Physicians*, 80:71–90.

104. Pearson, C. M., Kline, H. M., and Newcomer, V. D. (1960): Relapsing polychondritis. *N. Engl. J. Med.*, 263:51–58.
105. Perry, M. O. (1974): Fibromuscular dysplasia. *Surg. Gynecol. Obstet.*, 139:97–104.
106. Piers, A. (1977): Behçet's disease with arterial and renal manifestations. *Proc. R. Soc. Med.*, 70:540–544.
107. Pomerance, A. (1975): Cardiac involvement in rheumatic and collagen disease. In: *The Pathology of the Heart*, edited by A. Pomerance and M. J. Davies, pp. 279–306. Blackwell, Oxford.
108. Roberts, W. C. (1979): The aorta: Its acquired diseases and their consequences as viewed from a morphologic perspective. In: *The Aorta*, edited by J. Lindsey Jr. and J. W. Hurst, pp. 51–117. Grune & Stratton, New York.
109. Roberts, W. C. (1981): Aortic dissection: Anatomy, consequences and causes. *Am. Heart J.*, 101:195–214.
110. Roberts, W. C., McAllister, H. A., Jr., and Ferrans, V. J. (1977): Sarcoidosis of the heart: A clinicopathologic study of 35 necropsy patients (group I) and review of 78 previously described necropsy patients (group II). *Am. J. Med.*, 63:86–107.
111. Robinowitz, M., Virmani, R., and McAllister, H. A., Jr. (1980): Rheumatoid heart disease: A clinical and morphologic analysis of thirty-four autopsy patients. *Lab. Invest.*, 42:145–146.
112. Rose, A. G., and Dent, D. M. (1981): Inflammatory variant of abdominal atherosclerotic aneurysm. *Arch. Pathol. Lab. Med.*, 105:409–413.
113. Rosenberg, E. F., Bishop, L. F., Jr., Weintramp, H. J., and Hench, P. S. (1950): Cardiac lesions in rheumatoid arthritis. *Arch. Intern. Med.*, 85:751–764.
114. Schenk, E. A. (1973): Pathology of occlusive disease of the lower extremities. *Cardiovasc. Clin.*, 5:288–310.
115. Schlatmann, T. J. M., and Becker, A. E. (1977): Histologic changes in the normal aging aorta: Implications for dissecting aortic aneurysm. *Am. J. Cardiol.*, 39:13–26.
116. Schwartz, P. H., Wolfe, K. B., Bath, J. S., Ahluwalia, H. S., and Beuttas, J. T. (1976): Amyloidosis in human and animal pathology: A comparative study. In: *Amyloidosis*, edited by O. Wegelius and A. Pasternack, pp. 71–102. Academic Press, London.
117. Self, J., Hammersten, J. F., Lyne, B., and Peterson, D. A. (1967): Relapsing polychondritis. *Arch. Intern. Med.*, 120:109–112.
118. Silbergleit, A., Arbulu, A., Defever, B. A., and Nedwicki, E. G. (1965): Tuberculous aortitis: Surgical resection of ruptured abdominal false aneurysm. *JAMA*, 193:333–335.
119. Silberman, S., and Greenblatt, M. (1963): Primary mycotic aneurysm of the aorta: A complication of salmonellosis. *Angiology*, 14:372–376.
120. Sobin, L. H., and Hagstrom, J. W. C. (1962): Lesions of cardiac conduction tissue in rheumatoid arthritis. *JAMA*, 180:81–85.
121. Sokoloff, L. (1953): The heart in rheumatoid arthritis. *Am. Heart J.*, 45:635–643.
122. Sohn, D., and Levine, S. (1966): Luetic aneurysms of the aortic valve, sinus of Valsalva and aorta. *Am. J. Pathol.*, 46:99–102.
123. Symbas, P. N., Raizner, A. E., Tyras, D. H., Hatcher, C. R., Jr., Inglesby, T. V., and Baldwin, B. J. (1971): Aneurysms of all sinus of Valsalva in patients with Marfan's syndrome. *Ann. Surg.*, 174:902–907.
124. Thompson, J. R. (1966): Vascular changes in sarcoidosis. *Dis. Chest*, 50:357–361.
125. Tucker, C. R., Fowles, R. E., Calin, A., and Popp, R. L. (1982): Aortitis in ankylosing spondylitis: Early detection of aortic root abnormalities with two dimensional echocardiography. *Am. J. Cardiol.*, 49:680–686.
126. Tucker, D. H., Miller, D. E., and Jacoby, W. J., Jr. (1963): Ehlers-Danlos syndrome with sinus of Valsalva aneurysm and aortic insufficiency simulating rheumatic heart disease. *Am. J. Med.*, 35:715–720.
127. Volini, F. I., Olfield, R. C., Jr., Thompson, J. R., and Kent, G. (1962): Tuberculosis of the aorta. *JAMA*, 181:78–83.
128. Von Glahn, W. C., and Pappenheimer, A. M. (1926): Specific lesions of peripheral blood vessels in rheumatism. *Am. J. Pathol.*, 2:235–250.
129. Wagner, R. B., and Martin, A. S. (1973): Peripheral atheroembolism: Confirmation of a clinical concept, with a case report and a review of the literature. *Surgery*, 73:353–359.
130. Walker, D. I., Bloor, K., Williams, G., and Gillie, I. (1972): Inflammatory aneurysms of the abdominal aorta. *Br. J. Surg.*, 59:609–614.

131. Weinberger, H. W., Ropes, M. W., Kulka, J. P., and Baner, W. (1962): Reiter's syndrome, clinical and pathological observations. *Medicine (Baltimore)*, 41:35–91.
132. Wessler, S., Ming, S., Gurewich, V., and Freiman, D. G. (1960): A critical evaluation of thromboangiitis obliterans: The case against Burger's disease. *N. Engl. J. Med.*, 262:1149–1160.
133. Whelan, T. J., Jr., and Baugh, J. H. (1967): Non-atherosclerotic arterial lesions and their management. Parts I–IV. *Curr. Probl. Surg.*, 4–76 (February) and 3–47 (March).
134. Wilkins, R. F., Arnett, F. C., and Bitter, T. (1983): Reiter's syndrome—evaluation of preliminary criteria for definite disease. *Bull. Rheum. Dis.*, 32:31–34.
135. Wolinsky, H., and Glagor, H. (1964): Structural basis for the static mechanical properties of the aortic media. *Circ. Res.*, 14:400–413.
136. Wolinsky, H., and Glagov, S. (1967): A lamellar unit of aortic medial structure and function in mammals. *Circ. Res.*, 20:99–111.
137. Zvaifler, N. J., and Weintraub, A. M. (1963): Aortitis and aortic insufficiency in the chronic rheumatic disorders—a reappraisal. *Arthritis Rheum.*, 6:241–245.

Aortitis: Clinical, Pathologic, and Radiographic
Aspects, edited by A. Lande, Y.M. Berkmen, and
H.A. McAllister. Raven Press, New York © 1986.

Pathological Aspects of Takayasu's Arteritis

Renu Virmani, *Adam Lande, and †Hugh A. McAllister, Jr.

*Department of Cardiovascular Pathology, Armed Forces Institute of Pathology,
Washington, D.C. 20306; and Department of Pathology, Vanderbilt University, Nashville,
Tennessee 37232; *Department of Radiology, New York Medical College, Valhalla, New
York 10595, and Department of Radiology, Kingston Hospital, Kingston, New York 12401;
†Department of Cardiovascular Pathology, Texas Heart Institute, St. Luke's Episcopal
Hospital, Houston, Texas 77030; and Department of Pathology, Baylor University College
of Medicine, Houston, Texas 77025*

Takayasu's arteritis was first described by an ophthalmologist, Takayasu, in 1908
(36) in a 21-year-old woman with ocular changes. It was not until 1948, however,
that Shimizu and Sano (34) detailed the clinical features of this disorder, which in
1954 was termed Takayasu's arteritis. It is today believed to be an autoimmune
disease (4,6,8,26–28,35). It may begin with acute generalized signs and symptoms.
As originally described, its classical form consists of an early systemic and a late
occlusive phase. The early generalized prepulseless phase is characterized by such
diverse signs and symptoms as fever, night sweats, weakness, arthralgias, arthritis,
cough, hemoptysis, pleuritis, pericarditis, chest pain, and skin rashes (37). The
late occlusive, or pulseless, phase takes the form of various ischemic manifestations
secondary to arterial occlusions or stenosis.

As a rule the systemic generalized manifestations last for several weeks or
months, and as they subside signs and symptoms of occlusive manifestations appear.
Occasionally, however, a latent period of years or even decades separates the
prodromal systemic illness from the late ischemic manifestations. This "silent
interval" was observed in many of our patients and has been estimated by other
investigators to average 6.1 to 7.8 years (35,37).

The incidence and the severity of the early prepulseless phase of the disease is
highly variable. In a large series of patients with Takayasu's arteritis (TA) assembled
in the United States (see Lande and Berkmen, *this volume*), a history of a systemic
disease could be obtained in only 14 of 67 patients. The remainder came to clinical
attention during the late ischemic phase of the disease and displayed signs and
symptoms secondary to aortic or arterial stenosis. In the vast majority of patients
the onset of TA was insidious and the early systemic generalized manifestations
were either absent or were vague, abortive, and passed unrecognized. A similar
clinical background was observed in India (33).

The opinions or assertions contained herein are the private views of the authors and are not to be
construed as official or as reflecting the views of the Department of the Army or the Department of
Defense.

The incidence and clinical characteristics of the systemic generalized phase of TA are subject to marked geographic variations. The acute systemic phase appears to be common in the countries around the North and Baltic Seas, particularly England and the Scandinavian countries. The incidence of the systemic generalized symptoms is apparently less common in the United States and India. In Japan the percentage of patients presenting in the acute phase of the disease ranges from a small percentage to about 60% according to the sources consulted. It is, however, of crucial importance to recognize that in the United States very few patients are first seen by the clinician in the acute systemic phase of the disease. The over-whelming majority are seen in the late ischemic stage with signs and symptoms secondary to regional ischemia.

PATHOLOGY

The spectrum of histological changes in TA is closely related to the activity of the disease. After months or years the inflammatory activity tapers off or subsides, and the histology accordingly goes through a cycle of changes. In the old, inactive stage of the disease the inflammatory process has completely resolved. The adventia, media, and intima are replaced by fibrous tissue. This chapter describes the pathological aspects of TA in various stages of the disease ranging from an acute fulminating phase to an old scarred vessel with no evidence of inflammatory activity. The various synonyms used for this condition include idiopathic arteritis, pulseless disease, obliterative bronchiocephalic arteritis, panaortitis, idiopathic me-dial aortopathy and arteriopathy, arteritis of the aorta and its major branches, and occlusive disease of the abdominal aorta associated with panarteritis.

Gross Pathological Findings

The most striking feature of the aorta at gross pathological inspection is marked thickening and rigidity of the wall due to fibrosis of all three layers. Thickening and fibrosis of the adventitia may be limited to the aorta only; in most instances, however, there are extensive adhesions and fibrosis. Frequently fibrotic tissue penetrates the retroperitoneal fat, engulfing and constricting the adjacent structures. The inferior vena cava may be constricted or even occluded (33). In some instances the fibrotic tissue may be so extensive as to resemble retroperitoneal fibrosis and rarely may extend and involve the pericardium producing fibrinous pericarditis at first which later heals and gives rise to fibrosing pericarditis.

Although the lumen of the aorta is frequently narrowed or stenosed, the outer diameter of the vessel is not substantially affected. It is the enormous thickness of the aortic wall which is primarily responsible for luminal narrowings and occlusions (Fig. 1). In some patients, however, the outer diameter of the aorta is moderately to markedly narrowed. The reason for this discrepancy is not clear. It is suspected that the external narrowings may be the result of childhood aortitis with the damaged aorta unable to expand with progressive growth.

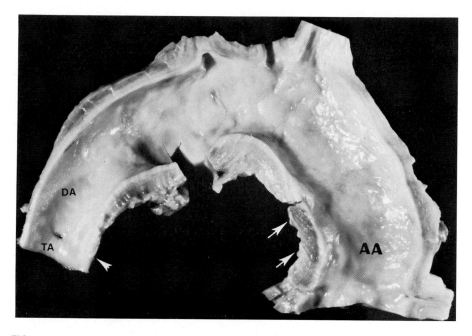

FIG. 1. A 51-year-old white female presented in severe congestive heart failure. Physical examination revealed aortic incompetence and pericarditis. Coronary angiography showed bilateral ostial stenosis. At autopsy there was marked thickening of the ascending aorta (AA), arch, and a portion of the descending (DA) thoracic aorta. Note the normal thickness of the wall of the distal thoracic aorta (TA).

"Skipped" areas of aortic involvement are quite characteristic for TA. The aortic narrowings are frequently multiple and may alternate with aneurysmal dilatation.

The incidence of aneurysmal dilatations in TA is variously reported to be approximately 10 to 33% (33). The aneurysms may be fusiform or saccular. A rapidly developing aneurysm is at times the cause of death leading to rupture and exsanguination (33). In other instances the aneurysms may be quite small ranging in size from several millimeters (Fig. 2) to several centimeters (6). In some patients the entire descending thoracic and/or the abdominal aorta may be irregularly dilated, or the dilatations may be uniform and smooth reminiscent of marked aortic ectasia (19,22).

The ascending aorta is frequently dilated in TA; we have not seen, however, any constrictions situated in the ascending thoracic aorta or the arch. These are usually located in the thoracic and abdominal aorta distal to the left subclavian artery.

On opening the aorta the discrepancy between the normal outer circumference and the luminal narrowings and coarctations becomes apparent. The marked thickening of the aortic wall comes to light. Aortic constrictions extend over variable segments of the vessel. Both the thoracic and the abdominal aorta may be affected in a "skipped" or diffuse fashion. The pathological anatomy of the aortic constric-

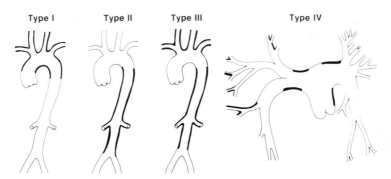

FIG. 2. Clinical classification of the TA as proposed by Ueda and associates (37) and modified by Lupi Herrera et al. (23a) Type I: TA is limited to the aortic arch and its branches. Type II: Lesions affect the descending thoracic and the abdominal aorta without involvement of the arch. Type III: Extensive lesions include the arch and the thoracic and abdominal aorta. Type IV: The features of types I, II, and III are incorporated and it affects the pulmonary arteries as well. The thickened lines represent the areas of involvement.

tions has been well depicted in schematic drawings and arteriographic illustrations published by Lande and co-workers (18,20–22).

The thoracic narrowings in TA may be of several types (3,23). Commonly the thoracic aorta tapers gradually with a definite tendency for the most severely constricted segment to be located at or slightly above the diaphragm. This creates a comma-shaped aorta, an appearance characteristic for TA. At times the entire thoracic aorta and the abdominal aorta are diffusely and severely narrowed. In other instances thoracic narrowings may be strictly localized and segmental.

Infradiaphragmatic narrowings may be supra-, inter-, or infra-renal in location. Again, they can be elongated or short and segmental. Abdominal narrowings are frequently diffuse and may involve the entire abdominal aorta down to the bifurcation (19). Branch vessels are usually affected with stenosis or occlusion of the visceral, renal, and iliac arteries (17) (Fig. 2). Whereas the stenotic forms of TA may be characteristic for this disease, the aneurysmal forms of TA are nonspecific in their appearance. Aneurysms of various etiologies may resemble each other closely.

The appearance of the aortic intima is closely related to the activity and duration of the disease. The intima shows round, well-circumscribed plaques of variable size or raised, smooth, gelatinous or pearly white patches with intervening normal or scarred intima. The plaques may be isolated or appear in crops. In chronic and old inactive forms of aortitis, patches of thickened, raised intima can be seen along with early changes of atherosclerosis. They are quite variable in number, size, and location and usually range in size from one to several centimeters (2,6,12,26). The surface of those patches of thickened intima is usually irregular or wrinkled.

Although patches and plaques of raised intima are frequently seen on the inner surface of the aorta, the most common manifestation is circumferential intimal thickening extending for short or long segments of the vessel. The intimal thickening may be several times the combined thickness of the adventitia and media and is primarily responsible for aortic and arterial narrowings and occlusions (26) (Fig. 3).

The thickened intima has a definite tendency for longitudinal wrinkling and ridging, and at times coarse longitudinal folds of intima extend over long segments of the vessel (6,24,26,33,38). In addition to the longitudinal ridging, transverse folds or ridges may appear, and the classical tree-bark appearance closely resembling syphilitic aortitis is formed (6,24,26,33,38). This tree-bark appearance of the intima appears to be quite characteristic for all forms of aortitis independent of underlying etiology.

The previously described patches of aortitis scattered haphazardly in the aortic intima are of significant pathological importance. When a patch of aortitis with a thickened intima is located in a neutral portion of the aorta, e.g., the descending thoracic aorta, it may be of limited clinical significance. However, if patchy intimal thickening settles near an orifice of vital artery, the clinical consequences may be dramatic. A patch of thickened intima situated at the orifice of the coronary artery may produce anginal symptoms or coronary occlusion (Fig. 4). A patch involving the orifice of the carotid artery may produce cerebrovascular symptomatology, whereas localized intimal thickening constricting the renal arteries may be responsible for severe renovascular hypertension (8,10,22). It is therefore like playing a "Russian roulette." When a patch of aortitis hits a vital artery, the patient may suffer serious consequences. When it is located in a neutral portion of the aorta, the patient may remain relatively asymptomatic.

The appearance of the intima is related to the phase of the inflammatory process. In acute florid inflammation the intima appears puffy, swollen, and wet. Swelling

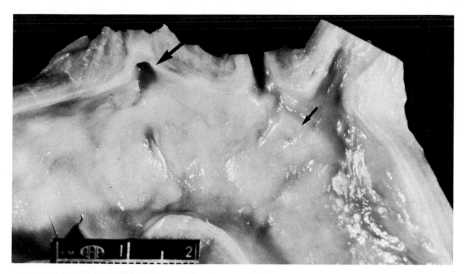

FIG. 3.   Note the irregularly thickened intima with raised pearly white plaques *(small arrow)* and intervening relatively normal intima. The arch vessels show intimal thickening with narrowing of the left subclavian artery *(large arrow).*

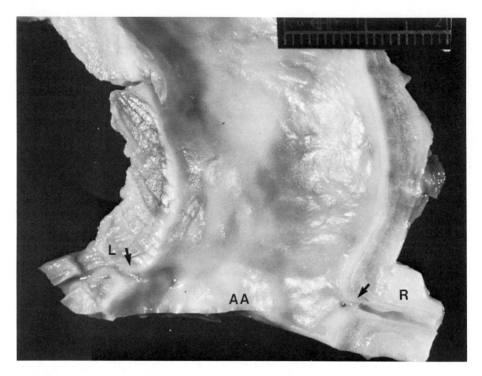

FIG. 4. Close-up view of the ascending aorta *(AA)* and both coronary ostia. Note the severe narrowing of the right *(R)* and left *(L)* coronary orifices.

of the intima in the region of the renal arteries constricts the vessels in a rather acute fashion causing severe renovascular hypertension and at times congestive heart failure (4–6,33). Because a postinflammatory intima predisposes to accelerated deposition of secondary atherosclerosis, variable degrees of atherosclerosis are usually seen intermixed with postinflammatory intimal changes. At times secondary atherosclerosis is so severe as to totally obscure underlying changes of aortitis (8). The aortas of young and middle-aged individuals with atherosclerotic deposits at unusual sites or of segmental distribution should be regarded with a high index of suspicion, as arteritis with superimposed degenerative changes may be easily mistaken for ordinary atherosclerosis (21).

As has been previously stated, after months or years the inflammatory activity of TA subsides and the destroyed muscular and elastic elements are replaced by fibrosis. In this stage identification of residual fibrosis as postinflammatory scar tissue may create difficulties because signs of active inflammation are absent. Under these conditions it is important to realize that hardening and fibrous sclerosis of the vessel wall is not synonymous with arteriosclerosis. On the other hand, the degree of secondarily engrafted atherosclerosis, meaning deposition of cholesterol esters and lipids, is quite variable. Nevertheless, careful microscopic analysis of the aortic wall may still permit differentiation of postinflammatory changes from secondary degenerative manifestations. Diagrammatic charts of the aortic intima with precise delineation of areas of postinflammatory intimal sclerosis with or without fibrous intimal thickening as well as regions of secondarily engrafted atherosclerosis were prepared by Klinge in 1933 for rheumatic aortitis (16). Following the same model, Yamada et al. in 1961 prepared charts of the aortic intima in TA, mapping out areas of postinflammatory fibrosis and secondary atherosclerosis (39). It is of utmost importance that plaques of secondary atherosclerosis and postinflammatory sclerosis of the vessel not be mistaken for ordinary atherosclerosis.

Microscopic Findings

The aortic lesions range from a florid inflammatory phase, with the infiltrate consisting predominantly of lymphocytes and plasma cells, to healed fibrotic lesions. Both types of lesions may be seen in the same patient, suggesting a chronic, recurrent process. Inflammatory changes in TA affect the adventitia and the media. The intima does not participate in the inflammatory process, and the marked intimal thickening is a secondary reactive phenomenon.

Changes in the Adventitia

As a whole, signs of florid inflammation are more pronounced in the media than in the adventitia. Diffuse sclerotic thickening is more severe in the adventitia (Fig. 5).

In the acute stage of inflammation there is cuffing of the vasa vasorum by lymphocytes, plasma cells, and mononuclear wandering cells (Fig. 6). The inflammatory infiltrate may extend into the adjacent fat. At the same time there is marked proliferation of connective tissue with new growth of blood vessels. With passage of time there is regression of the inflammatory activity with hyalinization and collagenization of the fibrous tissue. Similar changes are seen in large and medium-sized elastic arteries. The nutrient arteries of the adventitia show onion-skin-like thickening and intimal proliferation frequently leading to their obliteration (Fig. 7). Many are occluded by dense fibrosis. There is, however, no evidence of endarteritis obliterans or fibrinoid necrosis, or any changes suggestive of periarteritis nodosa.

Changes in the Media

The alterations in the medial layer are a reflection of the intensity of the inflammatory process. They undergo a cycle of alterations according to the duration and activity of the disease. In the acute phase there is evidence of vascularization of the tunica media. The capillaries originate at the transition zone of the adventitia and the media and subsequently fan out to incorporate the entire medial layer. Accompanying this neovascularization and invading the tunica media is diffuse productive inflammatory tissue consisting of lymphocytes, plasma cells, occasional giant cells, and young proliferating connective tissue (Fig. 8). The giant cells are

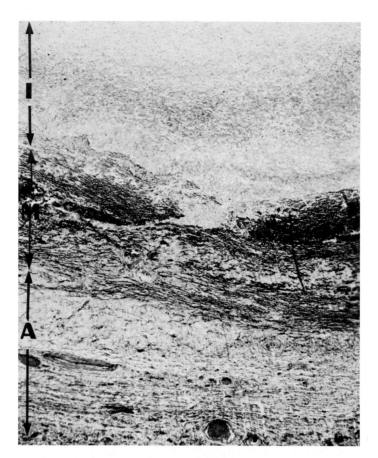

FIG. 5. Histological section of the ascending aorta showing diffuse sclerosis of the adventitia *(A)*, focal disruption of the media *(M)*, and moderate intimal *(I)* thickening. (Movat stain, ×25.)

primarily Langhan's type or foreign body giant cells; however, myogenous giant cells derived from smooth muscles of the media have also been described (26). In some instances a considerable number of foreign body giant cells can be seen congregating in the vicinity of disintegrated elastic tissue and therefore are functioning as elastophages (Fig. 9). Only rarely are giant cells present in large numbers, and they are never as numerous as in giant cell aortitis. In the acute phase of inflammation there are occasional patches of coagulation necrosis (Fig. 9) surrounded by epithelioid cells mingled with giant cells of various derivation. It must be emphasized, however, that they do not resemble tuberculoid or syphilitic mesoaortitis.

In advanced stages of the inflammatory process, fibrosis replaces the functional elements of the tunica media with thickening of the aortic wall. The degree of residual destruction of the tunica media varies from slight disruption of the elastic

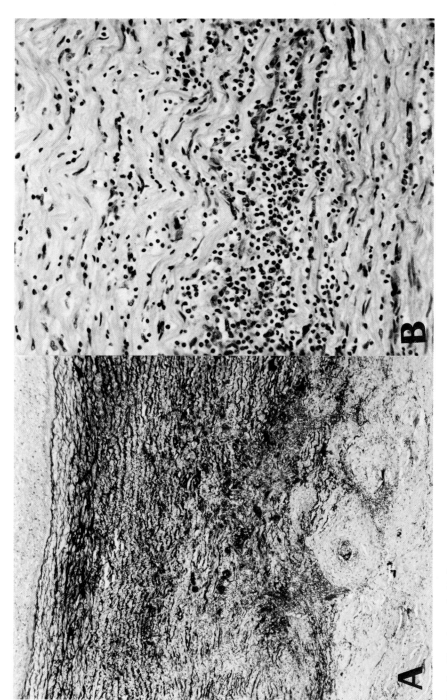

FIG. 6. Note the marked inflammatory exudate around the vasa vasorum consisting of lymphocytes, plasma cells, and mononuclear cells. (**A:** Movat stain, × 40. **B:** H&E, × 250.)

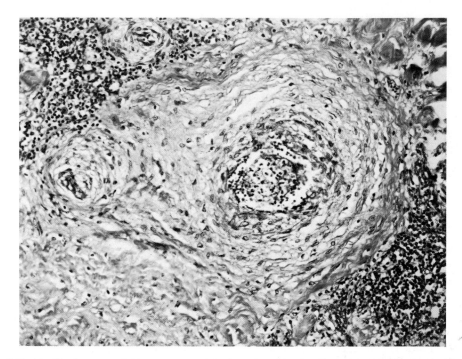

FIG. 7. Nutrient vessels (vasa vasorum) in the adventitia showing onion-skin-like thickening and luminal obliteration. (H&E, × 160.)

fibers to total disappearance of the elastic tissue with the adventitia directly over-lying the intima or with only remnants of the elastic tissue left between (17,21). When the aorta is affected in a "skipped-like" fashion, the normal elastic coat can be traced up to the edge of the lesion only to break up into a few shreds, or it completely disappears. At the opposite edge of the "skipped area" the changes stop quite abruptly with a transition to a relatively normal aortic wall (6,12). In older cases of TA with marginal inflammatory activity, fibrosis and scarring predominate and the infiltrate is scanty or absent. In burned-out vessels the cellular infiltrates are gone, and there is no microscopic evidence of inflammatory activity.

Changes in the Intima

As previously stated, thickening of the intima occurs at sites of active arteritis and is often very extensive. Frequently the thickened intima constricts the orifices of the branch arteries. In the thickened intima the basophilic ground substance is markedly increased. This ground substance is periodic acid-Schiff (PAS)-positive and shows metachromasia with toluidine blue (at pH 7.0 and 4.1). It stains blue by Alcian blue or by Hale's colloidal iron method and is rather unstable to the action of hyaluronidase. Therefore histochemically an increase of protein including acid mucopolysaccharides is present that is in a state of mucoid or gelatinous swelling (26).

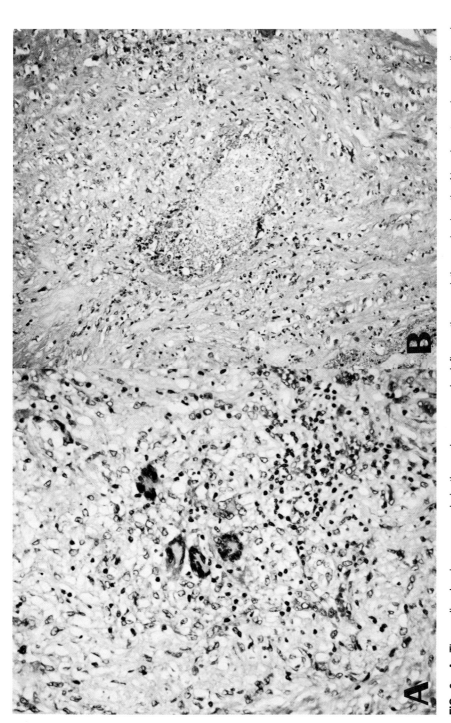

FIG. 8. A: The media, showing neovascularization and accompanying inflammation consisting predominantly of lymphocytes, plasma cells, and occasional giant cells. (H&E, ×250.) **B:** Area of necrosis with mild inflammation. (H&E, ×160.)

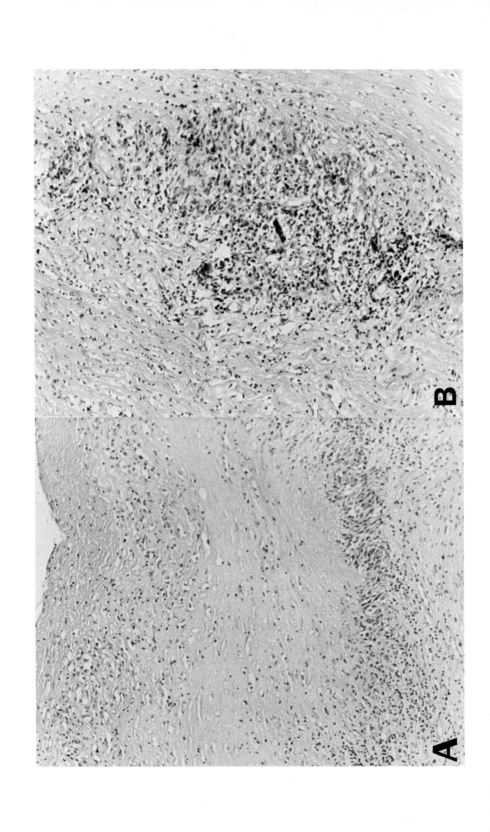

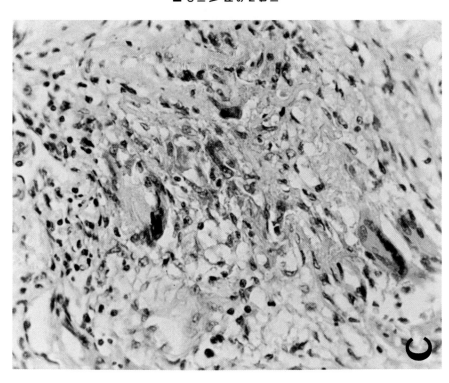

FIG. 9. Aortic wall, showing an extensive giant cell reaction and focal areas of coagulation necrosis in a 43-year-old female who presented with fever, weight loss, anemia, leukocytosis, and an increased erythrocyte sedimentation rate. While undergoing investigation for fever of unknown origin, she suddenly complained of chest pain and died. At autopsy her heart weighed 380 g. The intimal surface of the ascending aorta showed wrinkling and right coronary ostial narrowing. Histological sections of the aorta revealed focal coagulation necrosis of the media with marked histiocytic (**A,B**) and giant cell (**C**) reactions along with lymphocytic infiltrates. (H&E; **A** ×63, **B** ×85, **C** ×220.)

In the increased ground substance there is abundant proliferation of connective tissue cells and occasionally string-like proliferation of cells which may be considered smooth muscle cells because they show smooth muscle characteristics by the Mallory trichrome method, phosphotungstic acid hematoxylin, and Heidenhain's iron hematoxylin method. At times the smooth muscle cells may be so abundant as to be reminiscent of fibromuscular hyperplasia (38). In portions of the intima which are relatively old, there is frequently formation of delicate elastic fibers forming a lamellar structure with an attempt to recreate an internal elastic lamina. At times multiple layers of fine elastic fibers are seen (elastosis) (26). In old cases the intima shows marked fibrous sclerosis with hyalinization of the deeper layers. Dystrophic calcification of the hyalinized tissue is common. At x-ray examination the dystrophic calcium can be seen as a pencil-like calcification delineating the lumen of the aorta (19). The markedly thickened intima is not the result of intimitis but is a phenomenon secondary to the underlying inflammation of media and adventitia. There is no evidence in the intima of cellular infiltration with microabscesses or fibrinoid necrosis as seen in rheumatic fever and rheumatoid aortitis.

Coronary Arterial Narrowing in Takayasu's Arteritis

Initially Takayasu's arteritis was thought to be unique to the aortic arch; however, as described above, more diffuse involvement of the aorta and its major branches is common. The cardiac manifestations range from congestive heart failure to angina pectoris. Autopsy studies have documented ostial stenosis, coronary arteritis, and even aneurysm formation with myocardial infarction (30,32,40). Saito et al. (32) reviewed coronary arterial findings in 24 cases; ostial narrowing was found in 19 and obstruction in 1. The coronary arteries showed intimal thickening, adventitial fibrosis, and cellular infiltrates (lymphocytes and plasma cells) in the media and adventitia. Myocardial infarction was present in six cases. In a review of 16 cases by Rosen and Sinclair-Smith (30), epicardial coronary arteries were segmentally involved in three patients with coronary aneurysm formation in the right and left anterior descending coronary arteries in two. Thrombosis in one of the patients had caused myocardial infarction (30). Coronary angiography has documented the presence of ostial stenosis, and treatment with aortocoronary bypass grafting has been successfully tried in some patients.

Aortic Regurgitation

Aortic regurgitation was first described by Jervell (14) in Takayasu's disease. Since then, it has been documented by both auscultation and aortography (13). Pathologically, there is dilatation of the diseased ascending aorta with widening of the aortic commissures (Fig. 10) and thickening, fibrosis, and foreshortening of the valve cusps. There may also be some inflammatory infiltrates (lymphocytes, plasma cells) depending on the activity of the disease, and they have been reported to extend contiguously to involve the conduction system, causing a bundle branch block (1).

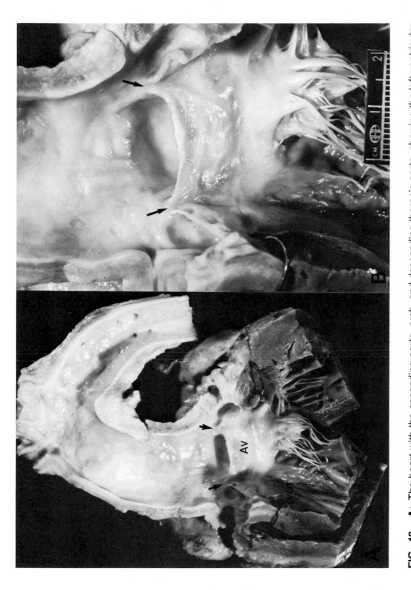

FIG. 10. A: The heart with the ascending aorta, arch, and descending thoracic aorta, showing the left ventricular outflow tract and the aortic valve *(AV)*. **B:** Note the thickened and fibrotic aortic valves but no commissural fusion; instead there is widening of the commissures *(arrows)*.

Pulmonary Artery Involvement

Pulmonary artery involvement has not only been confirmed at autopsy (26,32) but has also been detected by plain chest roentgenography, pulmonary arteriography, pulmonary arterial pressure measurements, and pulmonary perfusion scanning. Fifty percent or more of the patients have pulmonary artery involvement, but no relationship exists between severity and extent of involvement of the systemic and pulmonary arterial systems. The pulmonary involvement is similar to that seen in the aorta with marked thickening of the pulmonary wall, fibrosis and inflammation in the adventitia and media, with secondary sclerosis of the intima without inflammation (Fig. 11). A unique arteriopathy involving the small pulmonary arteries has been presented in patients with otherwise typical arterial lesions of TA (29). The arteriopathy is characterized by the formation of defects in the outer

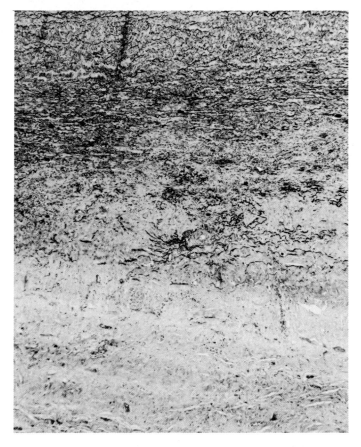

FIG. 11. Section of pulmonary artery, showing marked adventitial fibrosis and focal inflammation in the adventitia and media with secondary sclerosis of the intima. The changes in the pulmonary artery are similar to those seen in the aorta. (Movat stain, ×40.)

media of the arteries and an ingrowth of granulation-tissue-like capillaries. Also carbon pigment may be seen in the damaged media or intima suggesting pulmonary macrophage infiltration of the vessel wall. The intima is also greatly thickened by fibrosis, granulation tissue, and capillary proliferation. The newly formed capillary channels are prominently seen in the intima and media with dilatation of capillaries in the adventitia suggesting angiomatoid lesions seen in plexogenic arteriopathy. No fibrinoid change or vascular necrosis have been described in TA involving the lungs.

Our experience with 15 patients ranging in age from 20 to 49 years (10 females and 5 males) shows a wide range of changes and clinical presentations. The majority were symptomatic before death with acute onset of congestive heart failure, chest pain, and systemic hypertension. Only a few were presented with sudden death. At autopsy all patients had gross findings of aortitis with or without involvement of the arch and the renal vessels. Five had coronary ostial stenosis. The microscopic findings ranged from florid inflammatory infiltrates with areas of necrosis to minimal or no inflammation but marked elastic tissue destruction and fibrointimal proliferation. Aortic valve involvement was not infrequent, and two patients had myocarditis as well.

PITFALLS IN PATHOLOGICAL INTERPRETATIONS

In advanced stages of TA, when the activity of the disease has subsided, there are frequently no distinguishing signs to permit the crucially important differentiation of nonspecific fibrosis from postinflammatory scar tissue. Actually the proper expression would be to permit the identification of nonspecific fibrosis as due to previous inflammation and scarring. This statement applies to all three layers of the aorta. TA may heal leaving behind few specific identifying characteristics. Interpreting the presence of fibrosis as being secondary to a postinflammatory process is difficult. It is one of the primary reasons why old, healed cases of TA are so infrequently identified at pathological examinations.

Thickening and obliteration of the vasa vasorum is not sufficient evidence of previous aortitis. Of course when the characteristic cellular cuffing around the nutrient arteries is present the diagnosis of aortitis is easily made. In virtually all publications on TA cellular cuffing of the vasa vasorum is the characteristic histological sign of aortitis. However, obliteration of the nutrient arteries without evidence of a cellular infiltrate is of little diagnostic help. Because of these difficulties, the pathological identification of TA in advanced burned-out stages of the disease is usually inconclusive. The pathological diagnosis is frequently nonspecific fibrosis or, more often, arteriosclerosis; this simply indicates that the artery is hard and fibrotic, and it is a noncommittal and highly misleading statement.

The difficulties in pathological interpretation are further complicated by the fact that an injured intima, and particularly the postinflammatory intima, predisposes to secondary atherosclerosis. The rapidity of deposition of premature atherosclerosis depends on several factors, e.g., duration of disease and severity of hypertension (which many patients with TA have secondary to renal artery stenosis or suprarenal coarctation). It also depends on individual factors such as hyperlipidemia and the presence or absence of diabetes.

The degree of secondary atherosclerosis is at times so severe as to completely obscure the underlying changes of aortitis (2,8,19,21). When secondary atherosclerosis is present there is definite tendency toward description of the pathological changes in the aorta as only due to atherosclerosis. In the presence of secondary atherosclerosis, careful microscopic analysis, however, usually permits differentiation of both: atheromatous intimal changes from nonatheromatous postinflammatory intimal thickening and dystrophic from atherosclerotic calcifications (16,19,39). These changes have been elegantly displayed in schematic form by Klinge (16) for rheumatic fever and later by Yamada et al. (39) for TA. Their diagrams are very illustrative and should serve as guidelines when there is doubt about the pathological analysis. At the same time, strict adherence to the classical diagnostic criteria of atherosclerosis is mandatory in order to avoid misinterpretation.

In addition, there are several other pathological landmarks which strongly indicate the presence of aortitis. One of them is the appearance of the aortic intima. The intimal changes are sometimes nonspecific, in the form of well-circumscribed white or grayish plaques or irregular, patchy elevations. However, there is a definite inclination toward longitudinal wrinkling of the intima and formation of longitudinal folds and crevices. When transverse ridging is also present, the classical tree-bark appearance of aortitis is displayed. This configuration of the intima is a sign of previous aortitis.

Thus the combination of nonspecific fibrosis with destruction of elastic and muscular tissues, thickening and obliteration of the vasa vasorum, and fibrous thickening of the adventitia, as well as fibrous thickening of the intima with its characteristic appearance, are highly suggestive of previous aortitis in the absence of active inflammation. Secondary atherosclerosis may or may not be present. Aortography is frequently highly characteristic in advanced burned-out cases.

PERIPHERAL ARTERITIS

The pathological changes in TA may be confined to the aorta only or to the branch arteries. In the majority of cases, however, the aorta as well as the branch arteries are affected (15,25).

Narrowing of the orifices of the coronary, brachiocephalic, celiac, superior mesenteric, renal, and inferior mesenteric arteries is usually secondary to thickening, puckering, and swelling of the aortic intima. However, the ultimate occlusion of a branch orifice is usually accomplished by a thrombus. The occluding thrombus extends into the artery for a short distance, leaving only the proximal vessel patent. This may be of importance if surgical reconstruction is contemplated.

In addition to narrowing of the arterial orifices secondary to the intimal thickening of the aorta, aortitis may extend for a variable distance along the axis of the branch artery (Fig. 12). Histologically, the inflammatory changes in the wall of the

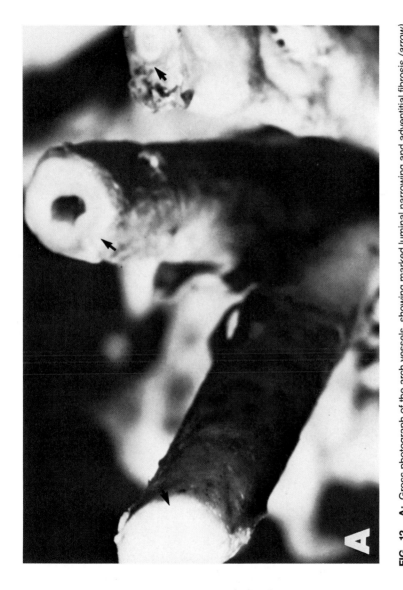

FIG. 12. A: Gross photograph of the arch vessels, showing marked luminal narrowing and adventitial fibrosis *(arrow).* **B–E:** Histological sections of the corresponding three arch vessels and the aorta demonstrate focal loss of the elastic tissue of the media. There is marked fibrosis of the intima and adventitia but an absence of cellular infiltration and active inflammation. (EVG stain; **B–D** ×15, **E** ×60.) (**B–E** on following pages.)

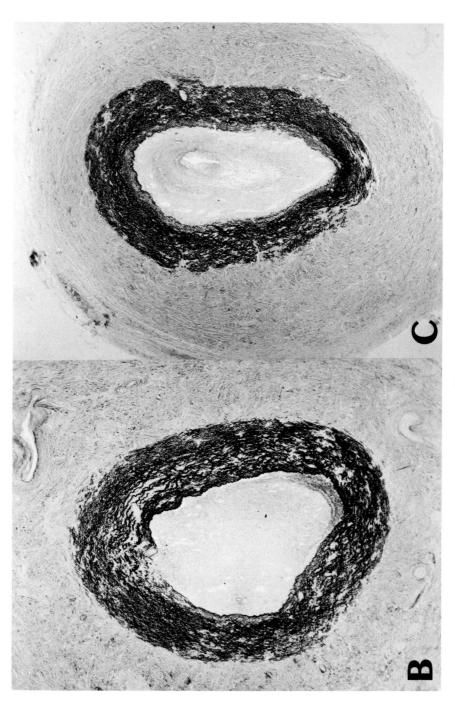

FIGS. 12 B and C

FIGS. 12 D and E

affected artery are similar to those seen in the aorta. The intima is thickened, and occlusion of the vessel may occur at any distance from the orifice. It must be stressed, however, that arteritis of peripheral vessels may occur at sites remote from the orifice of the vessel. This is an expression of independent peripheral localization of TA. It may occur with or without changes in the aorta. Under those circumstances the proximal segment of the artery usually remains well preserved. Two mechanisms therefore appear to be in operation: (a) extension of arteritis from the aorta along the axis of the arterial trunk; and (b) independent focal or diffuse peripheral arteritis. The former appears to be much more prevalent than the latter.

In the aortic arch the gamut of obliterative arterial occlusions may range from stenosis or occlusion of a single branchiocephalic trunk to total obliteration of all brachiocephalic vessels, creating the classical "bald aortic arch." Under those circumstances the blood supply to the head is maintained by collateral circulation only.

Carotid narrowings may be confined strictly to the origin of the vessel. In other instances, however, the narrowing may extend for a variable distance along the axis of the artery with a smooth symmetrical lumen. The wall of the affected artery is uniformly thickened. At times a marked reduction of the arterial lumen of the carotid artery creates a highly characteristic filiform narrowing extending from the orifice to the base of the skull. This can be best demonstrated at aortography. Similar uniform symmetrical thickening of the wall of the carotid artery, creating segmental narrowing, is an expression of focal arteritis at a site remote from the orifice of the vessel.

In addition to constrictions and occlusions, TA may cause diffuse or localized aneurysms of the brachiocephalic vessels as well.

In aortitis of the abdominal aorta the renal arteries are affected in the majority of patients. As a rule, narrowing or occlusion of the vessel takes place at or near their origin (19–22). The celiac, superior mesenteric, and inferior mesenteric arteries may be narrowed or occluded . Usually an abundant collateral circulation revascularizes the occluded trunk. Gastrointestinal complaints are rare in patients with TA. Occlusion of the celiac and superior mesenteric arteries may produce the syndrome of abdominal angina. Occlusive arteritis of Takayasu's type is apparently an insidious and gradual process. This permits development of the most abundant and variable collateral circulation.

In the ascending aorta various forms of aortitis, including Takayasu's disease, may present with similar pathological findings (11). The ascending aorta is thickened, ectatic, or aneurysmally dilated. The intima shows fibrous thickening with white or grayish plaques or patches. The aortic valves are usually incompetent. Virtually all forms of aortitis are capable of affecting the aortic valves. Aortic regurgitation may be caused by dilatation of the aortic ring, causing functional aortic insufficiency, or the aortic leaflets may be directly affected by extension of aortitis with foreshortening and separation.

AORTITIS, A COMMON PATHWAY

Any injury to the aorta—whether chemical, mechanical, infectious, toxic, autoimmune, or due to other causes—may produce a similar inflammatory response (7). The acute, chronic, and old healed stages of aortitis of various etiologies may resemble each other closely. Thus they seem to follow a common pathway.

During the late nineteenth century the histological and gross pathological aspects of syphilis were described in detail. For many decades the classical pathological changes described in syphilis, specifically plasma cell infiltration of the media and the highly characteristic "tree-bark" appearance of the intima, were considered pathognomonic for syphilitic aortitis. In 1936 Mallory first indicated that rheumatoid aortitis could not be distinguished from syphilitic aortitis (24). This nonspecificity of the microscopic and gross pathological appearance of various forms of aortitis was later confirmed by other investigators (7,33). It is now generally accepted that all forms of aortitis display striking gross pathological and histological similarities in the early and late stages of the disease. Apparently the aorta responds to various injuries in a similar fashion.

Despite the close similarities of various forms of aortitis, important differences do exist which permit differentiation of one form of aortitis from another. It appears that TA is the only form of aortitis capable of producing narrowings and coarctations of the aorta. Other forms of aortitis apparently cannot duplicate this phenomenon. In this manner all forms of aortitis may be conveniently subdivided into two major groups: The stenotic variety is synonymous with TA, whereas other forms of aortitis of known or unknown etiology producing dilatation of the aorta and aneurysms may include TA as well.

Although severe involvement of the aorta and the branch arteries in rheumatic fever is presently a rarity owing to early and extensive use of antibiotics in streptococcal infections of the throat, prior to the antibiotic era involvement of the aorta in rheumatic fever was common (16). There are many features of aortitis of rheumatic origin and TA which are strikingly similar, supporting the impression that TA is closely related to the broad spectrum of rheumatoid disorders. There are, however, substantial differences as well in the histological and gross pathological appearance of rheumatic fever and TA. The common features of both diseases are as follows: (a) "Skipped," segmental areas of aortic involvement. At the edges of the "skipped areas" the inflammatory changes stop short with abrupt transition to normal aortic tissue (4,6,12). This strictly segmental involvement of the aorta could affect short or long segments. (b) The gross appearance of the intima in rheumatic fever is strikingly similar to the appearance of the intima in TA. (16,17,19). (c) Both diseases have marked intimal fibrotic thickening with hyalinization of the deep layers and subsequent dystrophic deposition of calcium (6,19). (d) In both diseases there is evidence of secondary atherosclerosis superimposed on the arteritic intimal changes (16,39). (e) Both rheumatic fever and TA affect the pulmonary arteries in about 50% of patients (6,12,16). (f) Rheumatic fever and TA leave few recognizable stigmata of previous aortitis in the late advanced stages of the disease. In both diseases there is marked destruction of the tunica elastica and media with replacement fibrosis.

Despite those similarities there are also significant differences in the active as well as the late stages of the disease. The following morphological characteristics serve to differentiate rheumatic aortitis and probably also rheumatoid aortitis from TA. (a) There is aortic and pulmonary intimitis, with focal fibrinoid necrosis of the media that sometimes extends into the intima in both rheumatic and rheumatoid arthritis. (b) Rheumatic mesoaortitis may rarely produce extensive medial destruction (9) as seen in TA. (c) At gross inspection of the aorta and its branches there is no evidence of occlusion of the orifices of the branch arteries of the aorta in rheumatic fever and rheumatoid aortitis (12). This difference is of great significance as it provides an important differentiation of rheumatic fever and rheumatoid aortitis from TA at arteriography and at gross pathological inspection. Likewise, aneurysms are not a feature of rheumatic mesoaortitis. (d) As previously stated, narrowings and constrictions of the aorta appear to be an exclusive characteristic of TA.

REFERENCES

1. Akikusa, B., Kondo, Y., and Muraki, M. (1981): Aortic insufficiency caused by Takayasu's arteritis without usual clinical features. *Arch. Pathol. Lab. Med.*, 105:650–651.
2. Ask-Upmark, E., and Fajers, C. M. (1956): Further observations on Takayasu's syndrome. *Acta Med. Scand.*, 155:275–291.
3. Berkmen, M. Y., and Lande, A. (1975): Chest roentgenography as a window to the diagnosis of Takayasu's arteritis. *AJR*, 125:842–846.
4. Danaraj, T. J., and Ong, W. H. (1959): Primary arteritis of abdominal aorta in children causing bilateral stenosis of renal arteries and hypertension. *Circulation*, 20:856–863.
5. Danaraj, T. J., and Ong, W. H. (1960): Obliterative brachiocephalic arteritis (pulseless disease). *Am. J. Cardiol.*, 5:277–279.
6. Danaraj, T. J., Wong, H. O., and Thomas, M. A. (1963): Primary arteritis of aorta causing renal artery stenosis and hypertension. *Br. Heart J.*, 25:153–165.
7. DeTakats, G. (1959): Arterial injuries and arterial inflammation. In: *Vascular Surgery*, p. 130. Saunders, Philadelphia.
8. Ehrlich, A., Brodoff, B. N., Rubin, I. L., et al. (1953): Malignant hypertension in a patient with renal artery occlusions. *Arch. Intern. Med.*, 92:591–601.
9. Fassbender, H. G. (1975): *Pathology of Rheumatic Diseases*, pp. 57–62. Springer-Verlag, Berlin.
10. Fisher, E. R., and Corcoran, A. C. (1952): Congenital coarctation of the abdominal aorta with resultant renal hypertension. *Arch. Intern. Med.*, 89:943–950.
11. Heggtweit, H. A. (1964): Syphilitic aortitis: A clinicopathologic autopsy study of 100 cases, 1950 to 1960. *Circulation*, 29:346–355.
12. Heggtweit, H. A., Hennigar, R. G., and Morrione, G. T. (1963): Panaortitis. *Am. J. Pathol.*, 42:151–172.
13. Ishikawa, K. (1978): Natural history and classification of occlusive thromboaortopathy (Takayasu's disease). *Circulation*, 57:27–35.
14. Jervell, A. (1954): Pulseless disease. *Am. Heart J.*, 47:780–784.
15. Judge, R. D., Currier, R. D., Gracie, W. A., and Figley, M. M. (1962): Takayasu's arteritis and the aortic arch syndrome. *Am. J. Med.*, 32:379–392.
16. Klinge, F. (1933): Die rheumatische Narbe. *Ergebn. Allg. Pathd.*, 27:106.
17. Lande, A. (1976): Takayasu's arteritis and congenital coarctation of the aorta: A critical review. *AJR*, 127:227–233.
18. Lande, A., and Bard, R. (1976): Takayasu's arteritis in unrecognized case of pulmonary hypertension. *Angiology*, 27:114–124.

19. Lande, A., and Berkmen, Y. (1976): Aortitis: Pathologic, clinical and arteriographic review. *Radiol. Clin. North Am.*, 14:219–240.
20. Lande, A., and Gross, A. (1972): Total aortography in the diagnosis of Takayasu's arteritis. *AJR*, 116:165.
21. Lande, A., and LaPorta, A. (1976): Takayasu's arteritis, an arteriographic pathologic correlation. *Arch. Pathol.*, 100:437–440.
22. Lande, A., and Rossi, P. (1975): The value of total aortography in the diagnosis of Takayasu's arteritis. *Radiology*, 114:287–297.
23. Lande, A., Bard, R., Rossi, P., Passariello, R., and Castucci, A. (1976): Takayasu's arteritis, a worldwide entity (report of twelve Caucasian patients). *N.Y. State J. Med.*, 76:1477–1482.
23a. Lupi Herrera et al. (1977): Takayasu's arteritis: Clinical study of 107 cases. *Am. Heart J.*, 93:94–103.
24. Mallory, B. T. (1936): Case records of the Massachusetts General Hospital, case 22141. *N. Engl. J. Med.*, 214:690–696.
25. Nakao, K., Ikeda, M., Kimata, S., Niitani, H., Miyahara, M., Ishimi, A., Hashiba, K., Takeda, Y., Ozawa, T., Matashita, S., and Kuramochi, M. (1967): Takayasu's arteritis. *Circulation*, 35:1141–1155.
26. Nasu, T. Y. (1963): Pathology of pulseless disease. *Angiology*, 14:225–242.
27. Numano, F. (1979): Symposium on major histocompatibility antigens (HLA) and disease; Supplement: genetic factors in Takayasu disease. *Nippon Naika Gakkai Zasshi*, 68:1442–1448.
28. Numano, F., Maezawa, H., Aswada, S., Talal, N., and Theofilopoulos, A. N. (1980): Circulating immune complexes in Takayasu disease. *Jpn. Circ. J.*, 44:777–782.
29. Rose, A. G., Halper, J., and Factor, S. M. (1984): Primary arteriopathy in Takayasu's disease. *Arch. Pathol. Lab. Med.* 108:644–648.
30. Rosen, A. G., and Sinclair-Smith, C. C. (1980): Takayasu's arteritis: A study of 16 autopsy cases. *Arch. Pathol. Lab. Med.*, 104:231–237.
31. Rosen, N., and Gaton, E. (1972): Takayasu's arteritis or coronary arteries. *Arch. Pathol.*, 94:225–229.
32. Saito, Y., Hirota, K., Ito, I., Yamagachi, H., Takeda, T., Moroka, S., and Ueda, H. (1972): Clinical and pathologic studies of five autopsied cases of aortitis syndrome. *Jpn. Heart J.*, 13:107–117.
33. Sen, K. P. (1968): Obstructive disease of the aorta and its branches. *Indian J. Surg.*, 30:289–327.
34. Shimizu, K., and Sano, K. (1951): Pulseless disease. *J. Neuropathol.*, 1:37–47.
35. Strachan, R. W., Wigzell, F. W., and Anderson, J. R. (1966): Locomotor manifestations and serum studies in Takayasu's arteriopathy. *Am. J. Med.*, 40:560–568.
36. Takayasu, M. (1908): Case with unusual changes of the central vessels in the retina. *Acta Soc. Ophthalmol. Jpn.*, 112:554.
37. Ueda, H., Morooka, A., Ito, I., Yamacuchi, H., Takeda, T., and Saito, Y. (1969): Clinical observations on 52 cases of aortitis syndrome. *Jpn. Heart J.*, 10:227–288.
38. Vinijchaikul, K. (1967): Primary arteritis of the aorta and its main branches. *Am. J. Med.*, 43:15–27.
39. Yamada, H., Harumi, K., Ohta, A., Nomura, T., Okada, R., and Ishii, M. (1961): Aortic arch syndrome with cardiomegaly and aortic calcification. *Jpn. Heart J.*, 2:538–548.
40. Young, J. A., Sengupta, A., and Khaja, F. (1973): Coronary arterial stenosis, angina pectoris and atypical coarctation of the aorta due to nonspecific arteritis: Treatment with aortocoronary bypass graft. *Am. J. Cardiol.*, 32:356–360.

Aortitis: Clinical, Pathologic, and Radiographic Aspects, edited by A. Lande, Y.M. Berkmen, and H.A. McAllister. Raven Press, New York © 1986.

Radiologic Aspects of Aortitis

Adam Lande and *Yahya M. Berkmen

*Department of Radiology, New York Medical College, Valhalla, New York; and Department of Radiology, Kingston Hospital, Kingston, New York 12401; *Department of Clinical Radiology, Cornell University Medical College, and Section of Pulmonary Radiology, New York Hospital, New York, New York 10021*

The aorta reacts to various injuries in a limited manner and irrespective of the underlying etiology; the pathological alterations show similar gross and histological patterns. In aortitis the aortic wall may be weakened by the specific or nonspecific inflammatory process, and aortic ectasia or aneurysmal dilatation is a common sequela.

Takayasu's arteritis constitutes an exception to this rule since in addition to aneurysms it characteristically produces narrowings and coarctations of the aorta and its branches.

Hence, all forms of aortitis may be conveniently subdivided into two major groups: (a) The stenosing variety is synonymous with Takayasu's arteritis; (b) all other forms of aortitis including Takayasu's disease may produce aortic dilatations and aneurysms. Roentgenography of aortitis reflects the pathologic anatomy of the aorta and its branches. Several imaging modalities are currently available for the diagnosis and evaluation of aortic narrowings, coarctations, as well as aortic aneurysms. In evaluating aortic aneurysms, it is important to precisely determine their size, location, signs of infection, presence of bleeding, and evidence of compression or displacement of adjacent structures.

PLAIN CHEST ROENTGENOGRAPHY

Chest roentgenography plays an important part in the diagnosis of aortitis. It is a valuable screening test and provides several important radiographic signs indicating the presence of the disease. In some instances it permits identification of the disease prior to its clinical recognition. This is well illustrated in Fig. 6[1] which shows a 68-year-old man with sudden enlargement of the superior mediastinum. Since the patient had a staphylococcal septicemia, the diagnosis of a mycotic aneurysm was made. This was subsequently confirmed at surgery.

Aortic Calcifications

Dystrophic as well as secondary atherosclerotic calcifications are both parts of aortitis. Dystrophic calcification is produced by simple deposition of calcium in

---

[1]All figures discussed in this chapter are located at the end of the chapter, on pp. 97–139.

scarred intima and media. They are fine, sharp, and pencil-like in appearance (9). This type of calcification is highly suggestive of previous aortitis (49) (Figs. 1A, 2A, and 2B). Degenerative calcification is the result of secondary atherosclerosis which is engrafted upon the damaged intima. With secondary atherosclerosis the fine, pencil-like appearance of dystrophic calcifications changes in character and becomes rough, heavy, and irregular, as is usually seen in ordinary atherosclerosis. Prior to the use of antibiotics in the treatment of lues, 80 to 90% of patients with radiographically demonstrable calcifications of the ascending aorta were found to have syphilis (54). Consequently, calcification of the ascending aorta became radiographically synonymous with syphilitic aortitis (39,52,54,81,85). Because of the sharp decline in the incidence of untreated syphilis this trend has reversed, and currently atherosclerosis and nonsyphilitic aortitis are considered the most common causes of ascending aortic calcifications (33).

In ordinary atherosclerosis, calcifications of the ascending aorta are usually associated with calcifications in other portions of the vessel. Isolated calcification of the ascending aorta is still considered highly suspicious for syphilitic aortitis (Fig. 1A). Strictly segmental, fine dystrophic calcifications with abrupt terminations or heavy calcifications of the same segmental distribution should be strongly suspected as secondary to previous Takayasu's disease (5,9). In our series of patients strictly segmental calcifications of the thoracic aorta were associated with clinical symptoms of cerebral ischemia indicating brachiocephalic involvement in two patients. In one patient, there was evidence of severe diastolic hypertension suggesting renal artery involvement and clinical testing confirmed renal vascular component. In another patient there was associated claudication of the lower limbs. All four patients were subsequently proven to have Takayasu's arteritis.

Characteristic fine, pencil-like calcification of the dystrophic type is well illustrated in Fig. 2. Calcifications outlining long stenotic segments of the aorta are convincing evidence of long-standing Takayasu's arteritis (Fig. 3).

Rib Notching

Notching of the lower rib cage in Takayasu's arteritis usually indicates a severely coarcted segment of the upper abdominal aorta (4). The notching is an expression of collateral circulation bypassing a stenotic segment of the aorta. Characteristically, rib notching in congenital coarctations involves the upper thorax whereas rib notching due to coarctation of Takayasu's type affects the lower thorax (27). Notching of the first three ribs is an expression of subclavian artery occlusion and collateral circulation revascularising the distal portion of the vessel (38).

Bone Erosion and Destruction

Syphilitic aneurysms, by virtue of their chronicity and constant pulsatile thrust against adjacent bones, may produce erosions of the ribs, sternum, anterior margins of the vertebrae, and the clavicle. Association of tuberculous or suppurative spondylitis with aortic aneurysm is an indication of infectious aortitis (contiguous aortitis) (18,89).

Widening of the Ascending Aorta

Dilatation of the ascending aorta is common in aortitis and is secondary to aortic valve insufficiency or ascending thoracic aortitis. Virtually all forms of aortitis are capable of affecting the aortic valves. With the exception of rheumatic fever, where the cusps tend to fuse, the aortic leaflets in other forms of aortitis are foreshortened, spread apart, and retracted creating aortic insufficiency.

Dilatation of the ascending aorta in the presence of significant aortic regurgitation is very common in syphilitic aortitis, in aortitis complicating ankylosing spondylitis, and Takayasu's arteritis. It is infrequent in rheumatoid arthritis, giant cell arteritis, relapsing polychondritis, systemic lupus erythematosus, and Reiter's syndrome. In Takayasu's arteritis prominence of the ascending aorta is usually due to prestenotic dilatation or aortitis of this portion of the vessel (Fig. 4). The ascending aorta is commonly involved in the disease, and 10 to 20% of patients develop aortic insufficiency; aortic valvulitis, however, is uncommon (27).

Contour Irregularities of the Descending Aorta

Alternating narrowings and dilatations of the aorta may produce an undulating appearance of the descending aorta which is highly suggestive of Takayasu's arteritis (Fig. 4). This finding becomes diagnostic for Takayasu's arteritis if it is associated with other radiographic signs of the disease.

Aortic Aneurysms

As has been previously stated, various forms of aortitis may be associated with aortic aneurysms. Aortitis secondary to syphilis (Fig. 1A) (32), tuberculosis (Fig. 5) (80), bacterial infections (Fig. 6) (89), rheumatoid arthritis (35,87), giant cell arteritis (29,43,44,94), relapsing polychondritis (10,28,37,65), systemic lupus erythematosus (88), Behçet's syndrome (34,53) and occasionally Takayasu's arteritis (Figs. 50,51,53A,54), may be associated with aneurysms of the aorta. Sarcoidosis is an unusual form of aortitis causing saccular aneurysms (56).

In general, these aneurysms exhibit no morphological characteristics which would permit radiographic differentiation of one form of aneurysm from another (Figs. 5 and 6C). However, a few additional observations may provide some distinguishing features. Syphilitic aneurysms enlarge slowly. The ascending aorta and the aneurysm are commonly calcified (Fig. 1A). They may assume enormous proportions and may erode the adjacent skeleton. Sudden enlargment of a syphilitic aneurysm usually indicates bleeding and is a late complication. In contrast, aneurysms of nonsyphilitic nature appear more rapidly, show progressive enlargement, and have a high propensity for rupture. Fever and septicemia accompany mycotic aneurysms (Figs. 6A and B). Sudden enlargement of preexisting atherosclerotic aneurysms in a patient with fever and septicemia strongly suggests secondary infection and an infected atherosclerotic aneurysm. Miliary or cavitary tuberculosis is commonly present in tuberculous aortitis. Typical narrowing of the trachea (36) and a recently developed aneurysm may indicate relapsing polychondritis as an underlying cause of aortitis.

Thoracic aortic aneurysms have a variety of radiographic appearances, and their diagnosis in plain noncontrast chest roentgenography may be difficult. Their size may not be appreciated in absence of pulmonary interface, overshadowing massive atelectasis or ill-defined contours due to a surrounding inflammatory reaction (90). They mimic mediastinal, pulmonary, and pleural neoplasms (32,67). Conversely, pulmonary or mediastinal tumors contiguous with the aorta may be difficult to distinguish from aortic aneurysms (82). In uncertain cases, aortography and/or computed tomography will usually provide the correct diagnosis.

Aortic dissection can rarely complicate aortitis secondary to tuberculosis (58), giant cell arteritis (31,44,57,74), systemic lupus erythematosus (88), and relapsing polychondritis (28). Thickening of the aortic wall and sudden widening of the aortic diameter have been described as important radiographic signs indicating aortic dissection (1,17).

Changes in the Pulmonary Arteries

Involvement of the pulmonary arteries is an expression of the widespread systemic arteritis involving large and medium sized elastic arteries both in the systemic as well as in the pulmonary circulation. Similar to the systemic circulation, pulmonary arteritis may cause aneurysmal dilatation, stenosis, or occlusion of the pulmonary arteries.

Currently, mycotic aneurysms are the most common manifestations of pulmonary arteritis. They are usually a complication of intravenous drug abuse (40). They may be associated with bacterial endocarditis of the right heart chambers (7,40,41). On rare occasions, septic emboli may originate from the left heart, and at times pulmonary seeding through a patent ductus arteriosus may take place (7,40). In the past, syphilitic aneurysms (6,13) and gummatous lesions (77) of the pulmonary arteries had been found at autopsy with relative frequency. Other causes of pulmonary arterial aneurysms are rheumatic fever (6), giant cell arteritis (29,44), and Behçet's syndrome (14,25).

Arteritis of the pulmonary vessels in Takayasu's disease produces narrowings, stenosis, or occlusion of large, medium sized, and smaller elastic pulmonary arteries (56). Occasionally pulmonary vascular occlusions may cause diversion of pulmonary circulation and thus segmental or lobar hypo or hyper circulation. These may be severe enough to be recognized at plain noncontrast chest roentgenography. The hilum on the affected side may be small secondary to arterial occlusion or aneurysmally dilated (46).

At plain chest roentgenography mycotic aneurysms of the pulmonary arteries may appear as large densities indistinguishable from hilar or mediastinal masses or inflammatory lesions (7,40). Pulmonary angiography and computer tomography usually disclose the nature of the lesions.

NONCONTRAST ABDOMINAL RADIOGRAPHY

Abdominal aortic aneurysms are as a rule difficult to diagnose at noncontrast abdominal radiography. Plain abdominal roentgenograms may be unrevealing in spite of a clinically palpable, pulsating abdominal mass. Displacement of bowel loops by an aneurysmal sack occurs late and only after it has reached sizable proportions. Sudden lateral and anterior displacement of preexisting aortic calcifications may indicate presence of a developing or an enlarging aneurysm. Occasionally, discontinuity of the previously present abdominal aortic calcifications in association with an adjacent soft tissue mass obliterating the psoas margins or causing lateral displacement of the left kidney may indicate a ruptured abdominal aortic aneurysm and bleeding (11).

In Takayasu's arteritis typical dystrophic calcifications or thick irregular degenerative calcifications due to superimposed atherosclerosis may be seen outlining segments of the aorta (Fig. 7). As previously stated, they are frequently strictly segmental.

AORTOGRAPHY AND COMPUTERIZED TOMOGRAPHY (CT)

Once suspected, the diagnosis of aortic aneurysms must be further confirmed, and its size and location documented. Both aortography and CT provide the required information with a comparable high specificity (Figs. 6C–F) (22,68,91). The selection of diagnostic modality to be used depends largely on the availability of equipment, the expertise of the radiologist, and the personal preference of the surgeon (62). Each method has some advantages as compared with the other. Aortography demonstrates the aortic insufficiency, the site of bleeding, and the involvement of branch vessels which cannot be visualized by CT (62).

Computerized tomography, on the other hand, is better tolerated by sick patients, provides accurate measurement of the aneurysm (22,68,91), and is useful as a screening procedure and in the differential diagnosis of tortuous aorta, especially in the abdomen (22). Features not shown by aortography—such as periaortic bleeding, collection of fluid in the pericardial and pleural spaces and mediastinum, thickness of the laminated clot within the aneurysm, displacement and compression of the pulmonary arteries, superior vena cava, or bronchi—are clearly demonstrated by computerized tomography (10,62,73,91). Computerized tomography is a very reliable diagnostic modality and may obviate the necessity for aortography in many instances (62). It is also the method of choice for a follow-up of aneurysmal dissections (21,64).

The high mortality associated with infections of aortic grafts is well recognized. Clinically the diagnosis is based on the triad of bleeding from the gastrointestinal tract, previous aortic graft replacement, and fever (89). The method of choice is the diagnosis of infected aortic prosthesis. Multiple gas collections around the prostatic bed 10 days following surgery has been suggested as a diagnostic feature of prostatic infection (26).

Ultrasonography can be satisfactorily used for screening or diagnosis and follow-up examinations of abdominal aortic aneurysms. In general, however, it tends to underestimate the actual size of aneurysmal sacs, especially those containing large clots (22).

TAKAYASU'S ARTERITIS

In 1908 Takayasu, an ophthalmologist, described wreath-like anastomoses in the retina of a young female (84). The underlying cause of these collateral channels was not apparent to him, and he did not offer an explanation. In 1951 Shimizu and Sano described the clinical aspects of brachiocephalic arteritis and named the disease the "pulseless syndrome" (79). This appealing name became well entrenched in the world literature. In 1956 Ask-Upmark and Fajers were the first to report Takayasu's arteritis (TA) outside Japan, presenting a large series of patients from Sweden (2). In 1962 Inada et al. were one of the first groups to describe involvement of the descending thoracic aorta and the abdominal aorta in Takayasu's disease (38). Later in 1963 Nasu published a large autopsy series of patients with TA and clearly showed involvement of the descending thoracic and abdominal aorta by the inflammatory process (61). The pulmonary arteries were also involved in the majority of cases. During the following years numerous publications described the clinical aspects of the disease, with most of the papers originating in Japan (38,60,61,79,84,86,92). However, TA was identified rather early in Mexico, and a number of publications came from Mexico City (8,23,55,93). In the United States DeBakey and Cooley have treated many patients with obliterative aortic disease using bypass grafts, and they believed that the cases represented an inflammatory process somehow related to TA (12,59).

To date, TA has been reported from virtually all parts of the world without ethnic or geographic boundaries. Large series of cases have been published in the Scandinavian countries (4,15,20,63,75), western Europe (16,20,66,70–72,83), and South Africa (24,76), and the disease has been seen in Eskimos and Australian Aborigines as well.

In the United States, however, TA is rarely diagnosed, and there are several reasons for its infrequent recognition (45–51). First, the impression prevails that TA is an exotic disease of young females from the Orient. Second, there is still a popular belief that TA is limited to the aortic arch causing pulseless disease. It is not as yet widely recognized that it also involves the descending thoracic and abdominal aorta. Third, the symptomatology of TA is confusing and variable, as is described later in the chapter. Fourth, the pathology of TA is frequently misleading or inconclusive. The pathologic aspects of TA are discussed in a separate chapter. Fifth, the disease has been published under a variety of names, the most common of which are nonsyphilitic or nonspecific aortitis (69), aortitis syndrome (86), idiopathic arteritis (76), pulseless disease (79), aortic arch syndrome (75), middle aortic syndrome (78), and others. TA, however, is the most commonly used designation.

The International Athcrosclcrosis Project has shed some light on the probable incidence of TA in the United States and other countries (69). The primary interest of this study was investigation of the severity of atherosclerosis under various geographic and environmental conditions. As a by-product of this investigation nonspecific aortitis, which the investigators believed to be closely related to Takayasu's disease, was discovered in a certain percentage of patients. Conservative estimates indicated that at least 0.5% of the United States' population was affected by asymptomatic lesions of TA in the form of small patches scattered haphazardly in the aorta without symptoms attributable to TA. The lack of clinical manifestations has been attibuted to the sparing of ostia of the vital arteries. All lesions were located in neutral, insignificant portions of the aorta. Conversely, the literature provides several reports of small patches of aortitis involving the ostia of vital arteries causing severe hypertension (19), coronary occlusion (70), or cerebral ischemia (3), primarily in young individuals. Thus it is apparent that most of the cases reported in the literature, as well as those presented in our series, represent severe forms of the disease. Hence vascular involvement in TA may range from asymptomatic forms to extensive involvement of the aorta and its branches. Between these two extremes, there undoubtedly exists a large group of patients in whom moderately severe arterial involvement has escaped clinical identification.

The laboratory findings in TA support the impression of an autoimmune etiology. They are, however, nonspecific. The C-reactive protein is positive in a substantial proportion of patients. Protein electrophoresis shows elevation of alpha-2 and gamma globulins (51,60,63,86). The erythrocyte sedimentation rate (ESR) is an excellent indicator of activity of the disease. In the acute or active stage of TA the ESR is usually elevated and returns to normal after months or years. It is of interest that a mildly to moderately elevated ESR was seen in only 40% of our patients with TA when first admitted to the hospital. This indicates that the disease was of long duration and the ESR had returned to normal in the majority of patients.

The classic descriptions of TA stress the existence of two phases of the disease (60). The *prepulseless systemic phase* is characterized by such diverse signs and symptoms as fever, night sweats, weakness, weight loss, arthralgia, arthritis, myalgia, cough, hemoptysis, pleuritis, pericarditis, chest and abdominal pains, skin rashes, and erythemas. The *late occlusive* or *pulseless phase* of the disease takes the form of variable ischemic manifestations secondary to arterial occlusion. As a rule, the systemic manifestations last for several weeks or months; as they subside, signs and symptoms of occlusive arteritis appear. Occasionally a latent period of years or even decades separates the prodromal systemic illness from the late ischemic manifestations. This "silent interval" was observed in some of our patients and has been estimated by other investigators to average 6.1 to 7.8 years (83,86). This marked delay in appearance of the ischemic manifestations contributes to the difficulties in establishing the diagnosis of Takayasu's disease.

The incidence and severity of the early systemic phase of the disease is highly variable. In our series of 67 cases a definite history of a systemic illness could be obtained in only 14 cases. In the early years of our investigation absence of the systemic phase was perplexing, and it was difficult to reconcile with the classic Japanese papers describing a systemic phase of the disease followed later by a pulseless ischemic stage. During subsequent years, however, many sources have confirmed our original impression that the early constitutional phase of the disease may pass completely unrecognized (51,83,86). In the vast majority of our patients, the early constitutional symptoms were either absent or vague, abortive, and passed unnoticed (51). In our patients the presenting complaints were secondary to the late ischemic signs and symptoms, hypertension, or both in virtually all instances.

Not only the incidence but also the clinical characteristics of the systemic phase of TA is highly variable. This stage is apparently common in the countries around the North and Baltic seas (2,15,20,63,71,72,75,83). In the Scandinavian countries and England, polyarthritis is a frequently observed feature, and the disease closely resembles rheumatic fever or rheumatoid arthritis (2,15,20,63,75,83). However, in other European countries the clinical picture may simulate influenza with fever, myalgias, and similar disorders (16,66,71,72). The nonspecific flu-like illness is probably a common prodromal manifestation of Takayasu's disease.

In Japan the incidence of the generalized systemic symptoms ranges from a small number to 60% of patients depending on the sources consulted (60,86). The primary symptoms tend to center around the cardiopulmonary system, and polyarthritis is less common. There appears to be little doubt that geographic and climatic influences play a decisive role in the incidence and clinical characteristics of the prepulseless, systemic phase of the disease.

The difficulties in diagnosis of TA are well illustrated by the fact that the average interval from the onset of first symptoms to establishment of the diagnosis is approximately 8 years. These figures are reported by the Japanese and Mexican sources in whose areas TA is apparently relatively well known. As previously stated, the systemic phase of the disease is subject to marked variations. It may be mild and nonspecific or absent altogether. This further contributes to the difficulties in establishing the diagnosis of TA.

Although none of our patients at admission had the systemic form of the disease, reports from other countries indicate that TA frequently has a peculiar affinity to favor certain symptom complexes during the systemic illness which may dominate the clinical picture (e.g., a patient with erythema nodosum or multiforme may first seek the help of a dermatologist).

A similar situation exists in the chronic or inactive state of the disease when the symptomatology is caused by arterial occlusions and regional ischemia. When the ischemic changes are localized to a portion of the aorta only, they may cause very specific symptoms (e.g., cerebral ischemia or renovascular hypertension). When multiple portions of the aorta and its branches are affected, however, a variety of symptoms and clinical manifestations may coexist in a confusing array. All these factors may create highly variable signs and symptoms, and they highlight the difficulty of establishing the diagnosis (20,83).

The general physician may see a patient with fever of unknown origin or migratory arthralgias. Chest pain with or without hemoptysis may be present. The ESR may be persistently elevated, and there may be various forms of anemia. Frequently a combination of symptoms may simulate systemic lupus erythematosus or rheumatoid arthritis. Clinically TA may closely resemble other collagen diseases, indicating the close relationship of TA to the broad spectrum of rheumatoid disorders.

The cardiologist may see a patient with heart murmurs, effort angina, myocardial infarction, pericarditis, congestive heart failure, pulmomary hypertension, and other cardiac manifestations. Aortic aneurysms may become symptomatic. The neurologist may be faced with a variety of cerebral symptoms depending on the combination of brachiocephalic involvement. Because of occlusive arteritis the vascular surgeon is frequently consulted. The ophthalmologist may be faced with virtually the entire spectrum of ocular pathology. The psychiatrist may encounter a patient with constant fatigue, dizziness, and emotional instability. Three of our patients have been treated for anxiety neurosis. For more detailed information on various signs and symptoms, the reader is referred to the specific chapters in this volume on medical, neurologic, ophthalmologic, and surgical aspects of Takayasu's disease.

Takayasu's arteritis has been named one of the great imitators in medicine. The patients are often treated for a variety of complaints without exploration of the underlying etiology. Familiarity with the natural history of TA and its clinical presentation, pathologic aspects, and radiographic and arteriographic characteristics is essential. A high index of suspicion is of paramount importance if the diagnosis of TA is to be made.

Arteriography of Takayasu's Arteritis

In our series of 67 patients, the initial diagnosis of TA was made arteriographically in the majority of cases. The characteristic arteriographic appearance of the diseased aorta and its branches usually prompted further clinical and laboratory exploration. It is of interest that none of our patients was referred for arteriography with the presumptive diagnosis of Takayasu's disease. All patients were investigated for the secondary signs and symptoms of the late ischemic phase of the disease. The majority had cerebral ischemic manifestations or renovascular hypertension. This fact illustrates again the general lack of familiarity with the clinical aspects of Takayasu's disease.

Takayasu's arteritis may involve the aorta and its branches in a carpricious and unpredictable fashion. They may be narrowed, occluded, or aneurysmally dilated. The severity of involvement is subject to great variation. It may primarily involve the arch with little or no involvement of the remaining aorta. This type of Takayasu's disease has been named the *arch type*. When in addition to the arch the descending thoracic and/or abdominal aorta is involved, it is referred to as the *extensive type of TA*. In the third variety there is exclusive involvement of the descending thoracic and/or abdominal aorta without involvement of the arch. This type of TA has been named *atypical coarctation of the aorta* or *the middle aortic syndrome* (38,47,55).

During the last four decades approximately 150 cases of congenital coarctation of the descending thoracic and abdominal aorta have been reported in the United States and Europe. It has been shown that the majority represented unrecognized, old, inactive cases of acquired coarctation of the aorta secondary to Takayasu's disease (45). Involvement of the pulmonary arteries occurs in approximately 50% of patients, and it can be associated with any type of Takayasu's disease described (55).

When a large series of arteriograms of Takayasu's disease are tabulated, they can be arranged in such a fashion as to display the gradual transition of pathologic changes from the involvement of the arch only, to extensive involvement of the entire aorta, and finally to types of aortitis exclusively limited to the descending and abdominal aorta only (Fig. 8).

Three basic arteriographic patterns are observed in patients with TA: (a) varying degrees of aortic and arterial narrowings; (b) saccular and fusiform aneurysms; and (c) various combinations of the two. In the aorta, scarring, the sequela of arteritis, leaves its angiographically recognizable imprint in several patterns. The stenotic patterns of TA are displayed in Fig. 9 and 10. Each of the basic patterns presented may undergo modifications, but the principal configuration persists.

The earliest arteriographically detectable change in TA may be a localized narrowing or irregularity of the aortic wall (Fig. 23). Although TA has a distinct tendency toward segmental circumferential involvement (Fig. 26 and 27), asymmetrical eccentric irregularity of the aortic wall may occur (Fig. 25).

Moderate aortic narrowings may be completely asymptomatic. They represent, however, an important arteriographic landmark of Takayasu's disease. These aortic narrowings may progress to hemodynamically significant coarctations and occasionally total occlusions (Fig. 11). Coarctations and complete aortic blocks have been described to occur at various levels from the distal aortic arch down to the bifurcation. An excellent collateral circulation usually reconstitutes the distal vessel.

As shown in Figs. 9 and 10, aortic constrictions can be short and segmental, or long and diffuse. The most common findings are solitary or multiple segmental narrowings (Figs. 19, 20, 25A, 27A, and 28). Both the linear extent and the degree of narrowing are variable. Frequently a localized constriction is clearly demarcated with a sharp luminal surface (Figs. 26 and 27A). In other instances, however, the segmental constriction shows an irregular contour with gradual transition to a normal lumen proximally and distally (Figs. 20 and 21). At times the entire aorta is narrowed and irregular in outline with or without superimposed constriction (Figs. 17, 18, 30, and 31).

Takayasu's arteritis affects the aorta in an unpredictable fashion. Skipped areas of involvement are common. A localized narrowing of the descending thoracic aorta, for instance, may be associated with segmental constriction or aneurysmal dilatation of the more distal portions of the vessel (Figs. 20, 21, and 28). Dilatation of the ascending aorta is very common.

An outstanding feature of the thoracic coarctation is a predilection for the segment of severe constriction to be located at or slightly above the diaphragm. In the elongated form of thoracic coarctation, the aorta may have an irregular wall or a wavy contour or be perfectly smooth in outline. Usually the lumen tapers gradually toward the diaphragm (Figs. 12–15). The severity of the narrowing may or may not be hemodynamically significant. At times the proximal portion of the involved segment of the thoracic aorta tends to be sharply delineated, whereas the constricted segment is shaggy in outline (Figs. 14 and 21). This is especially true in older hypertensive patients in whom the appearance of secondarily engrafted atherosclerosis can be anticipated. Distal to the site of coarctation there is frequently an abrupt transition to a normally appearing aorta. A descriptive term of "rat-tail" aorta has been used for these elongated coarctations (Figs. 12–14).

Supra- and interrenal coarctations, as shown in Fig 10, are usually associated with severe diastolic hypertension. Infrarenal coarctations may be associated with claudication of the lower limbs. Abdominal narrowings are frequently long and diffuse, extending downward to the bifurcation (Figs. 30–32). In many instances the entire descending thoracic and abdominal aorta is diffusely and irregularly constricted.

In a 75-year-old patient, the abdominal aorta was severely contracted and buckled to the left as commonly seen in elderly patients (Fig. 22). The distal abdominal aorta and the bifurcation, commonly involved in ordinary atherosclerosis, were conspicuously spared. This observation indicated a different etiologic process rather than ordinary atherosclerosis. Corroborative evidence of TA in this 75-year-old female was further provided by the appearance of the descending thoracic and the upper abdominal aorta with a characteristic long, tapering, cone-like coarctation. Although this patient's TA undoubtedly took place in the early years, the imprint left was unmistakable and could not be distorted by secondary atherosclerosis. In some instances of thoracic coarctation, the thoracic aorta is diffusely narrowed whereas the abdominal aorta is well preserved and of normal caliber. In other instances the thoracic aorta is unaltered, whereas the abdominal aorta is severely contracted; at times the lumen is reduced to the size of a pencil (Fig. 32).

Aneurysm formation is common in TA. A combination of extensive destruction of the aortic wall and deficient production of the supporting fibrous tissue weaken the aortic wall, which balloons out. Aneurysms may develop in the acute systemic stage of the disease and may rapidly enlarge, rupture, and result in death. In other instances the arteritic process may leave the wall weakened and of borderline integrity. Over the years or decades, there is gradual dilatation of the vessel forming an aneurysm. This is especially true in the thorax where there is little surrounding supporting tissue (Figs. 54 and 55).

At times secondary atherosclerosis promotes weakening of the wall and contributes to aneurysm formation. At autopsy those aneurysms may, on gross inspection, look conspicuously atherosclerotic. In those instances, it is important to remember the natural history of atherosclerosis, with the distal abdominal aorta, the bifurcation, and the iliac and femoral arteries affected first. Atherosclerosis of the thoracic aorta associated with well-preserved abdominal aorta and the iliac arteries would be an unusual situation especially in a young or middle-aged individual. It would be contrary to the natural history of atherosclerosis, which primarily affects the distal abdominal aorta and bifurcation. In young and middle-aged individuals an isolated aneurysm of the thoracic aorta should be considered to be arteritic in origin, if syphilis, Osler-Weber-Rendu syndrome, mycotic aneurysms, pseudoaneurysms following trauma, and Marfan's syndrome can be excluded.

Aortic aneurysms may be fusiform or saccular. Frequently the aortic wall is diffusely dilated with irregular contours. The dilatation may involve long, contiguous segments of the aorta (Figs. 52 and 54). In some instances, the entire aorta may be irregularly dilated.

Aortic aneurysms similar to aortic coarctations can be sharply demarcated from the remaining normal aorta (Figs. 52 and 54). At times, multiple confluent aneurysms of the aorta suggest variable levels of origin (Fig. 54). Skipped areas of aortic involvement in which aneurysms and narrowings alternate with normal segments are most characteristic of TA.

When long segments of the aorta are dilated but the contours of the vessels remain smooth and symmetrical, the appearance is that of simple aortic ectasia. This appearance is usually an expression of extensive patchy involvement of contiguous segments of the vessel. Mild to moderate intimal irregularity often escapes arteriographic detection, and the contour of the vessel appears smooth (Fig. 50). At times there is diffuse ectasia of the thoracic and upper abdominal aorta (Fig. 50). In some patients, a saccular aneurysm may be superimposed on diffuse aortic dilatation (Fig. 51).

The pathologic process in TA may be confined to the aorta only or to the branch arteries, although both are usually affected. In our experience, occlusion of branch vessels is present in the majority of patients. The characteristic sites of involvement and the appearance of the occluded or narrowed arteries frequently indicate the nature of the disease.

Isolated involvement of a single branch artery with an otherwise normal arterial tree may represent a difficult diagnostic problem unless a characteristic clinical background and laboratory findings provide supporting diagnostic evidence. For instance, in one patient a localized arteritic occlusion of the subclavian artery was diagnosed as TA only after the history disclosed a prodromal systemic illness with characteristic features of this disease (Fig. 35).

In general, stenosis or occlusion of an artery at or near the point of origin from the aorta implies aortitis with extension of the inflammatory process into the branch artery. A cone-like narrowing or a flame-shaped occlusion of the vessel extending from the ostium of the artery appears to be characteristic for TA (Figs. 39, 41, and 44–47).

Arterial narrowings and occlusions may, however, be located at sites remote from the point of origin of the vessel. They are not simple extensions of aortitis but represent an independent arteritic process (Figs. 24, 33, and 38).

In the aortic arch the gamut of arterial obliterative changes may range from stenosis or occlusion of a single brachiocephalic trunk or its branch vessel to complete occlusion of all brachiocephalic trunks leading to the classic "bald aortic arch" of TA (Figs. 33, 34, and 49). Under these conditions, the blood supply to the head is provided by numerous collaterals originating from branches of the thyrocervical trunk, internal mammary artery, upper three intercostals, anterior spinal artery, and many unnamed vessels from the aorta.

When the brachiocephalic vessels are affected, the aortic arch is usually moderately dilated and has a smooth contour. The subclavian arteries are the most commonly affected vessels. The occlusion is usually at the point of origin of the vessel or just distal to the thyrocervical trunk. This is probably related to the fact that in subclavian occlusions the thyrocervical trunk assumes the major collateral pathway (Figs. 36, 37, and 42). When a subclavian artery is occluded, a subclavian steal syndrome with the occluded vessel revascularized by the vertebral artery is a common occurrence (Fig. 46). The well-entrenched name "pulseless disease" is an expression of stenosis or occlusion of the subclavian vessels, and clinically a difference in blood pressure between the right and left arm of more than 25 mm Hg in a young or a middle-aged patient is significant and suspicious for Takayasu's disease.

A unique situation arises in the presence of bilateral subclavian artery obstruction when there is associated severe coarctation of the distal thoracic aorta. This situation creates the famous "pulseless patient" in whom the high level of blood pressure is obscured by subclavian and aortic obstructions (Fig. 34). All four extremities show diminished blood pressure. In such a case, a direct recording of the aortic blood pressure may be the only means to obtain the actual level of the patient's hypertension.

Carotid narrowings may be strictly confined to the origin of the vessel. In other instances, the narrowing may extend for a variable distance along the axis of the artery with smooth symmetrical borders (Fig. 39). In some patients constriction of the carotid arteries is extreme, and a highly characteristic filiform smooth narrowing of the arterial lumen may extend from the aorta to the base of the skull (Fig. 40). On occasion, the stenotic lesion may be sharply demarcated with a symmetrical sharp lumen and be located at a site remote from the point of origin of the vessel. The appearance of this segmental constriction is unique (Fig. 38). The various forms of carotid constrictions just described are characteristic, virtually pathognomonic of TA.

In addition to the constrictions and occlusions, TA at times produces dilatations and aneurysms of the brachiocephalic vessels (Figs. 21, 29, and 43). The characteristic arteriographic appearance of the brachiocephalic vessels as well as the multiplicity of lesions and the clinical setting in a young or middle-aged individual should alert the radiologist to the possibility of a widespread arterial disorder. Familiarity with the arteriographic appearance and a high index of suspicion are of crucial importance. In 17 patients in this series, the diagnosis of TA was made or suspected at arch arteriography after the arteriographic appearance suggested systemic arteritis. This prompted extension of the study to include descending thoracic and abdominal arteriography, which usually further confirmed the diagnosis.

At the present time, *total* aortography is of paramount diagnostic importance in establishing the diagnosis of TA. The entire aorta and all its branches must be visualized in order to make a definite diagnosis of Takayasu's disease. It is the composite of the symptomatic and asymptomatic changes in the aorta and its branches which creates a highly characteristic arteriographic configuration. On occasion, the arteriographic findings in the arch closely mimics atherosclerotic occlusions, but, the clinical setting is usually quite different (Figs. 33 and 34).

It is important to recognize that Takayasu's disease may leave the arch and the brachiocephalic vessels totally unaffected with the pathologic changes concentrated in the distal aorta. Constriction of the renal arteries is very common in abdominal coarctations, and the resulting marked elevation of blood pressure may by itself produce variable neurologic manifestations.

Whereas aortitis of the descending thoracic aorta causes aortic narrowings, coarctations, and aneurysms, aortitis of the abdominal aorta usually has a devastating effect on the branch arteries with stenosis or occlusion of the renal and visceral vessels. The abdominal aorta itself at times preserves a smooth contour, usually indicating a patchy form of arteritis (Figs. 50 and 51A) or be coarcted in a segmental or elongated fashion (Figs. 10, 26A, 27A, and 29A). In other instances, the abdominal aorta displays an asymmetrical unilateral or diffuse irregularity of its contour (Figs. 24 and 25). In other patients the vessel may be ectatic or aneurysmally dilated (Figs. 51A, 52A, and 53). The effect on the branch arteries is similar: The vessels are stenosed or occluded at the point of origin or in close proximity to the orifice. Surprisingly, however, in some patients constrictive aortitis of the abdominal aorta may leave the branch arteries completely unaffected (Figs. 28 and 31). There is no good explanation for this phenomenon.

Frequently the arteritic process extends along the axis of the branch artery for a variable distance. The branch vessel under those circumstances shows a mildly irregular lumen or a beaded appearance (Figs. 26B, 29B, and 32A). Arteritis extending along the axis of the vessel may terminate in an occlusion at any point. At times the occlusion is at a distance from the point of origin. In addition, the arteritic process may cause obliteration or stenosis of branches ramifying from the main arterial trunk (Figs. 29B,C).

As in brachiocephalic arteritis, however, the arteritic process may be an independent manifestation, occurring at a site remote from the orifice of the vessel. In the abdomen, however, this focal arteritis causes occlusion rather than stenosis of the artery. The proximal segment of the artery usually remains well preserved. Two mechanisms therefore appear to be in operation: (a) extension of arteritis from the aorta along the axis of the arterial trunk; and (b) independent focal or diffuse arteritis. The former, however, appears to be much more prevalent than the latter. In abdominal aortitis the renal arteries are affected in the majority of patients. In most instances, the involvement is bilateral. As a rule, occlusion or stenosis of the renal arteries takes place at or in close proximity to the point of origin (Figs. 26A, 27A, and 29A). Poststenotic dilatation is common (Figs. 27A and 52A). When arteritis extends along the trunk of the renal artery, the vessel may have a beaded appearance (Fig. 26B). Severe renovascular hypertension is usually present. Because of excellent collateral circulation, the function is preserved in virtually all patients.

Gastrointestinal complaints are uncommon in the chronic stage of TA despite the frequently encountered obliteration of the visceral branches. Occlusion or stenosis of the celiac trunk appears to be much less common than occlusion of the superior and inferior mesenteric arteries. Extension of aortitis along the celiac artery trunk is frequently associated with occlusion of the ramifying arteries. The splenic artery, main branches of the hepatic artery, or gastroduodenal artery may in this fashion be obliterated (Fig. 29B). When the celiac artery is occluded, the pancreaticoduodenal arcade assumes an important collateral pathway (Figs. 51A and 53).

Occlusion or stenosis of the superior mesenteric artery is fairly common. It may occur at the point of origin or at any distance along the superior mesenteric artery trunk (Figs. 23, 27B, 29A, 51A, 52A, and 53). Excellent collateral circulation reconstitutes the distal vessel (Figs. 29C–E and 52A,B,D). The collateral pathways originate from the celiac or inferior mesenteric arteries. In some instances a mesh of small arterial colaterals in the mesentery helps to bypass the obstruction (Figs. 29C–E). The small intestinal mesenteric arcade extending along the small intestine is an important collateral pathway (Figs. 29C–E). Occlusion of the celiac and the superior mesenteric arteries causes the syndrome of abdominal angina (Fig 51). The inferior mesenteric is commonly occluded with revascularization from the superior mesenteric artery (Fig. 32) or from the internal pudendal artery via the rectal–superior hemorrhoidal anastomosis.

Occlusive arteritis of Takayasu's type is apparently an insidious and gradual process. This feature combined with the relatively young age of the patient permits the development of the most abundant and variable collateral circulation ever demonstrated angiographically. In our experience, evidence of abundant collateral circulation in the abdomen of a young or middle-aged individual usually indicates Takayasu's disease. Similarly, an extensive collateral circulation around a stenotic renal artery indicates TA or fibromuscular hyperplasia (Figs. 52A–C). A radiologist faced with this unusually well-developed collateral flow should be immediately alerted to the possibility of Takayasu's disease in other parts of the arterial tree.

Abdominal aortitis may extend into the iliac arteries causing irregularity of the lumen, narrowing or aneurysm formation of the iliac arteries, or at times occlusion (Figs. 29A, 32, 51A, and 53). Leriche's syndrome in young individuals is apparently one of the many faces of Takayasu's disease. Rarely, TA extends into the external iliac and superficial femoral arteries causing stenosis or occlusion (Fig. 24).

In the ascending aorta various forms of aortitides including Takayasu's disease may present with similar aortographic manifestations. The ascending aorta is ectatic or aneurysmally dilated, and the aortic valves are incompetent. Virtually all forms of aortitides are capable of affecting the aortic valves. In Takayasu's disease regurgitation may be caused by dilatation of the aortic ring leading to functional aortic insufficiency, or the aortic valves may be directly involved as an extension of the ascending thoracic aortitis with fibrosis and foreshortening. Usually the commissures are widened, and the aortic leaflets are separated from each other. Aortic valvular stenosis with fusion of the aortic cusps has not been reported in TA.

Coronary ostial stenosis is a serious complication of Takayasu's disease leading to angina or myocardial infarction in young and middle-aged women. The arteritic process in the ascending aorta extends into the ostia of the coronary arteries, or the intimal thickening of the aorta narrows the orifices without the artery being affected. The distal coronary arteries as a rule are not affected by TA. Several young and middle-aged women in our series presented with anginal pains and experienced myocardial infarction.

The pulmonary arteries are affected in the majority of patients with TA. Pulmonary arterial involvement is an expression of generalized arteritis. As in the systemic arterial tree, the main and large pulmonary arteries are affected. The sequela of pulmonary arteritis is stenosis or occlusion of the pulmonary arterial trunks. They are affected in an unpredictable fashion. At pulmonary arteriography there is evidence of a paucity of the pulmonary vessels usually in a lobar or segmental distribution (Fig. 56). Aneurysmal dilatation of the pulmonary arteries has been described. When obliteration of the pulmonary arteries is severe, the bronchial arteries take over the collateral blood supply. Pulmonary hypertension of mild to moderate degree is a late complication in the majority of cases.

As the preceding discussion indicates, aortography is a standard method of diagnosis in Takayasu's arteritis. Diagnostic potentials of computerized tomography and magnetic resonance imaging have not been explored. Our limited experience with both modalities has been encouraging, and it appears that they may offer valuable information about gross anatomic alterations of the involved vessels and perhaps be used in the future as an alternative to aortography (Figs. 57 and 58).

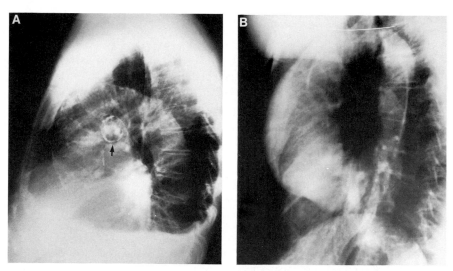

FIG. 1. Syphilitic aortitis. **A:** Lateral view of the chest shows combination of fine, pencil-line dystrophic calcifications of the ascending aorta and coarse, irregular calcifications due to atherosclerosis at the aortic arch. The ascending aorta is dilated. A small saccular aneurysm bulges from the inferior aspect of the proximal arch *(arrow)*. Note the lack of calcification of the distal aortic arch and the descending aorta. **B:** Aortography in a different patient. There is ectasia and a fusiform aneurysm of the ascending aorta.

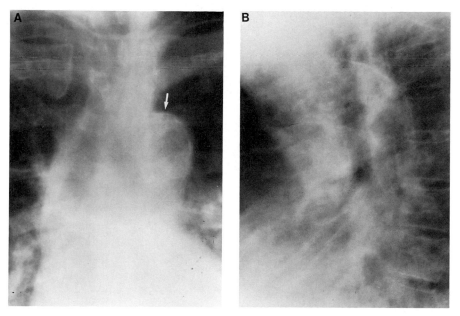

FIG. 2. Calcification of the aorta in Takayasu's arteritis. Same patient as in Figs. 17, 43, and 56. A mixture of pencil-line dystrophic *(arrow)* and atherosclerotic calcifications are seen in posteroanterior **(A)** and lateral **(B)** films.

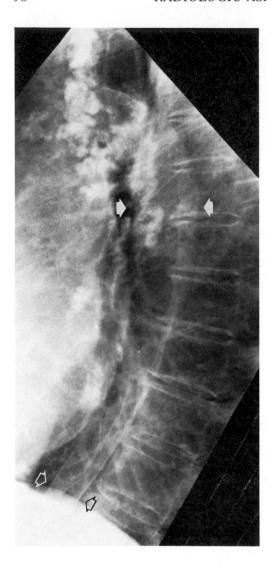

FIG. 3. A 63-year-old female with anginal pains and a history of myocardial infarction was admitted for breast surgery. The descending thoracic and upper abdominal aorta are smoothly narrowed *(arrows)* and outlined by fine pencil-line calcifications. There were no symptoms referable to the thoracic or abdominal narrowing. The calcification ended abruptly in the upper abdominal aorta as typically seen in TA. This pencil-line fine calcification is dystrophic in type and characteristic for aortitis.

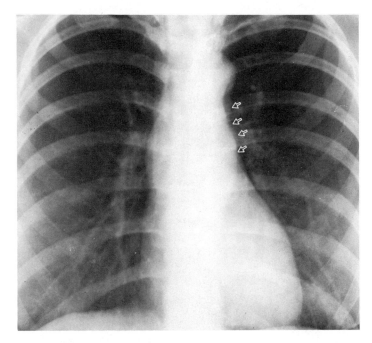

FIG. 4. An 18-year-old female had widespread involvement of the aorta by Takayasu's disease. Roentgenogram of the chest demonstrates indentation of the aortic contour in the region of the isthmus *(arrows)*, with a prominent aortic knob and ascending aorta. Irregularity of the descending aorta may provide clues indicating the presence of Takayasu's disease.

FIG. 5. False aneurysm of the upper abdominal aorta secondary to tuberculous aortitis. The aneurysm is indistinguishable from aneurysms associated with other forms of aortitis.

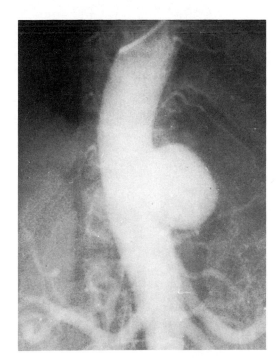

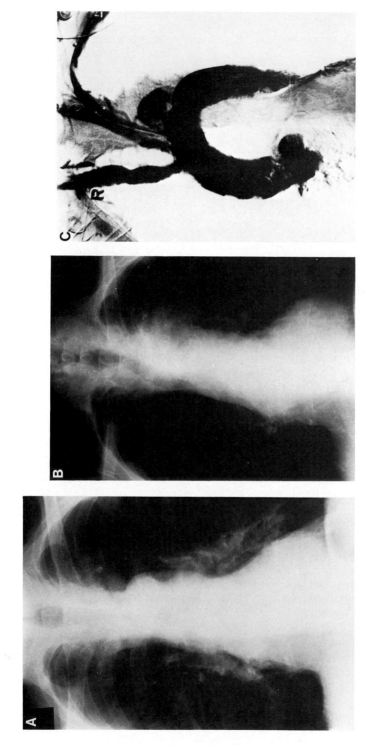

FIG. 6. Mycotic aneurysm in a 68-year-old male patient with *Staphylococcus aureus* septicemia. **A:** Normal posteroanterior chest roentgenogram 1 month prior to admission. **B:** Admission chest roentgenogram. There is obvious enlargement of the superior mediastinum, especially on the left side. The trachea is slightly deviated to the right side. The superior aspect of the aortic arch has lost its definition. **C:** Early filling of a false aneurysm during arch aortography. The aneurysm is immediately distal to the left subclavian artery. *(Continued.)*

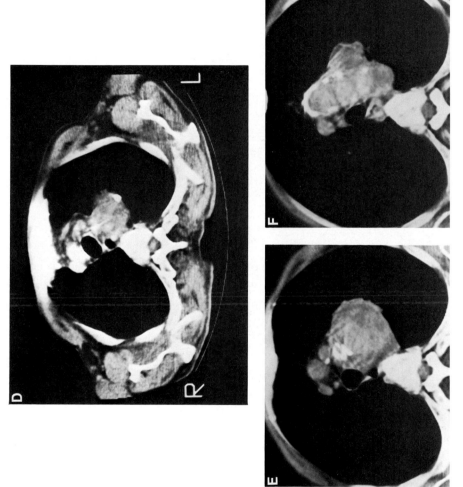

FIG. 6. *(Continued.)* **D–F**: CT study of the aneurysm. Sections through the top (**D**), middle (**E**), and neck (**F**) of the aneurysm.

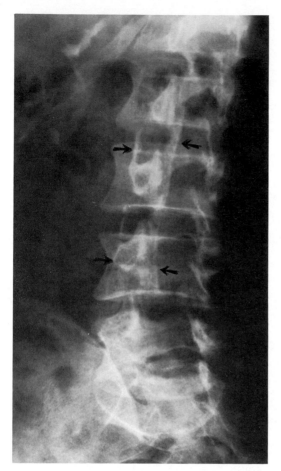

FIG. 7. A 28-year-old female with widespread involvement of the descending and abdominal aorta. There is segmental calcification of the distal abdominal aorta *(arrows)*. The calcification is thick and irregular suggesting secondary atherosclerosis rather than dystrophic calcification. However, segmental calcifications of this nature in a young or middle-aged individual are strongly suggestive of aortitis.

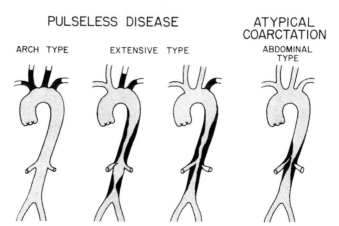

FIG. 8. Gradual transition of pathologic changes in TA, ranging from the arch type to the purely descending thoracic or abdominal type (atypical coarctation).

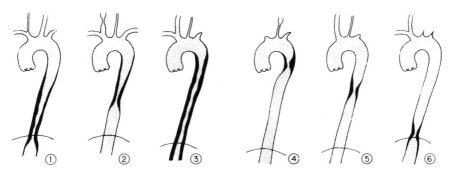

FIG. 9. Thoracic coarctations of Takayasu's type. Gradual tapering of the descending aorta creates a "rat-tail" or comma-shaped configuration (2,3). At times the entire descending thoracic aorta is diffusely constricted (4). Short, segmental narrowings may be located anywhere in the descending aorta (8,12.15).

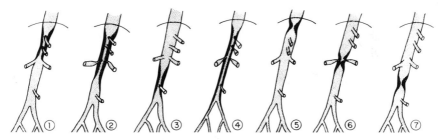

FIG. 10. Abdominal coarctations of Takayasu's type. Narrowings may be long and diffuse or short and segmental. Occasionally the entire abdominal aorta is constricted (8). Supra- and interrenal coarctations are frequently associated with severe hypertension (2,3,12.15). Infrarenal coarctations may cause claudication of the lower limbs (4,16).

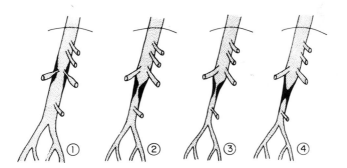

FIG. 11. Short segmental coarctations of Takayasu's type. *(1)* Minimal, hemodynamically insignificant aortic narrowing with involvement and constriction of the renal orifices. *(2)* Moderately severe constrictions with some narrowing of the distal aorta; common form. *(3)* Severe coarctation with marked narrowing of the distal aorta; terms such as "hypoplasia" and "atresia" of the abdominal aorta have been applied to this form of aortic constrictions. *(4)* Extreme forms of aortic constrictions which may culminate in total occlusion.

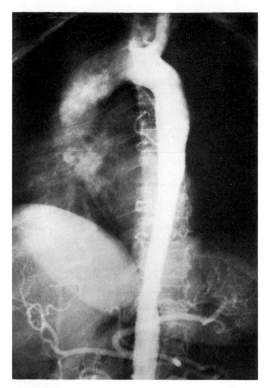

FIG. 12. Gradual tapering of the thoracic aorta of mild hemodynamic significance. This configuration of the descending thoracic aorta is frequently referred to as the "rat-tail" aorta. This is characteristic for TA. Arch aortography showed occlusion of the right subclavian artery.

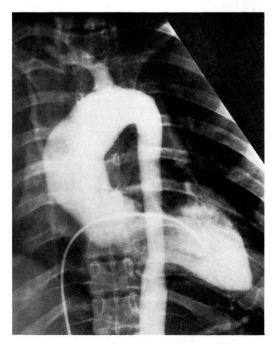

FIG. 13. An 18-year-old female had dilatation of the ascending aorta and arch with elongated smooth narrowing of the descending thoracic aorta. The point of maximal narrowing is several centimeters above the diaphragm. The arch was extensively affected.

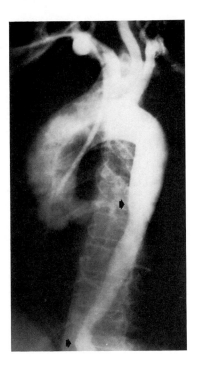

FIG. 14. A 52-year-old female had hypertension in both upper extremities. The thoracic aortogram shows diffuse coarctation of the descending aorta with gradual narrowing toward the diaphragm: "rattail" aorta typical for TA. The narrowing has irregular contours with a shaggy luminal margin *(arrows)* in the region of the maximal constriction, suggesting secondary atherosclerosis.

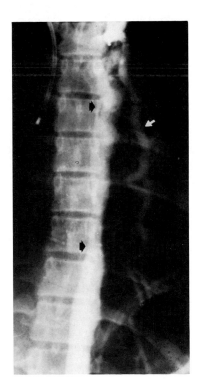

FIG. 15. Thoracic aortogram with the catheter tip at the orifice of the left subclavian artery. There is diffuse, marked narrowing of the descending thoracic aorta which tapers gradually *(black arrows).* The point of maximal narrowing is a few centimeters above the diaphragm. A large left mammary artery *(white arrow)* communicates with the interior epigastric artery in a collateral network.

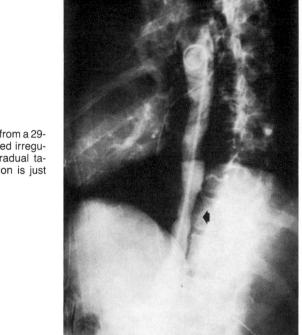

FIG. 16. Thoracic aortogram from a 29-year-old female. There is marked irregularity of the aortic wall with gradual tapering. The maximal constriction is just above the diaphragm *(arrow)*.

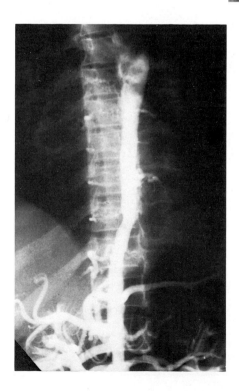

FIG. 17. Thoracic aortogram. Note the marked irregularity and narrowing of the descending thoracic aorta. The abdominal aorta was similarly affected in a contiguous fashion.

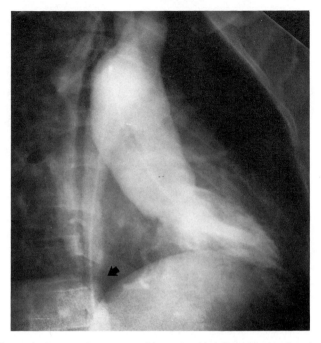

FIG. 18. Left ventriculogram shows a small hypertrophic left ventricular chamber with marked dilatation of the ascending aorta and the arch. Note the diffuse narrowings of the descending aorta and a short segmental constriction in the region of the diaphragm *(arrow)*. The abdominal aorta was diffusely constricted in a contiguous fashion. Branch arteries were not affected.

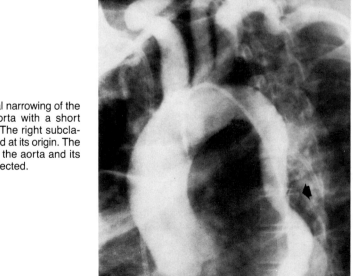

FIG. 19. Segmental narrowing of the proximal thoracic aorta with a short coarctation *(arrow)*. The right subclavian artery is occluded at its origin. The remaining portion of the aorta and its branches are not affected.

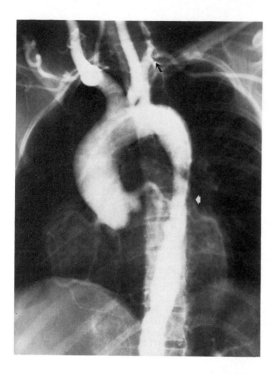

FIG. 20. Thoracic aortogram shows occlusion of the right subclavian artery and stenosis of the left subclavian artery *(black arrow)*. The entire descending thoracic aorta is diffusely irregular in outline with segmental constriction *(white arrow)*. The abdominal aortogram showed diffuse irregularity with a short area of segmental coarctation.

FIG. 21. Thoracic aortogram. The ascending aorta and arch are dilated. The aorta is markedly constricted just above the diaphragm *(open arrow)*. At the site of narrowing, the aortic lumen is irregular and shaggy. Poststenotic dilation of the upper abdominal aorta was present. Calcification outlines the aneurysm of the proximal left subclavian artery *(black arrow)*. Note the severe stenosis at the distal left subclavian artery *(black curved arrow)*. The right subclavian artery through which the catheter was advanced never visualized indirectly, indicating its near occlusion. There is segmental narrowing of the upper descending aorta *(white arrows)*. This is the typical "pulseless patient."

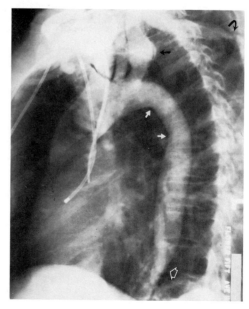

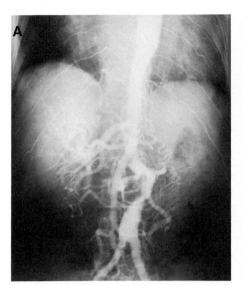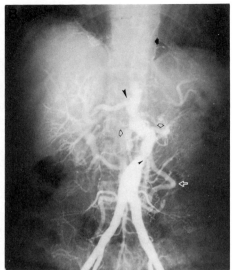

FIG. 22. **A:** A 75-year-old female with characteristic smooth cone-shaped coarctation of the descending thoracic aorta extending into the abdominal portion. The severely coarcted abdominal aorta buckles to the left. Shaggy contours of the abdominal aorta suggest secondary atherosclerosis. **B:** Below the level of the coarctation, the distal abdominal aorta and iliac arteries are unusually well preserved. The right renal artery *(large arrowhead)* and the inferior mesenteric artery *(small arrowhead)* are stenosed. The left renal artery is occluded. A large branch of the middle colic artery *(open arrows)* and the left colic artery *(white arrow)* create a prominent collateral channel contributing to the blood supply of the inferior mesenteric artery. The narrowed descending aorta is outlined by linear calcifications *(black arrow).*

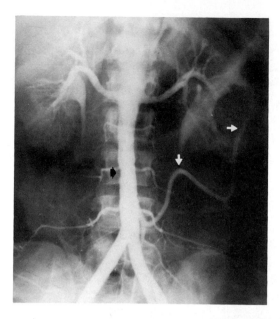

FIG. 23. At chest and abdominal roentgenography spotty calcifications outlined the descending and abdominal aorta. The abdominal aorta is narrowed with a slight constriction *(black arrow)*. Isolated irregularities of this nature can be easily overlooked. A large left colic artery *(white arrows)* revascularizes the occluded superior mesenteric artery. The brachiocephalic vessels were affected.

FIG. 24. Status of a 27-year-old female after splenorenal anastomosis (left renal artery severely constricted). The abdominal aorta is grossly irregular in contour *(upper two arrows)*. The left iliac artery is stenosed *(lower arrow)*.

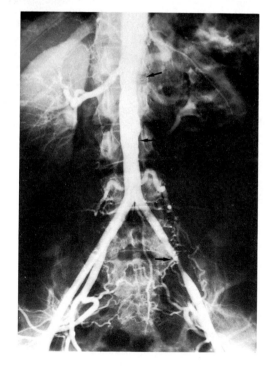

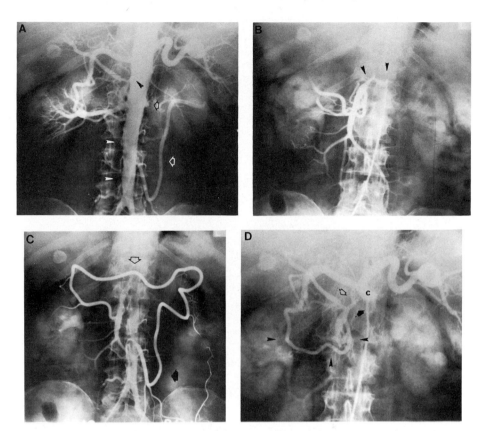

FIG. 25. A: A 38-year-old male with still active arteritis had a left-sided CVA 5 years prior to the present examination (Fig. 34). There is asymmetrical irregularity of the abdominal aortic wall. The right border has a grossly undulating contour *(white arrowheads)*. The left border is smooth. Note the occlusion of the left renal artery *(black open arrow)* and the long narrowing of the superior mesenteric artery at its orifice *(black arrowhead)*. The left colic artery *(white open arrow)* from the inferior mesenteric artery supplies the constricted superior mesenteric vessel. **B:** Selective superior mesenteric arteriogram. Note the long narrowing of the proximal superior mesenteric artery *(arrowheads)*. **C:** Selective inferior mesenteric arteriogram. Unusually well-developed collateral circulation is characteristic for TA. The stenotic superior mesenteric artery is revascularized by a prominent Riolan's anastomosis composed of the left colic artery *(black arrow)* and the left branch of the middle colic artery *(open arrow)*. The trunk of the superior mesenteric artery is beginning to visualize. **D:** Selective celiac arteriogram. The stenotic superior mesenteric artery is revascularized by a prominent pancreaticoduodenal arcade *(arrowheads)*. The superior mesenteric artery is opacified and shows a long constriction of the proximal segment *(black arrow)* with extension of the narrowing into the proximal segment of the replaced right hepatic artery originating from the superior mesenteric trunk *(open arrow)*. This Y-shaped segmental narrowing is characteristic for TA.

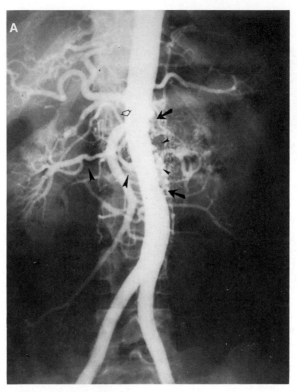

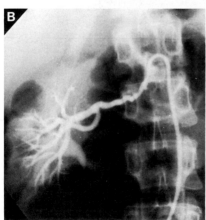

FIG. 26. A: Segmental constriction of the mid-abdominal aorta *(black arrows)*. The left kidney has a double blood supply, with the vessels occluded or severely stenosed *(small arrowheads)*. A rich collateral plexus is revascularizing the left kidney, which was only slightly smaller than the right. The patient's blood pressure was 220/130. The right renal artery is constricted throughout its length *(large arrowheads)*, the inferior mesenteric artery is occluded, and the left carotid artery was segmentally narrowed. **B:** A selective right renal arteriogram. Note the beaded appearance of the vessel.

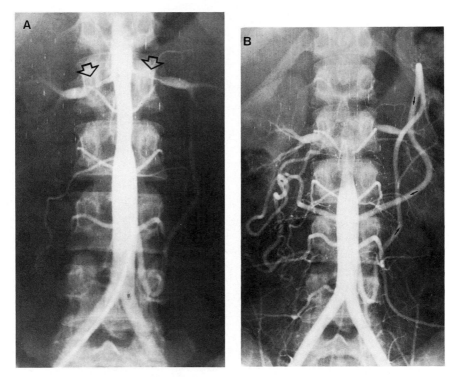

FIG. 27. **A:** Abdominal aortogram. Segmental interrenal coarctation with smooth symmetrical contours. Note the severe constriction of both renal arteries with poststenotic dilatations *(arrows).* **B:** The occluded superior mesenteric artery is reconstituted by an enlarged left colic artery.

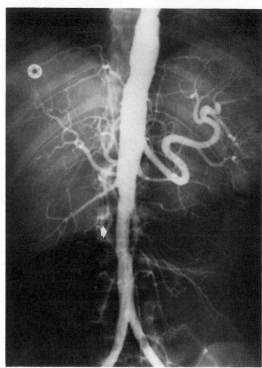

FIG. 28. Irregularity in the outline of the abdominal aorta with superimposed segmental narrowing *(arrow)*. Branch vessels are not affected. Arch aortography showed stenosis of the left carotid and occlusion of the left subclavian arteries. The descending thoracic aorta was also irregular in contour.

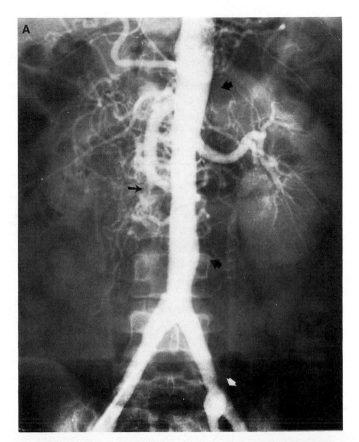

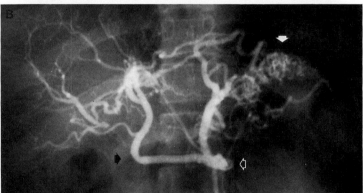

FIG. 29.   A: Abdominal aortography demonstrates segmental narrowing of the aorta *(thick black arrows)*. The right renal, inferior mesenteric, splenic, and right hepatic arteries are occluded. The superior mesenteric artery is obliterated at its midportion *(thin black arrow)*. Note the irregularity of the iliac arteries and the aneurysm at the origin of the hypogastric artery *(white arrow)*. **B:** Celiac arteriogram. The splenic artery is occluded *(open arrow)*, and the right branch of the common hepatic artery is obliterated *(white arrow)*. A cluster of small collateral vessels from the left gastric artery outlines the fundus of the stomach *(white arrow)* and proceeds to revascularize the splenic artery. *(Continued.)*

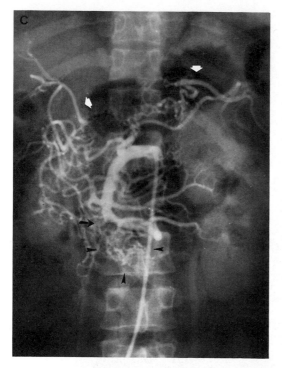

FIG. 29. *(Continued.)* **C:** Selective superior mesenteric arteriogram. Occlusion of the trunk of the superior mesenteric artery *(black arrow).* A rich network of fine collateral vessels appears in the small bowel mesentery *(black arrowheads).* The right hepatic and splenic artery are revascularized through collateral vessels *(white arrows).* **D:** The ileocolic artery is reconstituted by a collateral network in the small intestinal mesentery *(black arrowheads)* and the right colic artery *(white arrowheads). (Continued.)*

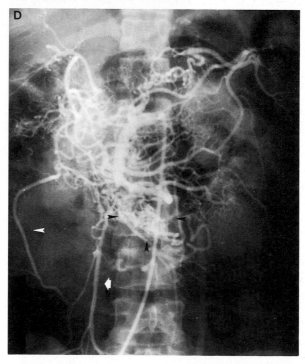

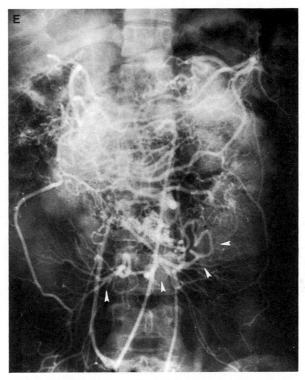

FIG. 29. *(Continued.)* **E:** The collateral anastomotic pathway in the small intestinal arcades extends in the mesenteric border parallel to the small intestine *(arrowheads)* and revascularizes the remaining trunk of the distal superior mesenteric artery.

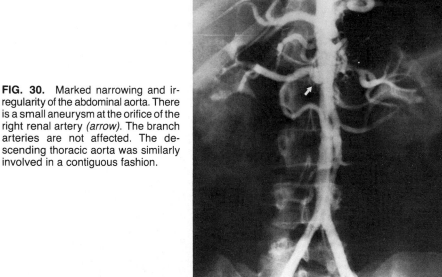

FIG. 30. Marked narrowing and irregularity of the abdominal aorta. There is a small aneurysm at the orifice of the right renal artery *(arrow)*. The branch arteries are not affected. The descending thoracic aorta was similarly involved in a contiguous fashion.

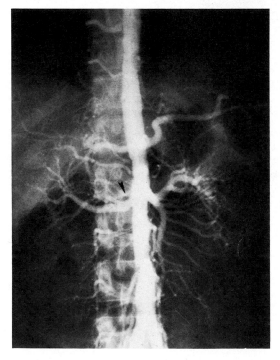

FIG. 31. Diffuse narrowing of the abdominal aorta with irregular contours. The origin of the right renal artery is slightly narrowed *(arrowhead)*. Branch vessels are otherwise not involved. The descending thoracic aorta was similarly narrowed. This is an example of contiguous involvement of the descending thoracic and abdominal aorta.

FIG. 32. This 37-year-old female had a long history of hypertension as well as a past and recent myocardial infarction. At arch aortography, the left subclavian artery was shown to be occluded. The interrenal abdominal aorta is moderately narrowed. The infrarenal aorta is seen to be severely and diffusely stenosed. The narrowing extends into the right iliac artery, which is also markedly constricted. The left iliac and inferior mesenteric arteries are occluded. A large collateral arcade (Riolan's anastomosis) revascularizes the inferior mesenteric artery *(white arrow).* A large lumbar artery *(open arrow)* contributes to the collateral blood supply of the left lower extremity. Note the fine irregularity of the contour of the superior mesenteric artery trunk *(arrowheads).*

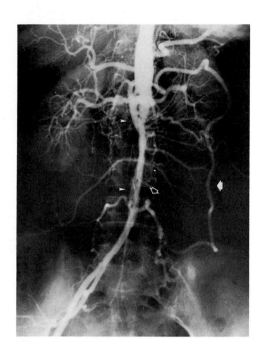

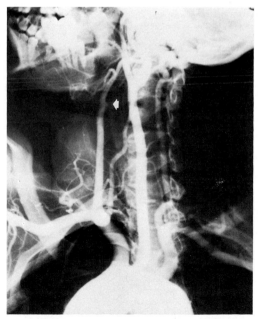

FIG. 33. In this 23-year-old female the right internal carotid artery is occluded at its origin *(arrow).* The abdominal aorta was segmentally coarcted with occlusion of the renal and visceral branches.

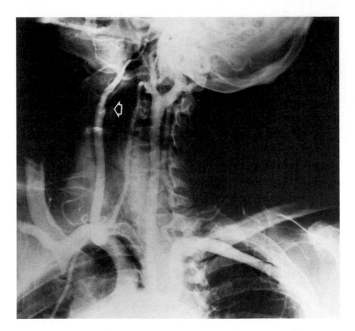

FIG. 34. This 38-year-old male veteran had had a left-sided CVA 5 years prior to admission with good recovery but residual symptoms. The right internal carotid artery is occluded at its origin *(arrow)*. Abdominal aortography showed the lumen of the abdominal aorta to be irregular with occlusion of the superior mesenteric artery. This patient's laboratory findings indicated a still active aortitis.

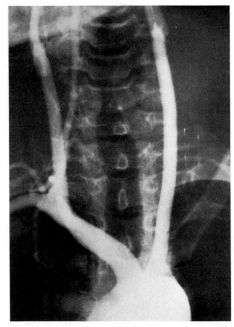

FIG. 35. This 21-year-old female had isolated occlusion of the left subclavian artery *(arrow)*. The abdominal aorta was also affected.

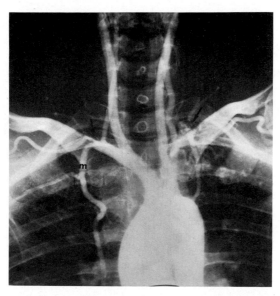

FIG. 36. This 32-year-old female had bilateral occlusion of the subclavian arteries just distal to the thyrocervical trunk *(arrows)*. There was associated involvement of the descending thoracic and the abdominal aorta.

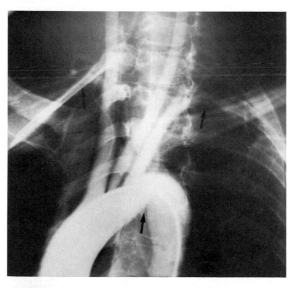

FIG. 37. This 31-year-old female had occlusion of the left subclavian artery just distal to the thyrocervical trunk *(arrow)*. The right subclavian artery is occluded at its point of origin.

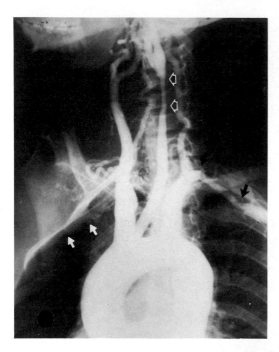

FIG. 38. The right subclavian artery is occluded in this 26-year-old hypertensive female. A rich collateral network revascularizes the right axillary artery. Coiling of the second intercostal artery produced a very fine notching of the adjacent rib *(white arrows)*. The left common carotid artery is constricted *(open arrows)*. The narrowed segment is well demarcated with a smooth luminal outline. This appearance is characteristic for TA. The left subclavian artery is segmentally narrowed *(black arrows)*. There was segmental involvement of the abdominal aorta.

FIG. 39. The right subclavian artery is occluded at its point of origin in this 28-year-old female. There is long segmental narrowing of the proximal left carotid artery *(open arrows)*. This type of long symmetrical narrowing is characteristic for TA. Note the flame-shaped occlusion of the left subclavian artery *(closed arrow)*. Serial arteriography showed a left vertebral subclavian steal.

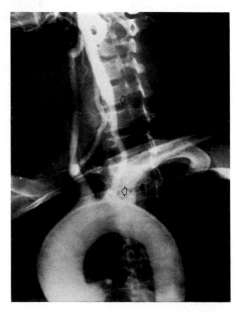

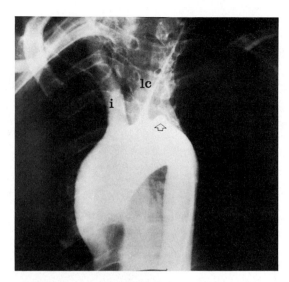

FIG. 40. Characteristic filiform narrowing of the left carotid artery *(lc)* and cone-shaped occlusion of the left subclavian artery *(arrow)* in a 32-year-old female. *i* = innominate artery.

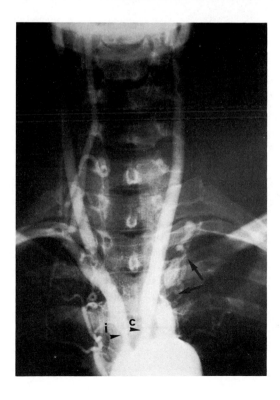

FIG. 41. This 35-year-old female has moderate narrowing of the origin of the innominate *(i)* and left common carotid *(c)* arteries. The left subclavian artery is occluded *(arrows)*. The abdominal aorta was not affected.

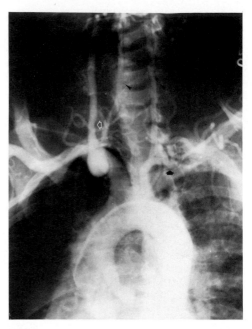

FIG. 42. Arch aortogram in which the left common carotid artery is occluded. The left subclavian artery is obliterated just distal to the thyrocervical trunk *(black arrow)*. Both vertebral arteries are prominent *(arrowheads)*. The right common carotid artery is slightly narrowed *(open arrow)*. There was associated involvement of the abdominal aorta.

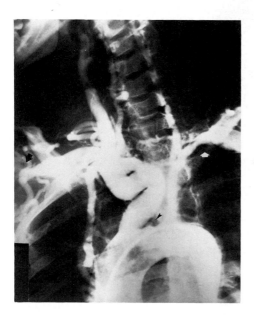

FIG. 43. A 24-year-old female had aneurysmal dilatation of the innominate, right common carotid, and right subclavian arteries with distal occlusion of the right subclavian artery *(black arrow)*. The stump of the occluded left carotid artery is shown *(arrowhead)*. Note the narrowing of the left subclavian artery *(white arrow)*. There was associated marked narrowing and irregularity of the descending thoracic and abdominal aorta.

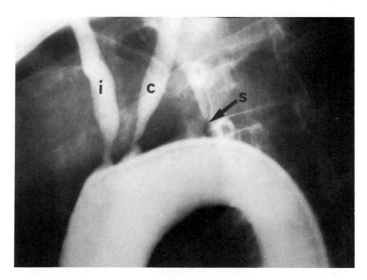

FIG. 44. This arch aortogram shows severe stenosis of the orifices of the innominate *(i)* and left common carotid *(c)* arteries in a 32-year-old female. The right and left subclavian arteries *(s)* are occluded.

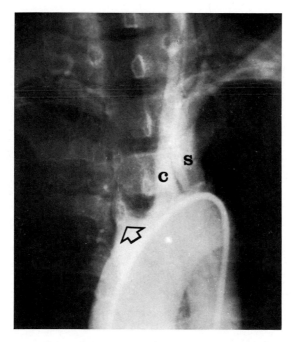

FIG. 45. This 34-year-old female had a flame-shaped occlusion of the innominate artery *(arrow)*. The left subclavian artery *(s)* is narrowed, and it was distally occluded. *c* = carotid artery.

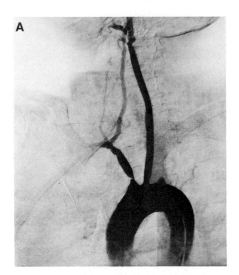

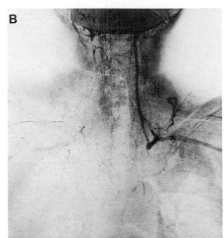

FIG. 46.   **A:** A 36-year-old male veteran had cone-like tapering of the innominate artery with severe stenosis at its apex. The right common carotid and right subclavian arteries are occluded. The right vertebral artery, however, is still patent. The left external carotid artery is occluded, and there is flame-shaped occlusion of the left subclavian artery. **B:** Sequential arteriography shows a left vertebral–subclavian steal.

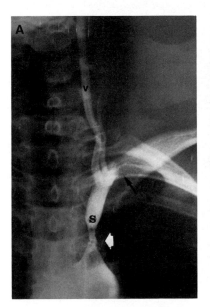

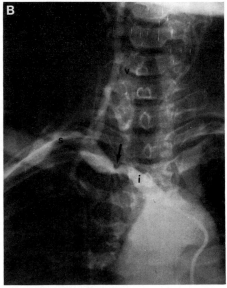

FIG. 47.   **A:** Markedly reduced blood supply to the head in a 36-year-old female. The origin of the left subclavian artery *(s)* shows a cone-like tapering with marked stenosis at the apex *(white arrow)*. There is associated occlusion of the left subclavian artery just distal to the thyrocervical trunk *(black arrow)*. **B:** There is marked stenosis *(arrow)* of the innominate artery *(i)*. The right and left common carotid arteries are occluded. The cerebral blood supply comes from the vertebral arteries. *s* = left subclavian artery.

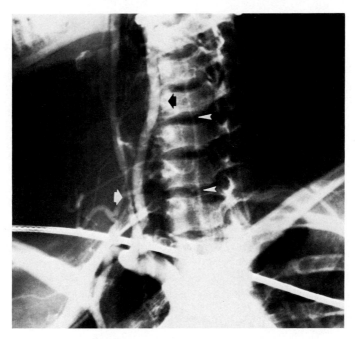

FIG. 48. This 18-year-old female had a critical cerebral perfusion deficit. Arch aortogram shows occlusion of the left common carotid and the left and right subclavian arteries. Note the marked narrowing of the origin of the right common carotid artery *(white arrow)*. The cerebral circulation is maintained by the right vertebral artery *(black arrow)*. On serial films, an anastomotic plexus of vessels was seen contributing to the blood supply to the brain. The anterior spinal artery participates in the collateral blood supply *(arrowheads)*.

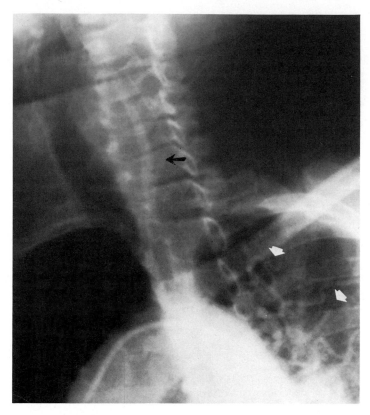

FIG. 49. In this 32-year-old female the left carotid artery is faintly opacified *(black arrow)*. All other vessels are occluded. This is the classical "bald aortic arch" of TA. Opacification of collateral vessels is beginning, originating from the intercostals and the arch of the aorta *(white arrows)*.

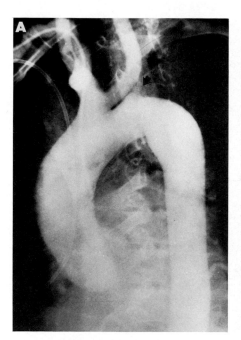 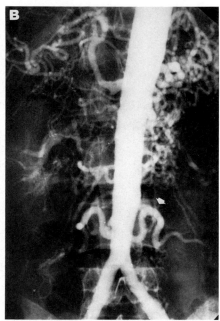

FIG. 50. A: Ectasia of the entire thoracic aorta and upper abdominal aorta. There is a flame-shaped occlusion of the left subclavian artery *(arrow)*. **B:** Tapered narrowing of the distal abdominal aorta returning to a normal caliber. The left kidney has been previously resected. The right renal artery is occluded. The splenic, gastroduodenal, right hepatic, and inferior mesenteric arteries are also occluded. The superior mesenteric artery is segmentally narrowed with occlusion of some of the jejunal and iliac branches. The large lumbar arteries *(arrow)* provide a collateral blood supply to the right kidney and other visceral organs.

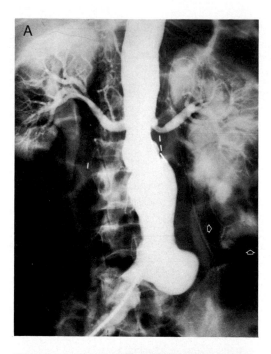

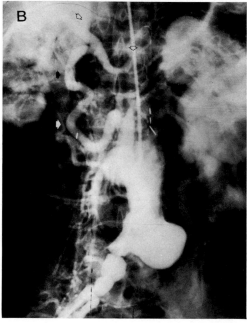

FIG. 51. The thoracic aortogram in this 44-year-old male showed a well-functioning aortic–left subclavian graft introduced 8 years prior to the present examination. The descending aorta was moderately ectatic with smooth contours. At autopsy the entire aorta showed diffuse aortitis. **A:** Note the conspicuous lack of opacification of the celiac and superior mesenteric arteries. A saccular aneurysm of the abdominal aorta is seen with occlusion of the left iliac artery and marked irregularity of the right iliac artery. The aneurysm compressed the left ureter causing distention and rupture of the superior calyx with pyelosinus backflow. There is extensive extravasation of the contrast material into the perirenal space *(arrows)*. **B:** Two seconds later the superior mesenteric artery opacifies through an aorticomesenteric graft (not visible because it overlies the aorta). A huge pancreaticoduodenal arcade *(closed arrows)* supplies the hepatic artery *(open arrows)*. The spleen was previously removed.

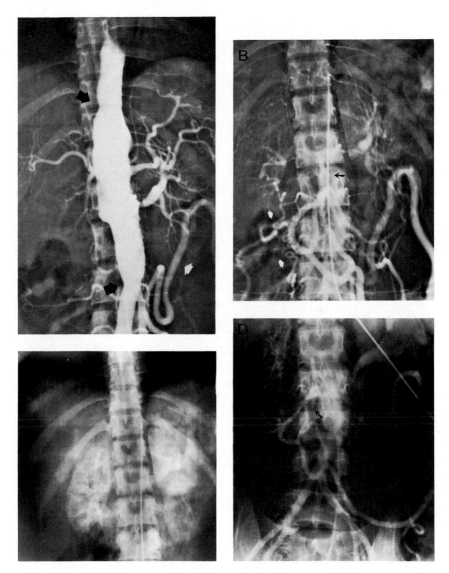

FIG. 52. A: A long segment of the abdominal aorta is aneurysmally dilated with multiple out-pouchings *(black arrows)* in this 18-year-old student nurse with TA. Interrenal aneurysms should make one suspect aortitis. The right renal artery is occluded, and the left renal artery is stenotic at its orifice. The superior mesenteric artery is occluded in close proximity to its point of origin. A large left colic artery *(white arrow)* is proceeding from the inferior mesenteric artery to revascularize the occluded superior mesenteric vessel. **B:** Abundant collateral flow is a hallmark of Takayasu's disease. An extensive network of collateral vessels originating from the lumbar arteries and forming a periureteric collateral plexus *(white arrows)* as well as collaterals arising from the intercostal arteries are revascularizing the right renal arterial tree. Through Riolan's anastomosis and the left branch of the middle colic artery a segment of the superior mesenteric trunk is reconstituted *(black arrow)*. **C:** Four seconds later a late nephrogram of the small atrophic right kidney is shown. **D:** Translumbar aortogram in the same patient. The visualized superior mesenteric artery is again occluded distally after giving off a few jejunal branches *(arrow)*. At sequential roentgenograms the opacification of the remaining superior mesenteric artery was accomplished by large collateral vessels.

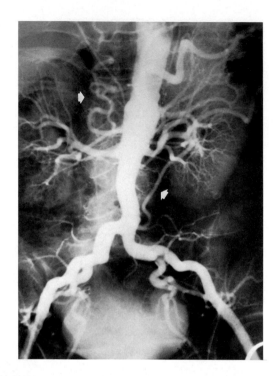

FIG. 53. Abdominal aortogram in this 26-year-old female demonstrates an irregular, fusiform aneurysm. The hepatic artery is occluded and is revascularized through the pancreaticoduodenal arcade *(upper arrow)*. The superior mesenteric artery is occluded, and a large left colic artery *(lower arrow)* ascends to supply the superior mesenteric territory. Marked tortuosity of the iliac arteries suggests previous arteritis.

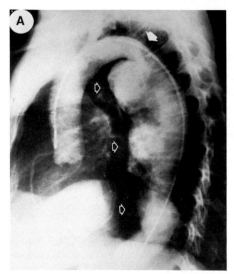

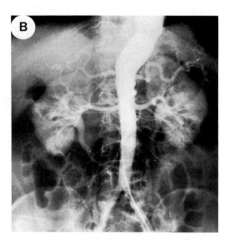

FIG. 54. **A:** This 44-year-old male veteran was admitted because of precordial pains. There are multiple aneurysms of the descending thoracic aorta *(open arrows)* and sharp demarcation of the aneurysmal aorta from the remaining aortic arch *(closed arrow)*. Confluent segmental aneurysmal outpouchings suggest multiple points of origin *(open arrows)*. The entire aneurysmal thoracic aorta was successfully resected and replaced with a Dacron graft. **B:** Abdominal aortogram. The proximal abdominal aorta is buckled and ectatic, but distally the vessel assumes a normal caliber.

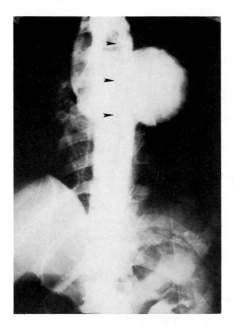

FIG. 55. This 27-year-old female has irregular narrowing of the descending thoracic aorta *(arrowheads)* with a broad-based eccentrically placed aneurysm. The lesion was resected and replaced with a graft.

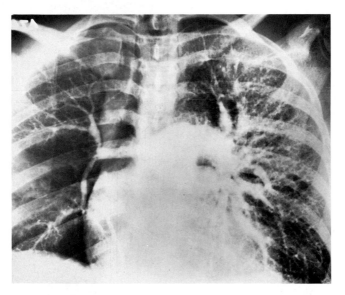

FIG. 56. This 24-year-old female has TA and widespread involvement of the aorta and its branches. The pulmonary arteriogram shows the right main pulmonary artery to be severely constricted with two slender branches preserved. At thoracic aortography the right lung was perfused by large bronchial collaterals. There was associated mild pulmonary hypertension of 40/20.

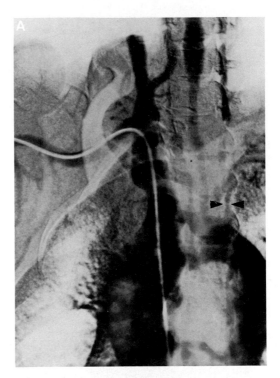

FIG. 57. Takayasu's arteritis in a 26-year-old female. **A:** Arch aortogram. There is a long segmental narrowing of the proximal left common carotid artery. The right and left vertebral arteries are enlarged. The left subclavian artery *(arrowheads)* is narrow at its origin and becomes larger distal to the left vertebral artery. The ascending aorta is dilated, and the posterior portion of the aortic arch is irregularly narrowed. **B:** Abdominal aortogram. There is severe stenosis of the aorta, and the intimal surface is irregular. Numerous mesenteric collaterals are shown by *arrowheads. (Continued.)*

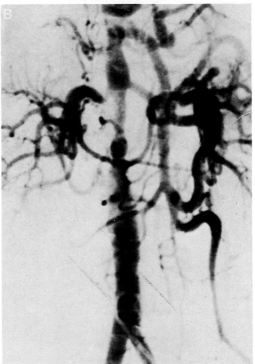

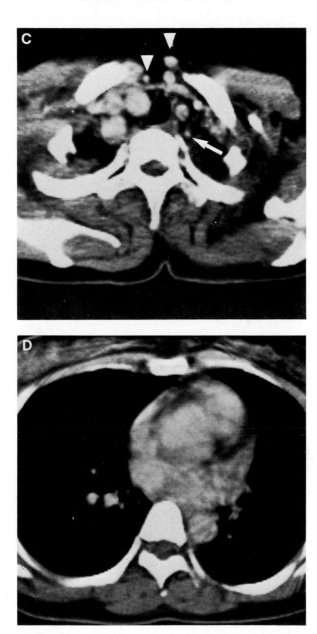

FIG. 57. *(Continued.)* **C:** CT scan at the thoracic inlet. The left common carotid artery is narrow, and the left subclavian artery is extremely stenosed *(arrow)*. In contrast, the right common carotid and subclavian arteries are considerably large. There are multiple collateral vessels *(arrowheads)*. **D:** Marked discrepancy between the external diameters of the ascending and descending aorta at a lower level. *(Continued.)*

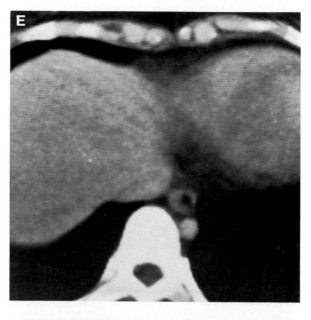

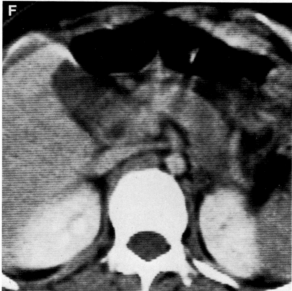

FIG. 57. *(Continued.)* **E:** Marked stenosis of the aorta as it crosses the diaphragm. **F:** Stenosis of the abdominal aorta is again well demonstrated. The outer diameter of the aorta approximates that of the superior mesenteric artery. *(Continued.)*

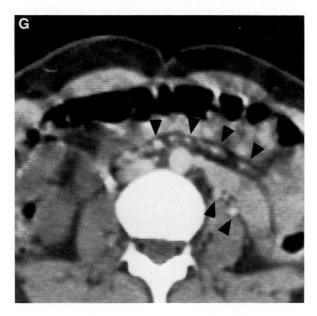

FIG. 57. (Continued.) **G:** The abdominal aorta returns to its normal size below the renal arteries. There are numerous retroperitoneal and mesenteric collaterals *(arrowheads).*

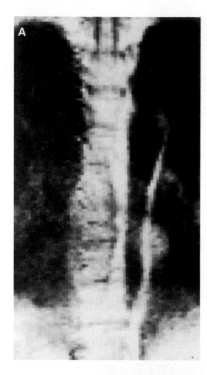

FIG. 58. Magnetic resonance imaging of Takayasu's arteritis (same case as in Figs. 2, 17, 43, and 56). A: Coronal section through the descending aorta. Note the tapered narrowing of the aorta as it approaches the diaphragm. The appearance is comparable to that in the aortogram in Fig. 17. B: Transverse section at the level of the diaphragm demonstrates marked narrowing of the aorta. (Continued.)

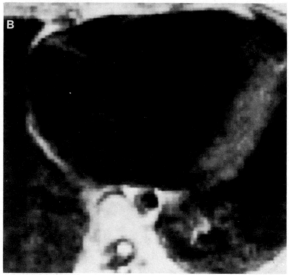

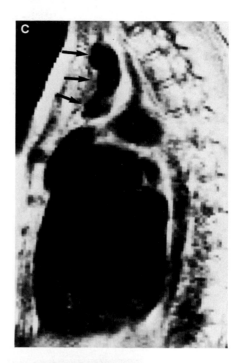

FIG. 58 *(Continued.)* **C:** Sagittal section through the right side of the sternum. Arrows point to the cross section of the markedly dilated and tortuous innominate artery. Compare with Fig. 43. **D:** Transverse section through the pulmonary artery. The marked narrowing of the right main pulmonary artery as it passes under the aortic arch extending to the right hilum is well demonstrated *(arrow)*. Compare with Fig. 56. The descending aorta is stenotic *(arrowheads)*. *AA* = ascending aorta; *RPA* = right main pulmonary artery: *SC* = superior vena cava; *IB* = intermediate bronchus; *LB* = left main bronchus.

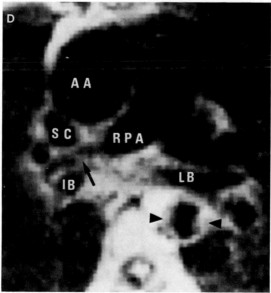

REFERENCES

1. Abrams, H. L. (1983): Dissecting aortic aneurysm. In: *Abrams Angiography: Vascular and Interventional Radiology*, Vol. I, 3rd Ed., pp. 441–446. Little, Brown, Boston.
2. Ask-Upmark, E., and Fajers, C-M. (1956): Further observations on Takayashu's syndrome. *Acta Med. Scand.*, 155:275–291.
3. Bahnson, H. T., Spencer, F. C., and Quattlebaum, J. K., Jr. (1959): Surgical treatment of occlusive disease of the carotid artery. *Ann. Surg.*, 149:711–719.
4. Berkmen, Y. M., and Lande, A. (1975): Chest roentgenography as a window to the diagnosis of Takayasu's arteritis. *AJR*, 125:842–846.
5. Bostrom, K., and Hassler, O. (1965): Takayasu's disease—postmortem examination of a previously published case. *Acta Med. Scand.*, 178:537–542.
6. Boyd, L. J., and McGovack, J. C. (1939): Aneurysm of the pulmonary artery—a review of the literature and report of two new cases. *Am. Heart J.*, 18:562–578.
7. Calenoff, L. (1964): Multiple mycotic pulmonary artery aneurysms. *AJR*, 91:379–384.
8. Cesarman, E., Cardenas, M., Escudero, J., et al. (1963): Arteritis de Takayashu, observaciones clinicas y anatamopathologicas. *Arch. Inst. Cardiol. Mex.*, 33:690–719.
9. Cheitlin, M. D. and Carter, P. B. (1965): Takayashu's disease—unusual manifestations. *Arch. Intern. Med.*, 116:283–288.
10. Cipriano, P. R., Alonso, D. R., Baltaxe, H. A., Gay, W. A., et al. (1976): Multiple aortic aneurysms in relapsing polychondritis. *Am. J. Cardiol.*, 37:1097–1102.
11. Clayton, M. J., Walsh, J., and Brewer, W. H. (1982): Contained ruptured of abdominal aortic aneurysms: Sonographic and CT diagnosis. *AJR*, 138:154–156.
12. Cooley, A. D., and DeBakey, E. M. (1955): Resection of the thoracic aorta with replacement by homograft for aneurysms and constrictive lesions. *J. Thorac. Surg.*, 19:66–104.
13. Deterling, R. A., Jr., and Clagett, O. T. (1947): Aneurysm of the pulmonary artery: Review of the literature and report of a case. *Am. Heart J.*, 34:471–499.
14. Durieux, P., Bletry, O., Huchon, B., Wechsler, B., et al. (1981): Multiple pulmonary arterial aneurysms in Behçet's disease and Hughes-Stovin syndrome. *Am. J. Med.*, 71:736–741.
15. Edling, N. P. G., Nystrom, B., and Seldinger, S. I. (1961): Brachial arteritis in the aortic arch syndrome: A roentgen and differential diagnostic study. *Acta Radiol.*, 55:417–432.
16. Engelsing, B. (1969): Die abdominale Koarktation der Aorta. *Z. Kreislaufforsch.*, 58:386–396.
17. Eyler, W. R., and Clark, M. D. (1965): Dissecting aneurysms of the aorta: Roentgen manifestations including a comparison with other types of aneurysms. *Radiology*, 85:1047–1057.
18. Felson, B., Akers, P., Hall, G. S., et al. (1977): Mycotic tuberculous aneurysm of the thoracic aorta. *JAMA*, 237:1104–1108.
19. Fisher, E. R., and Corcoran, A. C. (1952): Congenital coarctation of the abdominal aorta with resultant renal hypertension. *Arch. Intern. Med.*, 89:943–950.
20. Gillanders, L. A., and Strachan, R. W. (1965): The role of raddiology in the diagnosis of Takayasu's arteriopathy ("pulseless disease"). *Clin. Radiol.*, 16:119–129.
21. Godwin, J. D., Turley, K., Herfkens, R. J., et al. (1981): Computed tomography for follow up for chronic aortic dissections. *Radiology*, 139:655–660.
22. Gomes, M. N., Schelling, D., and Hufnagel, C. A. (1979): Abdominal aortic aneurysms: diagnostic review and new technique. *Ann. Thorac. Surg.*, 27:479–488.
23. Gonzalez-Cerna, J. L., Villavicencio, L., Molina, B., et al. (1967): Non-specific obliterative aortitis in children. *Ann. Thorac. Surg.*, 4:193–204.
24. Gotsman, M. S., Beck, W., and Schrire, V. (1967): Selective angiography in arteritis of the aorta and its major branches. *Radiology*, 88:232–248.
25. Grenier, P., Bletry, O., Cornud, F., et al. (1981): Pulmonary involvement in Behçet's disease. *AJR*, 1337:565–569.
26. Haaga, J. R., Baldwin, G. N., Reich, N. E., et al. (1978): CT detection of infected synthetic grafts: Preliminary report of a new sign. *AJR*, 131:317–320.
27. Hachiya, J. (1970): Current concepts of Takayasu's arteritis. *Semin. Roentgenol.*, 5:245–259.
28. Hainer, J. W., and Hamilton, G. W. (1969): Aortic abnormalities in relapsing polychondritis—report of a case with dissecting aneurysm. *N. Engl. J. Med.*, 280:1166–1168.
29. Hamrin, B. (1972): Polymyalgia arteritica. *Acta Med. Scand. [Suppl.]*, 533:1–33.
30. Harrell, J. E., and Manion, W. C. (1970): Sclerosing aortitis and arteritis. *Semin. Roentgenol.*, 5:260–266.

31. Harris, M. (1968): Dissecting aneurysm of the aorta due to giant cell arteritis. *Br. Heart J.*, 30:840–844.
32. Heggveit, H. A. (1964): Syphilitic aortitis—a clinicopathology study of 100 cases, 1950 to 1960. *Circulation*, 29:346–355.
33. Higgins, C. B., and Reinke, R. T. (1974): Nonsyphilitic etiology of linear calcification of the ascending aorta. *Radiology*, 113:609–613.
34. Hills, E. A. (1967): Behçet's syndrome with aortic aneurysms. *Br. Med. J.*, 4:152–154.
35. Hope-Ross, P., Bien, E. J., Palladino, V. S., and Graham, G. (1960): Rheumatoid arthritis—report of an unusual case. *Ann. Intern. Med.*, 52:682–693.
36. Horns, J. W., and O'Loughlin, B. J. (1962): Tracheal collapse in polychondritis. *AJR*, 87:844–846.
37. Hughes, R. A. C., Berry, C. L., Seifert, M., and Lessof, M. H. (1972): Relapsing polychondritis—three cases with a clinico-pathological study and literature review. *Q. J. Med.*, 41:363–380.
38. Inada, K., Shimizu, H., Kobayashi, T., et al. (1962): Pulseless disease and atypical coarctation of the aorta. *Arch. Surg.*, 84:306–311.
39. Jackman, J., and Lubert, M. (1945): The significance of calcification in the ascending aorta as observed roentgenographically. *AJR*, 53:432–438.
40. Jaffe, R. B., and Condon, V. R. (1975): Mycotic aneurysms of the pulmonary artery and aorta. *Radiology*, 116:291–298.
41. Jaffe, R. B., and Koschmann, E. B. (1970): Intravenous drug abuse—pulmonary, cardiac, and vascular complications. *AJR*, 109:107–120.
42. Kaufman, L., Crooks, L. E., Sheldon, P. E., et al. (1983): The potential impact of nuclear magnetic resonance on cardiovascular diagnosis. *Circulation*, 67:251–259.
43. Kent, D. C., and Arnold, H. (1967): Aneurysm of the aorta due to giant cell aortitis—successful surgical correction. *J. Thorac. Cardiovasc. Surg.*, 53:572–577.
44. Klein, R. G., Hunder G. G., Stanson, A. W., and Sheps, S. G. (1975): Larger artery involvement in giant cell (temporal) arteritis. *Ann. Intern. Med.*, 83:806–812.
45. Lande, A. (1976): Congenital coarctation of the descending thoracic and the abdominal aorta: A critical review. *AJR*, 27:227–233.
46. Lande, A., and Bard, R. (1976): Takayasu's arteritis: An unrecognized cause of pulmonary hypertension. *Angiology*, 27:114–121.
47. Lande, A., and Berkmen, Y. M. (1976): Aortitis—pathologic, clinical and arteriographic review. *Radiol. Clin. North. Am.*, 14:219–240.
48. Lande, A., and Gross, A. (1972): Total aortography in the diagnosis of Takayasu's arteritis. *AJR*, 116:165–178.
49. Lande, A., and La Porta, A. (1976): Takayasu's arteritis: An arteriographic pathologic correlation. *Arch. Pathol.*, 100:437–440.
50. Lande, A., Bard, R., Bole, P., and Guarnaccia, M. (1978): Aortic arch syndrome (Takayasu's arteritis): Arteriographic and surgical considerations. *J. Cardiovasc. Surg.*, 19:507–513.
51. Lande, A., Bard, R., Rossi, P., Passariello, R., and Castrucci, A. (1976): Takayasu's arteritis, a worldwide entity (report on twelve Caucasian patients). *N.Y. State J. Med.*, 776:1477–1482.
52. Leighton, R. S. (1948): Calcification of the ascending aorta as a sign of syphilitic aortitis. *Radiology*, 51:257–259.
53. Little, A. G., and Zarins, C. K. (1982): Abdominal aortic aneurysm and Behçet's syndrome. *Surgery*, 91:359–362.
54. Lodwick, G. S., and Gladstone, W. S. (1957): Correlation of anatomic and roentgen changes in arteriosclerosis and syphilis of the ascending aorta. *Radiology*, 69:70–78.
55. Lupi, H. E., Sanchez, T. G., Marcushamer, J., et al. (1977): Takayasu's arteritis—clinical study of 107 cases. *Am. Heart J.*, 93:94–102.
56. Maeda, S., Murao, S., Sugiyama, T., Utaka, I., et al. (1983): Generalized sarcoidosis with "sarcoid aortitis." *Acta Pathol. Jpn.*, 33:183–188.
57. Magarey, F. R. (1950): Dissecting aneurysm due to giant-cell aortitis. *J. Pathol. Bacteriol.*, 62:445–446.
58. Meehan, J. J., Pastor, B. H., and Torre, A. V. (1957): Dissecting aneurysm of the aorta secondary to tuberculous aortitis. *Circulation*, 16:615–620.
59. Morris, C. G., DeBakey, E. M., Cooley, A. D., and Crawford, E. S. (1960): Subisthmic aortic stenosis and occlusive disease. *Arch. Surg.*, 80:87–104.
60. Nakao, K., Ikeda, M., Kimata, S., et al. (1967): Takayasu's arteritis: Clinical report of eighty-four cases and immunological studies of seven cases. *Circulation*, 35:1141–1155.

61. Nasu, T. (1963): Pathology of pulseless disease. *Angiology*, 2:225–242.
62. Oudkerk, M., Overbosch, E., and Dea, P. (1983): CT recognition of acute aortic dissection. *AJR*, 141:671–676.
63. Paloheimo, J. A. (1967): Obstructive arteritis of Takayasu's type: clinical roentgenological and laboratory studies on 36 patients. *Acta Med. Scand. [Suppl.]*, 468:7–45.
64. Parienty, R. A., Couffinhal, J-C., Wellers, et al. (1982): Computed tomography versus aortography of aortic dissection. *Cardiovasc. Intervent. Radiol.*, 5:285–291.
65. Pearson, C. M., Kroening, R., Verity, M. A., and Getzen, J. H. (1967): Aortic insufficiency and aortic aneurysm in relapsing polychondritis. *Trans. Assoc. Am. Physicians*, 80:71–90.
66. Perrin, A., Berthou, J., Gonin, A., et al. (1970): Les arteriopathies de type Takayasu. *Ann. Cardiol. Angeiol. (Paris)*, 19:315–326.
67. Phillips, P. L., Amberson, J. B., and Libby, D. M. (1981): Syphilitic aortic aneurysm presenting with superior vena cava syndrome. *Am. J. Med.*, 71:171–173.
68. Randall, P. A., and Jarmowski, C. R. (1983): Aneurysms of the thoracic aorta. In: *Abrams Angiography: Vascular and Interventional Radiology*, Vol. 1, 3rd Ed., pp. 417–440. Little, Brown, Boston.
69. Restrepo, C., Tejeda, C., and Correa, P. (1969): Nonsyphilitic aortitis. *Arch. Pathol.*, 87:1–12.
70. Rosen, N., and Gaton, E. (1972): Takayasu's arteritis of coronary arteries. *Arch. Pathol.*, 94:225–229.
71. Rykowski, H., and Bednarski, Z. (1969): Is acquired coarctation of abdominal aorta with arterial hypertension and asymptomatic occlusion and stenosis of aortic branches a separate vascular syndrome? *Pol. Tyg. Lek.*, 24:363–366 [in Polish].
72. Rykowski, H., Liszka, W., Lasocki, J., et al. (1968): Coarctation of the abdominal aorta with stenosis of renal arteries. *Pol. Przegl. Chir.*, 40:1034–1038 [in Polish].
73. Sagel, S. S., Siegel, M. J., Stanley, R. J., et al. (1977): Detection of retroperitoneal hemorrhage by computed tomography. *AJR*, 129:403–407.
74. Salisbury, R. S., and Hazleman, B. L. (1981): Successful treatment of dissecting aortic aneurysm due to giant cell arteritis. *Ann. Rheum. Dis.*, 40:507–508.
75. Sandring, H., and Welin, G. (1961): Aortic arch syndrome with special reference to rheumatoid arteritis. *Acta Med. Scand.*, 170:1–19.
76. Schire, V., and Asherson, R. A. (1964): Arteritis of the aorta and its major branches. *Q. J. Med.*, 33:439–463.
77. Segal, A. J. (1940): Syphilitic (gummatous) pulmonary arteritis with rupture into the bronchial tree. *Arch. Pathol.*, 30:911–915.
78. Sen, P. K. (1968): Obstructive disease of the aorta and its branches. *Indian J. Surg.*, 30:289–327.
79. Shimizu, K., and Sano, K. (1951): Pulseless disease. *J. Neuropathol. Clin. Neurol.*, 1:37–47.
80. Silbergleit, A., Arbulu, A., Defver, B. A., et al. (1965): Tuberculous aortitis—surgical resection of ruptured abdominal false aneurysm. *JAMA*, 193:333–335.
81. Smith, W. G., and Leonard, J. C. (1959): The radiological features of syphilitic aortic incompetence. *Br. Heart J.*, 21:162–166.
82. Sos, T. A., Sniderman, K. W., and Wixson, D. (1979): Pitfalls in the plain film evaluation of the thoracic aorta: the mimicry of aneurysms and adjacent masses and the value of aortography. Part II. Descending thoracic aorta. *Cardiovasc. Radiol.*, 2:77–83.
83. Strachan, R. W., Wigzell, F. W., and Anderson, J. R. (1966): Locomotor manifestations and serum studies in Takayasu's arteriopathy. *Am. J. Med.*, 40:560–568.
84. Takayasu, M. (1908): Case with peculiar changes in retinal vessels. *Acta Soc. Ophthalmol Jpn.*, 12:554.
85. Thorner, M. C., Carter, R. A., and Griffith, G. C. (1949): Calcification as a diagnostic sign of syphilitic aortitis. *Am. Heart J.*, 38:641–653.
86. Ueda, H., Morooka, S., Ito, I., et al. (1969): Clinical observation of 52 cases of aortitis syndrome. *Jpn. Heart J.*, 10:277–288.
87. Valaitis, J., Pilz, C. G., and Montgommery, M. M. (1957): Aortitis with aortic valve insufficiency in rheumatoid arthritis. *Arch. Pathol.*, 63:207–212.
88. Walts, A. E., and Dubois, A. L. (1977): Acute dissecting aneurysm of the aorta as a fatal event in systemic lupus erythematosus. *Am. Heart J.*, 93:378–381.
89. Wilson, S. E., Van Vagenen, P., and Passaro, E., Jr. (1978): Arterial infection. *Curr. Probl. Surg.*, 15:6–89.
90. Wixson, D., Baltaxe, H. A., and Sos, T. A. (1979): Pitfalls in the plain film evaluation of the

thoracic aorta: the mimicry of aneurysms and adjacent masses and value of aortography. Part I. Transverse aortic arch. *Cardiovasc. Radiol.*, 2:69–76.

91. Wolk, L. A., Pasdar, H., McKeown, J. J., Jr., et al. (1981): Computerized tomography in the diagnosis of abdominal aortic aneurysms. *Surg. Gynecol. Obstet.*, 153:219–232.

92. Yamada, H., Harumi, K., Ohta, A., et al. (1961): Aortic arch syndrome with cardiomegaly and aortic calcification. *Jpn. Heart J.*, 2:538–548.

93. Zajarias, S., Rotberg, T., Stevens, H., et al. (1969): Arteriopathia tipo Takayasu con localizacion renovascular. *Arch. Inst. Cardiol. Mex.*, 39:490–499.

94. Zumbro, G. L., Henley, L. B., and Treasure, R. L. (1975): Saccular aneurysm of ascending aorta caused by granulomatous aortitis in a child. *J. Thorac. Cardiovasc. Surg.*, 69:397–401.

Aortitis: Clinical, Pathologic, and Radiographic Aspects, edited by A. Lande, Y. M. Berkmen, and H. A. McAllister. Raven Press, New York © 1986.

Medical Aspects of Rheumatoid Diseases

Harry Spiera and Leslie D. Kerr

Department of Medicine, Division of Rheumatology, Mount Sinai School of Medicine and Mount Sinai Hospital, New York, New York 10029

The concept of the diffuse disorders of connective tissue arose from the studies of Klemperer and his associates (13). Since then study of the "collagen" diseases has evolved. For the most part the connective tissue diseases include rheumatoid arthritis, the spondyloarthropathies, psoriatic arthritis, the rheumatoid variants, systemic lupus erythematosus, scleroderma, dermatomyositis, polymyositis, and the various vasculitic syndromes. All of these diseases are illnesses of unknown etiology. The exception is polyarteritis, which is sometimes caused by the hepatitis B virus (9). Their pathogenesis is presumed to involve abnormalities of the immune system. These are diseases with rather variable clinical courses and a tendency toward exacerbations and remissions. There is a wide spectrum of disease severity within each subtype. In many of these syndromes, various types of autoantibodies are found. The use of corticosteroids and other anti-inflammatory medicines form a cornerstone in their treatment. There is considerable overlap within many of these syndromes.

The reasons for grouping these diseases into one category seems to be the diffuse involvement of the connective tissue, the frequent presence of rheumatic complaints, the presence of autoantibodies, and the overlap that occurs in these various syndromes. Obviously, a logical classification of these illnesses depends on a better understanding of their etiology and pathogenesis.

It is important to recognize that arteritis, with a varying degree of frequency, is seen in many of these conditions and may be the underlying pathogenic feature of many of them. The following are brief clinical descriptions of the various connective tissue diseases with some emphasis on their possible relationship to aortitis. The vasculitic syndromes are discussed elsewhere in this book.

RHEUMATOID ARTHRITIS

Rheumatoid arthritis is a disease of unknown etiology in which the major clinical feature is chronic synovitis (15). It occurs frequently, affecting 1 to 2% of the general population with a female/male predominance of 2:1. It may occur at any age from early childhood to extreme old age. It may begin acutely or insidiously. In the classic variety, joint involvement is symmetrical with the major predilection for the second and third metacarpal (MCP) joints, wrists, elbows, shoulders, knees, ankles, and feet, though any joint or combination of joints may be involved.

Histopathologically, it is characterized by a proliferative synovitis in which the synovial tissue become infiltrated with acute and chronic inflammatory cells including lymphocytes and plasma cells. The inflamed synovium, which is called pannus, invades the articular cartilage, subchondral bone, and the surrounding ligamentous structures leading to joint destruction and deformity. It is this destructive process which is responsible for the serious crippling of rheumatoid arthritis.

The clinical course is extremely variable. Some patients have a pauciarticular involvement and a benign course, whereas others have a fulminating disease with rapid joint destruction. Exacerbations and remissions are frequent, though in most cases the disease eventually becomes progressive. Laboratory manifestations include the presence of mild anemia, polyclonal hyperglobulinemia, elevated erythrocyte sedimentation rate (ESR), and other acute-phase reactants. Circulating rheumatoid factor is found in about 70% of patients. Rheumatoid factor is an immunoglobulin M (IgM) which reacts with aggregated gamma globulin. The presence of rheumatoid factor in the serum is assayed by the latex fixation test. The presence of rheumatoid factor is not necessary for the diagnosis of rheumatoid arthritis, but it is associated with more severe disease and thus is of some prognostic significance (19). The etiology of rheumatoid arthritis is unknown. A number of infectious organisms have been proposed as putative etiologic agents, but none has been found consistently.

The pathogenesis of the chronic joint inflammation is believed to be due to an immunologic reaction occurring within the synovial space. It is believed that immune complexes are formed, and these in turn activate the complement cascade. This results in an influx of inflammatory cells that ingest the immune complexes and release lysosomal enzymes which destroy the cartilage and surrounding structures. Whether the antigen in this proposed schema is an autoantigen or an antigen resulting from some microbacterial organism is not known at the present time (11).

There is no known cure for rheumatoid arthritis, though it may remit spontaneously. Treatment of early rheumatoid arthritis includes analgesics, anti-inflammatory medicines, rest, and physiotherapy. If the disease is prolonged and progressive, there are a group of other agents, known as long-acting agents, which seem to have the properties of possibly inducing a remission of the disease and halting the progression of the destructive change. Drugs in this category include gold, antimalarials, penicillamine, and the immunosuppressive medicines. The use of any of these is associated with significant potential toxicity. Corticosteroids are often helpful in suppressing the inflammatory response but do not seem to alter the natural history of the disease.

Associated with rheumatoid arthritis are extra-articular manifestations. These include fever, anemia, skin rash, pulmonary fibrosis, pulmonary nodules, pleural effusion, pericarditis, hypersplenism, iritis, uveitis, and amyloidosis. Vasculitis may complicate rheumatoid arthritis. It is believed by some that the synovitis itself is a vasculitis. There is some evidence that the subcutaneous nodules found in about 20% of patients also are vasculitic in origin (22). A small number of patients with rheumatoid arthritis, however, develop a more significant vasculitis. This clinical syndrome usually is characterized by fever, peripheral neuropathy, skin ulcers, bowel perforation, and other consequences of inflammatory arterial disease. Small to medium-sized blood vessels are involved. Histopathologically and clinically, this illness resembles polyarteritis with the exception that renal involvement and hypertension are very infrequent in rheumatoid vasculitis. The thinking is that the arteritis is the result of immune complex deposition. The arteritis complicating rheumatoid arthritis has a potentially serious prognosis. Treatment usually involves steroids, immunosuppressive drugs, and penicillamine, though spontaneous remission may occur (24).

Myocarditis and cardiac valvular disease may be associated. Although histologically some infiltration of inflammatory cells in the aorta may be found on postmortem examination, clinically significant aortitis is not seen. Aortic valvular disease occasionally occurs.

ANKYLOSING SPONDYLITIS

Ankylosing spondylitis (AS) (18) is a form of synovitis of unknown etiology in which the major areas of involvement are in the axial rather than the peripheral skeleton. In contrast to rheumatoid arthritis, a disease with which it was initially identified, AS is a disease predominantly associated with males, with a male/female ratio of 8:1. Onset is usually during the third to fifth decades. It is characterized by severe pain and stiffness in the lower back, dorsal spine, and cervical spine with progressive pain and rigidity of the spine. Calcification of the spinal ligaments may occur. In about 25% of patients, peripheral arthritis resembling rheumatoid arthritis occurs. This illness is not associated with subcutaneous nodules, and rheumatoid factor is not found. Laboratory abnormalities include an increased ESR and the presence of other acute-phase reactants. Autoantibodies are rarely found. Genetically, it is characterized by a predisposition for people who carry the HLA-B27 antigen (2). Approximately 90% of patients with this disorder have the HLA-B27 antigen in contrast to 5 to 10% of the general population. It is speculated that the combination of the genetic predisposition afforded by the HLA-B27 antigen and some external infectious organism may interact to produce this chronic inflammatory disease. This is inferred by implication from other diseases in which HLA-B27 positivity is found, e.g., Reiter's syndrome, *Salmonella* arthritis, and *Yersenia* arthritis (collectively referred to as reactive arthritis). In these patients who have the HLA-B27 antigen, exposure to certain strains of *Shigella, Salmonella,* and *Yersinia enterocolitica* interact to result in a chronic inflammatory disease of the joints.

Histopathologically in AS there is proliferative synovitis involving predominantly the apophyseal joints leading to destruction, ankylosis, and eventually calcification. Like rheumatoid arthritis, this disease is characterized by exacerbations and remissions. The majority of patients do eventually have some degree of remission. On the basis of the data accumulated, there is some evidence that this disease may be much more common than heretofore thought. This results from prospective studies on patients who are found to have HLA-B27 positivity. Many of these patients have musculoskeletal symptoms involving the spine, although they lack the classic clinical and radiographic findings of AS. Whether these patients have a "mild" form of AS is unknown. The distinction may be semantic.

Treatment is mainly supportive. The nonsteroidal anti-inflammatory agents are often extremely effective in relieving the symptoms of this condition. Physiotherapy is vitally important to maintain function and posture. In contrast to rheumatoid arthritis, the "long-acting" drugs, e.g., gold, antimalarials, penicillamine, and immunosuppressants, do not have a place in management.

Ankylosing spondylitis patients have relatively high incidence of inflammatory bowel disease, both Crohn's disease and ulcerative colitis. Similarly, there seems to be a high incidence of coincident psoriasis. Extra-articular complications include iritis, prostatitis, and amyloidosis. Aortic valvular disease occurs frequently in patients with AS (10). Clinically, this is manifested primarily by aortic insufficiency. There is some controversy as to the percentage of patients who have this complication. In some series, up to 10% of patients may have some clinical involvement. The pathology of the aortic valve in AS consists of sclerosis with fusion of the commissures. There may be some infiltration of inflammatory cells in the aorta near the valve, but it tends not to be very extensive. Aortic valve disease may be apparent before the clinical AS. Arterial occlusive disease is not seen in AS.

REITER'S SYNDROME

Reiter's syndrome (21) is a clinical entity which in the full-blown picture includes arthritis, urethritis, conjunctivitis, and mucocutaneous abnormalities. In some patients only some of the features are present. It is found more frequently in males and, similar to AS, is associated with a high incidence of the HLA-B27 genome. The precipitating factor of the syndrome initially described was *Shigella* dysentery, but often it follows nonspecific urethritis. It seems to be the result of an interaction of a predisposed host with some microbiologic organism. In most patients the exact nature of the organism is not identified. The clinical picture is usually dominated by an arthritis which tends to predominate in the lower extremities, although almost any joint can be involved. A certain percentage of patients have spondylitic involvement with sacroileitis and spondylitis. A distinction of Reiter's syndrome from ankylosing spondylitis radiographically is that in ankylosing spondylitis the radiographic process seems to ascend from the sacroiliac joints, whereas in Reiter's syndrome there may be more skip areas. There is, however, a considerable amount of overlap. The eye involvement usually consists of conjunctivitis, though at times iritis or a uveitis may occur. The urethritis is nonspecific, and no organisms are cultured consistently. In the female trigonitis and cystitis may occur. Skin lesions include hyperkeratotic lesions of the nails of the hands and feet, psoriatic type skin lesions, balinitis circinata of the penis, and lesions on the bottom of the feet referred to as keratoderma blennorrhagicum. Painless mouth ulcers are also frequently seen.

The arthritis of Reiter's syndrome may be acute and self-limited, though in many patients it goes on to chronic and destructive synovitis with a tendency toward bony ankylosis (8). Attacks may recur. The histopathology is that of a chronic, nonspecific synovitis which has no unique histopathologic features. Laboratory findings are usually nonspecific, revealing an elevated ESR and occasionally mild anemia. Autoantibodies such as rheumatoid factor and antinuclear antibody are absent. In contrast to rheumatoid arthritis, wherein the synovial fluid complement is found to be low, complement in the synovial fluid of Reiter's syndrome tends to be elevated.

Treatment of Reiter's syndrome is supportive and nonspecific, though many clinicians use broad-spectrum antibiotics when the patient has urethritis. This is to be sure that the patient does not have gonococcal infection. The patient is usually treated with nonsteroidal anti-inflammatory agents. Gold does not seem to have a place in the management of Reiter's syndrome. Occasionally in progressive disease immunosuppressive agents such as methotrexate and azathioprine (Imuran) are good, but their use is considered to be experimental.

Aortic valvular disease very similar to that seen in ankylosing spondylitis occurs among patients with Reiter's syndrome. Once again occlusive arterial disease is not seen as part of the picture of Reiter's syndrome.

PSORIATIC ARTHRITIS

Psoriatic arthritis (27) is considered to be a "variant" of rheumatoid arthritis. In this disease patients with psoriasis develop an arthritis with predominant involvement of the distal interphalangeal (DIP) joints of the hands and feet, asymmetrical synovitis elsewhere, and the absence of rheumatoid factor. These patients do not have rheumatoid factor or subcutaneous nodules and do not develop the extra-articular manifestations of rheumatoid arthritis. An exception is a relatively high incidence of eye inflammation. This histopathology is similar to that seen in rheumatoid arthritis though with a lesser tendency toward lymphoid follicle formation. The psoriasis may be mild or severe. At times the arthritis antedates the psoriasis, making diagnosis difficult.

Treatment is very similar to that of rheumatoid arthritis, though long-acting agents are less frequently used, as patients with psoriatic arthritis seem to have a higher incidence of remission. Aortic disease does not occur in psoriatic arthritis.

SYSTEMIC LUPUS ERYTHEMATOSUS

Systemic lupus erythematosus (SLE) is a chronic disease of unknown etiology in which many systems are involved and in which the patient displays multiple immunologic abnormalities (6). It is a disease of unknown etiology. The pathogenesis is thought to involve hyperactivity of the immune system wherein the body produces antibodies to its own constituents and in which immune complexes circulate resulting in tissue damage. It is a disease predominantly of women in that 90% of patients are female. Although it can be seen in the very young and very old, it occurs most frequently in women of childbearing age.

Clinical manifestations are variable and widespread. Most common are fatigue, fever, skin rash, arthralgias, arthritis, hematologic abnormalities, myositis, hair loss, mouth ulcers, Raynaud's phenomenon, renal disease, central nervous system (CNS) disease, and myocardial and pulmonary disease. The severity of the disease varies. Some patients may have nothing more than arthralgias, fatigue, and a skin rash which may not progress to more substantial disease. On the other hand, patients are seen who have a fulminant disease which may be rapidly fatal with multiple organ failure. At one time lupus was considered to be a uniformly fatal disease. However, our understanding of the disease has expanded, and it is clear that many patients do quite well. The prognosis depends more on the organ system involved than it does on the label of lupus.

Little is known of the etiology of SLE, though there is some speculation that it may be some type of chronic viral infection. Evidence for this stems from the observation that in some of the murine models of SLE, e.g., NZB/NZW mice, viruses seem to play somewhat of a role (28). Furthermore, on kidney biopsy of patients with lupus, myxovirus-like structures are often seen. To date no consistent viral infection has been found.

The diagnosis of lupus is made on the basis of a combination of clinical findings (Table 1) in association with serologic abnormalities. The American Rheumatism Association has proposed criteria for the diagnosis of lupus (26); these are primarily for purposes of communication, but their existence tells us that there is no absolutely certain diagnostic test. Patients with lupus have various serologic abnormalities. Anemia, leukopenia, and thrombocytopenia are frequent and seem to be related, at least partially, to antibodies to the various blood constituents. Anti-red blood cell antibodies may cause hemolytic anemia, and antibodies to platelets induce thrombocytopenia. There is some evidence that antibodies to white blood cells cause leukopenia. An elevated ESR is common. Hypocomplementemia is often seen, and it is thought to result from circulating immune complexes which cause activation of the complement cascade and depletion of complement. Some patients with lupus seem to have a congenital absence of some of the components of complement, particularly C2, which seems to predispose to some of the manifestations of the disease.

The most common autoantibody found is the antinuclear antibody, which is present in about 90 to 98% of patients with SLE. The specificity of this antibody for SLE is low. It is often found in other connective tissue diseases, infectious diseases, neoplasm, and in a certain percentage of the population at large. Other commonly found antibodies include rheumatoid factor, antithyroglobulin antibody, various antibodies against tissue components, and antibody reacting with reagents. An antibody against double-stranded DNA seems to be fairly specific for SLE and is commonly used as a test, but the sensitivity is not very high. Another antigen, the SM antigen, is also found to be characteristic in SLE. Circulating anticoagulants may be found and are often associated with thrombotic disease.

The clinical findings in the individual patient depend on which systems are involved. As mentioned before, fatigue is very common. Arthralgias and arthritis are frequent, the former being more common. Patients with lupus may have severe joint pain and yet have very little in the way of objective synovitis. This is in

TABLE 1. *1982 Revised criteria for classification of SLE*

Criterion	Definition
Malar rash	Fixed erythema, flat or raised, over the malar emitnences, tending to spare the nasolabial folds
Discoid rash	Erythematous raised patches with adherent keratotic scaling and follicular plugging: atrophic scarring may occur in older lesions
Photosensitivity	Skin rash as a result of unusual reaction to sunlight, by patient history or physician observation
Oral ulcers	Oral or nasopharyngeal ulceration, usually painless, observed by a physician
Arthritis	Nonerosive arthritis involving two or more peripheral joints, characterized by tenderness, swelling, or effusion
Serositis	Pleuritis—convincing history of pleuritic pain or rub heard by a physician or evidence of pleural effusion *or* Pericarditis—documented by ECG or rub or evidence of pericardial effusion
Renal disorder	Persistent proteinuria greater than 0.5 g per day or greater than 3+ if quantitation not performed *or* Cellular casts—may be red blood cell, hemoglobin, granular, tubular, or mixed
Neurologic disorder	Seizures—in the absence of offending drugs or known metabolic derangements, e.g., uremia, ketoacidosis, electrolyte imbalance *or* Psychosis—in the absence of offending drugs or known metabolic derangements, e.g., uremia, ketoacidosis, or electrolyte imbalance
Hematologic disorder	Hemolytic anemia—with reticulocytosis *or* Leukopenia—less than 4,000/mm³ total on two or more occasions *or* Lymphopenia—less than 1,500/mm³ on two or more occasions *or* Thrombocytopenia—less than 100,000/mm³ in the absence of offending drugs
Immunologic disorder	Positive LE cell preparation *or* Anti-DNA: antibody to native DNA in abnormal titer *or* Anti-Sm: presence of antibody to Sm nuclear antigen *or* False-positive serologic test for syphilis known to be positive for at least 6 months and confirmed by *Treponema pallidum* immobilization or fluorescent treponemal antibody absorption test
Antinuclear antibody	An abnormal titer of antinuclear antibody by immunofluorescence or an equivalent assay at any point in time and in the absence of drugs known to be associated with "drug-induced lupus" syndrome

The proposed classification is based on 11 criteria. For the purpose of identifying patients in clinical studies, a person shall be said to have systemic lupus erythematosus if any four or more of the 11 criteria are present, serially or simultaneously, during any interval of observation.
From Tan et al. (16).

contrast to what is observed in rheumatoid arthritis. At other times an active synovitis can be seen. This synovitis tends not to be destructive. Narrowing of the joint spaces or erosive changes seen on x-ray films are infrequent, in contrast to rheumatoid arthritis. In some patients with chronic lupus arthritis, a ligamentous weakness occurs leading to reducible deformities of the joints unaccompanied by radiologic changes. This is referred to as "Jaccoud's arthritis," which has heretofore been described as being present in some patients with chronic rheumatic fever (4).

The skin rash classically seen is that of an erythema on the bridge of the nose and cheeks referred to as a "butterfly erythema." This may be associated with atrophy and hyperkeratosis. There may be other types of skin rash of a nondescript nature elsewhere. Alopecia is very common. Patients with lupus often manifest symptoms and signs of pleuritis, pericarditis, and peritonitis which may be associated with effusions. Myositis may occur during the course of SLE with proximal muscle weakness and findings indistinguishable from those seen in polymyositis. Raynaud's phenomenon is seen in a high percentage of patients. This may be manifested by blanching, bluish discoloration, or reddish discoloration of the distal extremities during exposure to the cold. On rare occasions this leads to finger ulcers and gangrene.

Various types of renal involvement occur including glomerulonephritis manifested as a nephrotic syndrome or as a rapidly progressive glomerulonephritis. Kidney involvement is a major cause of morbidity and mortality of the disease. Before the advent of hemodialysis and renal transplantation, renal disease was the most frequent cause of death in SLE.

Cardiac involvement is frequent including pericarditis, myocarditis, valvulitis, and coronary arteritis. In patients with long-standing lupus, particularly those who have been hypertensive, an increased incidence of atherosclerotic coronary artery disease is also seen.

Disease of the nervous system is also quite frequent. Virtually every type of neurologic picture can be seen including seizures, psychosis, peripheral neuropathy, dystonic syndromes, chorea, aseptic meningitis, diffuse encephalopathy, and vascular occlusive disease. CNS disease is a common cause of death. Eye manifestations include scotomas, optic neuritis, retinitis, and migraine-like syndromes.

Gastrointestinal manifestations include peritonitis, vasculitis of the bowel, and protein-losing enteropathy.

Pulmonary manifestations include pleuritis, interstitial pulmonary fibrosis, pulmonary hemorrhage, and nonspecific pneumonitis. In essence, any type of inflammatory manifestation involving almost any tissue of the body may be seen. Patients with SLE are highly susceptible to infections. This is due to the disease itself and is also a result of steroid and immunosuppressants used in the treatment of this disease.

Treatment depends on its manifestation and involves the whole gamut of techniques available for treatment of medical patients in general. Specific treatment for lupus usually involves anti-inflammatory drugs and corticosteroids. In patients in whom the major manifestations are cutaneous, articular, or associated with serous membranes, the antimalarials such as hydroxychloroquine sulfate (Plaquenil) and chloroquine are often efficacious. In disease that is life-threatening or in which the side effects of steroids become unacceptable, immunosuppressive drugs seem to be effective, though clear-cut prospective evidence of their efficacy is lacking. The treatment of renal lupus usually involves the use of corticosteroids and immuno-suppressive medicines. Most investigators have the impression that these are effective in controlling the disease and possibly preventing its progression. Hard data demonstrating the efficacy of these agents, however, are difficult to obtain. When patients develop irreversible renal failure, chronic hemodialysis and transplantation are lifesaving. Plasmapheresis is an experimental treatment used in an attempt to remove immune complexes, but its efficacy is also not proved.

Vasculitis is commonly seen as a complication of SLE; it is most commonly a small vessel vasculitis causing skin lesions, palpable purpura, ulceration, and sometimes frank gangrene. Occasionally large vessel vasculitis of a rather severe nature is present, and sometimes there are changes similar to those of polyarteritis nodosa. There have been reports of aortic insufficiency complicating SLE (3). At autopsy the aortic valve is dilated with perforation of the cusps. We have seen a patient with long-standing SLE develop cystic medial necrosis of the aorta with a dissecting aneurysm (H. Spiera, *unpublished observation*). To my knowledge no occlusive disease of the aorta or its branches have been described in SLE.

SCLERODERMA

Scleroderma is one of the few true "collagen" diseases. It is an illness characterized by increased deposition of collagen in the cutaneous and subcutaneous tissues and in multiple organ systems. The etiology and pathogenesis are unknown. Scleroderma is characterized by progressive thickening and tightening of the skin. The skin becomes bound down over the entire body with special predilection for the fingers, feet, face, and chest wall. Similar fibrosis occurs in the pulmonary parenchema causing interstitial pulmonary fibrosis. Involvement of the gastrointestinal tract leads to swallowing difficulty and small and large bowel dysfunction. Arthralgias and arthritis are common. There is also thickening of the tendons about the joints (16).

In addition to the increased deposition of connective tissue there are various vascular abnormalities in scleroderma. Raynaud's phenomenon is seen in over 90% of patients. Rapidly progressive renal disease resembling malignant hypertension may occur. Cardiac involvement is frequent.

Though the etiology and pathogenesis of scleroderma are unknown, there is some speculation that endothelial vascular thickening with resultant ischemia could lead to the fibrotic changes (12). Autoantibodies are sometimes found, particularly antinuclear antibodies. Their presence seems to have no diagnostic specificity. In some of the subsets of scleroderma such as the CREST syndrome—characterized by calcinosis (C), Raynaud's (R) phenomenon, esophageal motility disturbances (E), sclerodactyly (S), and telangiectasias (T)—patients often manifest an anticentromere antibody. This type of scleroderma seems not to result in pulmonary fibrosis, myocardial disease, renal disease, or major gastrointestinal disturbance. However, these patients are particularly prone to develop pulmonary hypertension.

Some forms of scleroderma are limited to the skin. These patients have only local skin lesions or linear areas of skin involvement referred to as morphea or linear scleroderma. These are not associated with systemic manifestations.

Treatment for the various manifestations of scleroderma are purely symptomatic. Analgesics and anti-inflammatories are used for the articular problems. Physiotherapy and range-of-motion exercises are employed to prevent contractures; antacids and H_2 blockers are employed for esophageal reflux symptoms; antibiotics are used for the bacterial overgrowth phenomenon seen in small bowel involvement; and various vasodilators are used for Raynaud's phenomenon. The hypertensive renal crisis may be successfully treated with captopril. There is some evidence that pencillamine may retard the progression of scleroderma, though this is far from proved (25). Inflammatory vascular disease, on the other hand, is infrequent, though it has been described. Some patients with scleroderma have been described with inflammatory disease of the vessels similar to polyarteritis nodosa (5). Aortic disease and disease of its major branches are not a feature of progressive systemic sclerosis.

DERMATOMYOSITIS/POLYMYOSITIS

Dermatomyositis/polymyositis (DM/PM) is an acquired disease of the muscle characterized by muscle weakness which is predominantly proximal (23). It occurs at all ages including childhood and old age. In some patients it is associated with an underlying malignant neoplasm. It has a slight female predominance. There is often a characteristic skin rash consisting of a "heliotrope" erythema about the eyelids and V-area of the neck with some hyperpigmentation over the extensor surfaces of the joints. The association of this rash with muscle weakness defines the symptoms of DM.

Nothing is known of its etiology and pathogenesis, though there are some claims that autoimmunity may play a role. Antibodies against a cytoplasmic antigen called PM-1 has been described in some patients. DM/PM may occur as a single disease entity or in association with another connective tissue disease such as lupus, scleroderma, and rarely rheumatoid arthritis. Patients may have Raynaud's phenomenon and arthralgias and arthritis, but these are usually not the primary features. Patients are seen who have muscle inflammation in addition to features of scleroderma and SLE. This is called "mixed connective tissue disease" (MCTD). This designation is based on the overlap features of these patients and its association with an antibody to an extractable nuclear antigen (20). Whether this indeed is a separate syndrome is not clear. Most patients with MCTD have the prognosis of either scleroderma or SLE.

The diagnosis of polymyositis is based on the presence of an acquired myopathy in which there is evidence of muscle inflammation manifested by an elevation of creatine phosphokinase (CPK) and aldolase, electrodiagnostic abnormalities, and characteristic though not diagnostic changes on biopsy. It must be distinguished from other situations that can simulate this such as hyper- and hypothyroidism, hyperparathyroidism, hypokalemic myopathy, and occasionally acute muscular dystrophy.

Treatment of polymyositis usually involves the use of corticosteroids to suppress the inflammation, though sometimes cytostatic agents such as azathioprine or methotrexate are used. Essential in the work-up of a patient with polymyositis is a search for a neoplasm which might not be clinically manifest.

Vasculitis occasionally accompanies dermatomyositis, particularly in children. In adults this is not a frequent association. Disease of the aorta and its branches are not a feature of PM/DM.

BEHÇET'S SYNDROME

Behçet's syndrome is an illness of unknown etiology and pathogenesis characterized by the presence of recurrent oral and genital ulcerations. It is accompanied by iritis, skin lesions, arthritis, superficial phlebitis, major vessel thrombosis, CNS disease, gastrointestinal disease, and glomerulonephritis (7). There is no single diagnostic test for this syndrome, and the diagnosis depends on a combination of clinical findings. Minimal criteria seem to be the presence of recurrent oral and genital ulcerations. The disease was initially described in Turkey. It occurs frequently in Japan and is a major cause of morbidity there. Sporadic cases are seen in the United States and western countries, and its true incidence is not known. There seems to be a slight female predominance. The association with thrombophlebitis, nephritis, and recurring pauciarticular arthritis may cause it to be confused with other connective tissue diseases, particularly SLE. A distinguishing feature is the absence of any characteristic autoantibody.

Thrombophlebitis is characteristically seen and is sometimes so severe as to cause thrombosis of the vena cava. Arteritis of major arteries is sometimes noted, though lesions of the aorta are not seen.

There is no specific treatment for the disease, though some workers believe that the use of colchicine may be effective in preventing some of the acute attacks and the skin lesions (17). Corticosteroids are often used in the life-threatening aspects of the disease but sometimes are ineffective. Cytostatic agents are used including azathioprine, cyclophosphamide (Cytoxan), and chlorambucil, the latter believed to be the most effective though objective evidence is lacking. Prognosis of the disease depends on its manifestations. Because of severe eye involvement, patients may develop blindness. Vasculitis may result in gangrene and indeed loss of an extremity. Vasculitis involving the CNS can lead to a fatal outcome. Glomerulonephritis is an infrequent concomitant but at times may be rapidly progressive (14).

RELAPSING POLYCHONDRITIS

Relapsing polychondritis is an illness characterized by inflammation of the cartilaginous structures of the body, particularly the ears, nose, tracheobronchial tree, and articular cartilage (1). It is an infrequent disease occurring most commonly during middle age, though it can occur during childhood and old age. Its course tends to be recurrent and episodic, consisting of intermittent painful swelling of the pinna of the ears, swelling of the nose, arthritis, and often inflammation of the trachial rings. The disease may be life-threatening, as collapse of the tracheobronchial tree due to dissolution of the supporting cartilaginous structures leads to airway obstruction. Another common cause of mortality is aortic insufficiency resulting from a widening of the aortic ring.

It is a disease of unknown etiology. Pathogenesis is believed to be immunologically mediated. Evidence for this is the deposition of immunoglobulin in affected cartilage. It may be associated with other connective tissue diseases particularly SLE. It may cause deafness due to involvement of the external and internal auditory apparatus, and it may cause blindness due to progressive eye inflammation. The arthritis is usually episodic and self-limited and rarely leads to permanent joint deformity. Laboratory features include elevation of the ESR and the presence of other acute-phase reactants. Rheumatoid factor and antinuclear antibody are not usually found, though on occasion they are present in low titers.

Treatment includes the use of corticosteroids, particularly when there is life-threatening involvement of the tracheobronchial tree. When only ear inflammation, nose inflammation, or arthritis is present, nonsteroidal anti-inflammatory agents may be helpful. Steroids do not seem to have any influence on the aortic insufficiency that may develop. When patients with aortic insufficiency become symptomatic, they must be treated surgically as patients with aortic insufficiency of any other cause. Diagnosis is based on the characteristic clinical picture of recurrent cartilaginous inflammation, and it must be distinguished from other diseases with cartilage destruction, e.g., Wegener's granulomatosis, Cogan's syndrome, and syphilis. The multiple areas of cartilaginous involvement are so characteristic of this disease that it is usually easy to diagnose. Confusion may exist when it is associated with any other connective tissue diseases such as SLE.

RHEUMATIC FEVER

Though not classically considered one of the "connective tissue diseases" rheumatic fever is often considered in the differential diagnosis of the various rheumatic diseases. Virtually all attacks of rheumatic fever are preceded by evidence of an infection with a Group A beta hemolytic streptococcus. It is a disease that used to be quite common but now occurs infrequently in the highly industrialized countries. Its incidence seems to be related to poor socioeconomic conditions, particularly in newly industrialized societies where there is over-crowding.

Though the development of acute rheumatic fever is related to an antecedent streptococcal infection, there is no evidence that the streptococcus itself invades the involved tissues. Joint fluid and tissue cultures of patients dying of rheumatic fever are sterile. Nor is there evidence that the toxin released by the streptococcus causes injury to the various tissues. A postulated mechanism whereby streptococcal infection may eventually lead to rheumatic fever is the development of antibody initially directed against the streptococcus or one of its products which cross-reacts with cardiac or joint tissue. A Group A streptococcal membrane antigen has been found which is cross-reactive with human heart. Whether this indeed is the mechanism for rheumatic fever is speculative. The arthritis of rheumatic fever may be immunologically mediated. Evidence for this is that complement components in synovial fluid are decreased in rheumatic fever. Immunoglobulins are found deposited in myofibers of patients with rheumatic heart disease. These include IgG, IgA, IgM, and complement components.

The primary clinical features of rheumatic fever are migratory polyarthritis, chorea, carditis, erythema marginatum, and subcutaneous nodules. The arthritis is usually evanescent with the entire duration lasting about 6 weeks. There is no permanent joint damage. Carditis is characterized by the presence of congestive heart failure, appearance of new systolic or diastolic murmurs, pericarditis, or cardiomegaly. The carditis may be fatal or, more commonly, lead to residual rheumatic valvular disease, particularly the mitral valves. This may not become manifest until later in the course after recurrent attacks of rheumatic carditis. Chorea is a late manifestation of rheumatic fever and often occurs as late as 2 to 3 months after the streptococcal infection; in fact, serological evidence of a streptococcal infection may no longer be evident. The rash of erythema marginatum and subcutaneous nodules are infrequently seen.

The treatment of rheumatic fever includes initial eradication of any streptococcalinfection present with penicillin. Aspirin is usually dramatically effective in alleviating joint symptoms. When carditis is severe and life-threatening, corticosteroids are often used even though unequivocal proof of their efficacy is lacking.

When the diagnosis of rheumatic fever is made, the patient is then given penicillin prophylactically to prevent further recurrence of rheumatic fever, as rheumatic fever will not recur without a preceding streptococcal infection. The most effective prophylactic treatment is 1.2 million units of benzathine penicillin G intramuscularly every 4 weeks. Alternate prophylactic regimens are oral penicillin 250,000 units twice a day, sulfadiazine 500 mg once daily, or erythromycin 500 mg daily. Long-term bed rest, which was once used in the treatment of rheumatic fever, is now thought to be unnecessary and is prescribed only in the setting of active carditis. The treatment of chorea includes mild sedation and tranquilizers such as chlorpromazine or phenobarbital. Subcutaneous nodules and erythema marginatum usually need no treatment as they are self-limited.

The diagnosis of rheumatic fever is at times extremely difficult to establish. There are no diagnostic tests for rheumatic fever, and the diagnosis is made on the basis of the entire clinical picture. The modified Jones criteria were introduced because there was a tendency to over-diagnose rheumatic fever. The major manifestation are carditis, polyarthritis, chorea, erythema marginatum, and subcutaneous nodules. Minor manifestations include previous rheumatic fever or rheumatic heart disease, arthralgias, fever, elevated ESR, elevated C-reactive protein, or prolonged PR interval on electrocardiogram. In order for these criteria to apply, there must be evidence of preceding streptococcal infection as indicated by an increased titer of antistreptolycin O antibody, other streptococcal antibodies, positive throat culture for Group A streptococcus, or recent scarlet fever. It must be recognized that these criteria are for communication purposes and basically serve as minimum criteria for the diagnosis of rheumatic fever. For the diagnosis of rheumatic fever it is necessary to have evidence of preceding streptococcal infection, two major manifestations or one major and two minor manifestations. It must be recognized that since streptococcal infections are so frequent these criteria are not specific. Thus, patients with lupus who have evidence of preceding streptococcal infection may easily meet the Jones criteria. Thus the Jones criteria are not diagnostic but rather serve as guidelines. It is important to recognize this fact in order to avoid the over-diagnosis of rheumatic fever, which may needlessly stigmatize the patient and subject the patient to long-term prophylaxis.

The prognosis of rheumatic fever depends almost exclusively on the presence of carditis and residual rheumatic heart disease. With the rare exception of a nonerosive deforming arthritis of the hands, referred to as Jaccoud's arthritis, chronic arthritis does not occur in rheumatic fever. The most frequent valve involved in rheumatic fever is the mitral valve; second in frequency is the aortic valve. The deformity of the aortic valve results from a fusion of the cusps, rigidity and shortening of the cusps, and sometimes calcification. Aortitis with a resultant pulseless disease syndrome has, to our knowledge, not been reported in rheumatic fever.

REFERENCES

1. Arkis, C. R., and Masi, A. T. (1970): Relapsing polychondritis: Review of current status and case report. *Semin. Arthritis Rheum.*, 5:41.
2. Aryo, K., Ahvonen, P., Sassu, S. A., Sievers, K., and Tillikainen, A. (1973): HL-A antigen 27 reactive arthritis. *Lancet*, 2:157.
3. Bernhard, G. C., Lange, R. C., and Hensley, G. T. (1960): Aortic disease with valvular insufficiency as the principal manifestation of systemic lupus erythematosus. *Ann. Intern. Med.*, 71:81–87.
4. Bittl, J. A., and Perloff, J. K. (1983): Chronic postrheumatic fever arthropathy of Jaccoud. *Am. Heart. J.*, 105:515.
5. D'Angelo, W. A., Fries, J. F., Masi, A. T., and Schulman, A. E. (1969): Pathologic observations in systemic sclerosis (scleroderma): A study of 58 autopsy cases and 58 matched controls. *Am. J. Med.*, 46:428–440.
6. Dubois, E. L. (1974): *Lupus Erythematosus*. University of Southern California Press, Los Angeles.
7. Ehrlich, G. E. (1985): In: *Arthritis and Allied Conditions*, 10th Ed., edited by D. J. McCarty, pp. 891–896. Lea & Febiger, Philadelphia.
8. Fox, R., Calin, A., Gerbo, R. C., and Gibson, D. (1979): The chronicity of symptoms and disability in Reiter's syndrome: An analysis of 131 consecutive patients. *Ann. Intern. Med.*, 91:190.
9. Gocke, D. F., Morgan, C., Lockshin, M., Hsu, K., Bombardieri, S., and Christian, C. L. (1970): Association between polyarteritis and Australia antigen. *Lancet*, 2:1149–1153.
10. Graham, D. C., and Smythe, H. A. (1958): The carditis and aortitis of ankylosing spondylitis. *Bull. Rheum. Dis.*, 9:171.
11. Harris, E. D., Jr. (1981): Pathogenesis of rheumatoid arthritis. In: *Textbook of Rheumatology*, edited by W. N. Kelly et al. Saunders, Philadelphia.
12. Kahaler, M. B., Sherer, G. K., and LeRoy, E. C. (1979): Endothelial injury in scleroderma. *J. Exp. Med.*, 149:1326.

13. Klemperer, P. (1947): Diseases of the collagen system. *Bull. N.Y. Acad. Med.*, 23:581–588.
14. Landwehr, D. M., Cooke, D. L., and Rodriquez, G. E. (1980): Rapidly progressive glomerulo-nephritis in Behçet's syndrome. *JAMA*, 244:1709–1711.
15. McCarty, D. J. (1985): *Arthritis and Allied Conditions*, 10th Ed., pp. 557–785. Lea & Febiger, Philadelphia.
16. Medsger, T. A. (1985): In *Arthritis and Allied Conditions*. 10th Ed., Lea & Febiger, Philadelphia.
17. Miyachi, Y., Taniguchi, S., Ozaki, M., and Horio, T. (1981): Colchicine in the treatment of cutaneous manifestations of Behçet's disease. *Br. J. Dermatol.*, 104:67–69.
18. Moll, J. M. H. (1980): *Ankylosing Spondylitis*. Churchill Livingstone, New York.
19. Ragan, C., and Farrington, E. (1967): The clinical features of rheumatoid arthritis. *JAMA*, 181:663–667.
20. Sharp, G. C., Irvin, W. S., Tan, E. M., Gould, R. G., and Holman, H. R. (1972): Mixed connective tissue diseases: An apparently distinct rheumatic disease syndrome associated with a specific antibody to an extractable nuclear antigen (ENA). *Am. J. Med.*, 52:148–159.
21. Sharp, G. T. (1985): Reiter's syndrome (reactive arthritis). In: *Arthritis and Allied Conditions*, 10th Ed., edited by D. J. McCarty, pp. 841–849. Lea & Febiger, Philadelphia.
22. Sokoloff, L., McCloskey, R. T., and Bunim, J. J. (1953): Vascularity of the early nodule of rheumatoid arthritis. *A.M.A. Arch. Pathol.*, 55:475–495.
23. Spiera, H. (1977): Polymyositis and other diseases of muscle. In: *Rheumatic Diseases, Diagnosis and Management*, edited by W. A. Katz. Lippincott, Philadelphia.
24. Spiera, H. (1985): Rheumatoid vasculitis in rheumatoid emergencies. *In preparation*.
25. Steen, V. D., Medsger, T. A., Jr., and Rodnan, G. P. (1982): D-Penicillamine therapy in progressive systemic sclerosis (scleroderma). *Ann. Intern. Med*, 97:652–659.
26. Tan, E. M., Cohen, C. S., Fries, J. F., Masi, A. T., McShane, D. J., Rothfield, N. F., Shalle, J. G., Talal, N., and Winchester, R. J. (1982): Revised criteria for the classification of systemic lupus erythematosus. *Arthritis Rheum.*, 25:1271–1277.
27. Wright, V., and Moll, J. M. J. (1976): *Seronegative Polyarthritis*. North Holland, Amsterdam.
28. Yoshiki, T., Mellors, R. C., Strand, M., and August, J. T. (1974): The viral envelope glycoprotein of murine leukemia virus and the pathogenesis of immune complex glomerulonephritis in New Zealand mice. *J. Exp. Med.*, 140:1011–1027.

Aortitis: Clinical, Pathologic, and Radiographic Aspects, edited by A. Lande, Y. M. Berkmen, and H. A. McAllister. Raven Press, New York © 1986.

Medical Aspects of Infectious Aortitis

Yahya M. Berkmen

Department of Clinical Radiology, Cornell University Medical College, and Section of Pulmonary Radiology, New York Hospital, New York, New York 10021

Reference to infectious aortitis was first made during the sixteenth century by Ambroise Paré who associated syphilis with aortic aneurysms. Two hundred years later Lancisi again called attention to the relationship between aortic aneurysms and syphilis, and emphasized the cardiovascular complications of the disease.

During the late nineteenth century pathologic and clinical aspects of syphilis were well studied, and aortitis emerged as its most common and serious complication. Meanwhile pyogenic infections and tuberculosis were being recognized as significant factors in the etiology of infectious aortitis (71).

In 1885 Sir William Osler used the term "mycotic" in his historic and often quoted Gulstonian lecture in reference to vegetations of endocarditis. Although soon after its introduction the wrong connotation of the term "mycotic" became evident, it is now well entrenched in the medical literature, and its place in the vocabulary of aortitis appears to be unshakable.

Epidemiology, bacteriology, and pathogenesis of mycotic aneurysms have changed dramatically within the hundred years since Sir William Osler's lecture. This required constant revision and reclassification of the entity. In 1887 Eppinger introduced the term "embolomycotic" to indicate the causal relationship between mycotic aneurysms and subacute bacterial endocarditis which remained as a most prevalent cause of these aneurysms until 1945. In fact, in 1923 Stengel and Wolforth found endocarditis to be responsible for 86% of mycotic aneurysms, and only 14% were due to other causes, i.e., pneumonia and osteomyelitis (65).

In 1926 Rappaport described acute pyogenic infection of the aorta caused by *Streptococcus viridans* in a patient with syphilitic aortitis and collected other similar cases from the literature. The source of infection was extravascular in all these cases, and organisms cultured were pneumococci, gonococci, *Streptococcus hemolyticus*, and even the anthrax bacillis in one case. He referred to them as "primary acute aortitis" and applied the term to "acute inflammation of the aorta in which the infection is not attributable to an associated or preceding infection of the heart valves or of the adjacent mediastinal structures" (55).

Crane in 1937 popularized the term "primary mycotic aneurysms" referring to "lesions not associated with intravascular inflammatory focus as bacterial endocarditis, or with any inflammatory process in the surrounding tissues" (21). Aneurysms caused by endocarditis were called "secondary."

By this time different aspects of nonsyphilitic aortitis were well studied and published. In contrast to resistance of intact intima to infection, susceptibility of previously injured aorta to bacterial colonization was already established. Many investigators showed that organisms could reach the aortic wall from an extravascular and distant source through the intraluminal bloodstream, via the vasa vasorum, by contiguity, and rarely through the lymphatics.

However, primary infections of the aorta were still uncommon as demonstrated by Revell in 1945 (56). He found only 23 cases of primary mycotic aneurysms in the literature and added a case of his own.

After 1945 the addition of antibiotics to the medical armamentarium resulted in a dramatic and simultaneous decline in the incidence of subacute bacterial endocarditis and secondary mycotic aneurysms. Paradoxically, however, this was followed by a sharp rise in the occurrence of primary mycotic aneurysms.

Antibiotics not only changed the relative frequency of primary and secondary forms of aortitis but also influenced its bacteriology. Whereas before 1945 nonhemolytic streptococci, staphylococci, pneumococci, gonococci, and *Hemophilus influenzae* were the most common causes of mycotic aneurysms, during the years following the introduction and wide use of antibiotics salmonellae and staphylococci have become the most prevalent organisms (4,18,73).

Blum and Keefer in 1962 applied the term "cryptogenic" to those "mycotic aneurysms arising in the absence of endocarditis or other local or systemic infection" (7). Two years later the same authors called attention to the antibiotic resistance of the bacteria cultured from these patients (8).

In 1977 Patel and Johnston emphasized the importance of including both preexisting conditions of the vessel (normal or atherosclerotic, aneurysm, arterial prosthesis) and the source of infection [(a) intravascular: embolism, septicemia, extension of adjacent endocardial infection, erosive; and (b) extravascular: spread from adjacent infection, iatrogenic] to the classification of mycotic aneurysms (52).

Wilson et al. in 1978 discussed the broad subject of arterial infections, including aortitis, in two groups: (a) spontaneous and (b) postoperative graft infections. They classified spontaneous infections under six main categories: (a) *mycotic aneurysms*: used as a specific definition of Osler to indicate endocardial origin; (b) *infected aneurysm*: secondary infections of an established aneurysm; (c) *microbial arteritis*: includes "primary," "secondary," and "cryptogenic" infections; (d) *traumatic infected aneurysm*: includes traumatic, iatrogenic, and self-induced infections; (e) *contiguous arterial infection*; and (f) *septic arterial emboli* (71). A modified version of this classification has been provided by Ewart et al. (27).

CLINICAL ASPECTS

Of all the classifications of infectious aortitides, that of Wilson et al. is the most up to date, all-inclusive, and easily comprehensible. Therefore it has been adopted in the following discussion.

Spontaneous Infections

Mycotic Aneurysm

Prevention and early treatment of bacterial endocarditis has markedly lowered the incidence of mycotic aneurysms of intravascular origin, whereas that of aortitis due to extravascular causes has sharply risen. During the postantibiotic era, the average age of patients with endocarditis has significantly increased. However, patients presenting with mycotic aneurysms are younger than those with atherosclerotic aneurysms. Approximately one-fourth of mycotic aneurysms occur within the second decade of life and one-third during the third decade (71). There is a distinctive male predominance over females: The ratio varies from 2:1 to 5:1 in different series (43).

Staphylococcus and *Streptococcus* are responsible for bacterial endocarditis in 88.4% of patients (43). Other commonly cultured organisms are *Salmonella*, *H. influenzae*, enterococci, diphtheroids, and *Serratia* (43,71). Fungal infections are rare; they occur in immunosuppressed patients, after protracted administration of antibiotics, and in intravenous drug abusers. *Candida*, *Histoplasma*, and *Aspergillus* are the most common offenders; however, *Blastomyces*, *Coccidioides*, *Cryptococcus*, and *Mucor* have been found in occasional cases (19,43,71).

Aortitis with mycotic aneurysm formation may result from subacute, and less commonly from acute, bacterial endocarditis. The source of infection may not be apparent in a significant percentage of patients with subacute bacterial endocarditis. Occasionally, a history of recent trauma or dental manipulation can be elicited. Its clinical manifestations are insidious and usually consist of fever, malaise, easy fatigability, anorexia and weight loss, night sweats, arthralgias, etc. Previously damaged valves of the left side of the heart are more prone to be the seat of subacute bacterial endocarditis. Sinuses of Valsalva (52,54) and coronary arteries (22) may be involved by direct extension of the infection from the diseased valves. Septic emboli arising from the valves can reach the aortic wall via the bloodstream and through the vasa vasorum. The most common sites of involvement are the aortic root and ascending aorta.

Acute bacterial endocarditis occurs about 50% of the time in intravenous drug abusers. Skin infections, burns, insect bites, instrumentation of the urinary tract, abortion, or parturition are other recorded causes of acute bacterial endocarditis. The onset of symptoms are sudden, and the course is fulminant (71). Acute bacterial endocarditis almost exclusively attacks previously healthy tricuspid valves. Pulmonary valves, as a rule, are spared. Aortic or mitral valves are rarely involved in acute bacterial endocarditis (37).

Whereas clinical recognition of bacterial endocarditis is easy, the development of a mycotic aneurysm may not be suspected. Sudden rupture of the aneurysm with fatal hemorrhage before it is clinically diagnosed is unfortunately not uncommon. The clinical symptoms are usually related to the systemic manifestations of the infection and, if the aneurysm is large enough, to its local pressure effects. Thus cough, chest pain, hoarseness, and dysphagia in thoracic aneurysms, and epigastric and/or lumbar pain in abdominal aneurysms, may be present. The sudden appearance of a pulsatile mass in the abdomen or radiographic demonstration of mediastinal widening in a patient with known bacterial endocarditis is diagnostic. Mycotic aneurysms are usually true aneurysms. Dissecting aneurysms are rare.

Immediate diagnosis and initiation of vigorous therapy are more critical in acute bacterial endocarditis than in subacute endocarditis, as overall mortality is higher in the acute form (43). Although high-dose intravenous antibiotic therapy is essential, the heart valves cannot be completely "sterilized" until the aneurysm is totally resected (71).

Infected Aneurysm

Bacterial colonization of a preexisting aortic aneurysm results in an infected aneurysm. Seventy-four percent of infected aneurysms are atherosclerotic and are frequently located in the abdomen (5). They may also be syphilitic (5,12,73) or traumatic (5) in origin. The tuberculous aortitis reported by Kline and Durant was probably a traumatic pseudoaneurysm secondarily infected during miliary dissemination of tuberculosis (41). Another case of infected aneurysm due to *Mycobacterium* was reported by Jarrett et al. (38). Fungal infections are rare (47).

Infection spreads either hematogenously from a distant source or through lymphatics of a contiguous infectious process (38). In about half of the cases the source of the infection cannot be determined (5).

Salmonella accounts for most of the secondary infections of aortic aneurysms, *Staphylococcus* being second in frequency. *Escherichia coli* and other Gram-negative bacilli are responsible for infected aneurysms in about 20% of cases (71).

Specific clinical signs directly referable to infected aneurysms are often lacking, subtle, or overshadowed by local or systemic manifestations of primary infection (5). Thus early diagnosis is rarely made, which accounts for the high mortality rate seen in these cases. Fever of unknown origin in a patient with known aortic aneurysm should be considered highly suspicious for infected aneurysm (5,38).

Frequent rupture of the aorta accounts for the high mortality rate associated with infected aneurysms. There is an even higher incidence of aortic rupture in infections with Gram-negative bacteria.

Microbial Aortitis

Infection of the aortic wall during transient bacteremia results in microbial aortitis, a classic example of which is syphilitic aortitis (discussed separately). Previously damaged or atherosclerotic aortic wall is particularly susceptible to bacterial seeding. The segment of the aorta distal to a congenital coarctation is also prone to infection (9,36,50).

Microbial aortitis is a frequent complication of intravenous drug abuse. *Salmonella*, *Staphylococcus*, and *E. coli* are the most common offenders. *Aspergillus* has been implicated in a few cases (48,60). Because of subtle and insidious clinical manifestations, the diagnosis is often not suspected and the necessary surgical intervention is delayed until fatal or near-fatal hemorrhage occurs. Sudden appearance of a palpable pulsatile abdominal mass or radiographic demonstration of rapid enlargement of the mediastinum in a patient with fever is diagnostic.

Although pseudoaneurysm is a common complication of microbial aortitis, the intermediate stages prior to formation of aneurysm have been demonstrated. Cohen found endothelial infection in 25% of patients over 50 years of age with *Salmonella* bacteremia (43). Bardin et al. (3) reported two patients who suffered from suppurative aortitis without aneurysm. In the first patient, there was necrosis and rupture of the aorta secondary to beta-hemolytic *Streptococcus* infection. The second patient had *Salmonella* aortitis and was treated successfully by surgical intervention. The authors suggested careful evaluation of atherosclerotic patients with sepsis, particularly if it is due to *Salmonella*.

Traumatic Infected Pseudoaneurysms

The infection may be self-inflicted (drug abuse) or iatrogenic (arterial catheters, arteriography, arteriovenous fistulas, vascular contamination during surgery) or may be introduced through penetrating trauma. Commonly peripheral arteries are affected, and aortitis is rare.

Contiguous Aortic Infection

Tuberculosis of the aorta is a classic example of contiguous aortic infection and is discussed separately. Infection may originate from the lung (61) or mediastinum (6), bones, or retroperitoneal organs (71). *Salmonella* is the most common offender, and *Staphylococcus* is next in frequency. Fungal infections are rare (61).

Extension of suppuration from a contiguous inflammatory process erodes the aortic wall, and pseudoaneurysm is formed. Diagnostic difficulties arise from obscure clinical manifestations. Sudden and unexplained bacteremia and local pain are suggestive evidence of aortitis; the sudden appearance of a bruit or murmur and a pulsatile abdominal mass is diagnostic.

Infected Arterial Emboli

Today septic emboli originating from vegetations of subacute bacterial endocarditis are extremely rare. They are almost exclusively secondary to intravascular drug abuse. Cardiac valvular prostheses, pacemakers, and intravenous catheters are responsible for a small percentage of cases. Extravascular but adjacent infections may rarely be the source of septic emboli (71).

Postoperative Infections

Vascular Graft Infections

Vascular grafts are highly susceptible to infection caused by either intraoperative contamination, postoperative bacteremia, and/or extension from a contiguous source.

Ernst et al. obtained positive cultures from contents of surgically removed aneurysms of the abdominal aorta without evidence of infected aneurysm. The authors believed that these aneurysms pose a potential danger for development of graft infection and strongly suggested prophylactic use of antibiotics after graft procedures (26).

Staphylococcus accounts for most of the infections after aortofemoral and aortoiliac grafts. Abdominal aortic grafts, on the other hand, are frequently infected by *E. coli* and *Klebsiella* species. Although it apears that infection is seeded during surgery, its manifestations are commonly delayed, occurring within 6 months in the majority of cases (26).

Infected grafts carry a high mortality rate—more than 50% for retroperitoneal grafts (71). They present with a low clinical profile. Fever and leukocytosis are commonly absent. Back pain has been the most constant finding (71).

Infected vascular grafts have a high propensity for rupture into the gastrointestinal tract. Aortoduodenal fistulas occur 80% of the time. Next in frequency are fistulas to the ileum and jejunum.

Fistulous communications occur more frequently from the proximal side of the graft. The catastrophic outcome may be signaled about 24 hr earlier by melena and hematemesis. Fever of unknown origin, evidence of bacteremia, or evidence of gastrointestinal bleeding in a patient with a previous graft procedure should be enough to alert the clinician to the need for immediate surgical intervention.

Prosthetic Cardiac Valves

Infection of prosthetic cardiac valves is found within 60 days after operation in most cases, and *Staphylococcus aureus* and *S. epidermidis*, *Diplococcus diphtheriae*, Gram-negative bacilli, and *Candida* are commonly found (13). The source of infection is the heart–lung machine in a high percentage of cases (13). *Aspergillus* and *Candida* infections are uncommon (13,14).

Syphilitic Aortitis

For centuries syphilis had been one of the most prevalent infectious diseases and common causes of death. During the postantibiotic era the incidence of primary syphilis precipitously declined until 1950; however, it increased three times between 1950 and 1960 and has leveled off at the same rate since then (16,45). Penicillin obviously did not eradicate the disease, and syphilis today continues to be a public health problem in the United States.

Clinically untreated syphilis evolves through four stages (51):

1. *Primary*: After an average incubation period of 3 weeks (which may vary, however, from 10 to 90 days) a chancre appears at the site of inoculation and lasts 1 to 5 weeks.

2. *Secondary*: Two to ten weeks later generalized cutaneous and mucosal eruptions appear associated with malaise, fever, adenopathy, and less commonly alopecia, hepatitis, and nephrotic syndrome. This stage lasts 2 to 6 weeks.

3. *Latent*: This is a silent period and is divided into early and late phases. The *early latent stage* is the period 2 years from onset of the infection during which intermittent eruptions similar to those seen in the secondary stage occur. The *late latent stage* starts 2 years after the beginning of infection, with the disease progressing to organs other than the skin without clinical manifestations. This period may last 20 years or more.

4. *Tertiary*: Late manifestations occur in the skin, bones, central nervous system, and cardiovascular systems.

The disease is continuously infectious in the primary and secondary stages, intermittently infectious in the early latent stage, and noninfectious in the late latent period.

The outcome of untreated syphilis has been well studied in three classic works: the Oslo, Tuskegee, and Rosahn studies (17,58,59). These studies produced remarkably similar conclusions. The probability of dying as a direct result of syphilis was 17.1% in males and 8% in females; and cardiovascular syphilis (14.9% in males and 8% of females) was more prevalent than neurosyphilis (9.4% in males and 5% in females) (17).

Syphilic aortitis starts just above the aortic ring and, in order of frequency, involves the ascending aorta, aortic arch, and descending aorta (42). It is associated with aortic aneurysm, aortic valvulitis, and coronary ostial stenosis, or it may remain uncomplicated.

Syphilitic Aortic Aneurysm

The majority of luetic aneurysms are located at the thoracic aorta; according to Kampmeier, the frequency of occurrence at various sites is less than 1% at the sinus of Valsalva, 36% at the ascending aorta, 24% at the transverse arch, 5% at the descending aorta, and 4% at multiple sites (39).

Syphilitic aneurysms may gradually enlarge and attain enormous size. These large aneurysms may erode the adjacent bones (40) and produce symptoms by compressing the contiguous mediastinal structures, i.e., cough, shortness of breath, hemoptysis, atelectasis, pneumonia, Horner's syndrome, hoarseness, dysphagia (12,53), and superior vena cava syndrome (2,53).

The prognosis in symptomatic syphilitic aneurysm is guarded, and death by rupture within a short period is an anticipated outcome (40). Dissecting aneurysm of the aorta usually does not occur in syphilitic aortitis because of extensive fibrosis of the media. Miliary aneurysms of the aorta are rarely observed (44).

Syphilitic aneurysms of the sinuses of Valsalva may occur as isolated pathology. Dilatation is asymmetrical, and no sinus is favored, in contrast to cystic medial necrosis in which dilatation of the sinuses is symmetrical, resembling a "tulip bulb" (20). Congenital aneurysms, on the other hand, affect primarily the right coronary sinus and less frequently the noncoronary sinus. The left coronary sinus is rarely involved.

Syphilitic aneurysms of the sinuses of Valsalva have a strong tendency to rupture outside the heart rather than into the pericardium or cardiac chambers. A syphilitic aneurysm may become an "infected aneurysm" with colonization by pyogenic bacteria (12,73).

Aortic Regurgitation

Approximately 60% of patients with cardiovascular syphilis present with aortic insufficiency (34). This common complication is due to valvulitis, relaxation of the aortic ring, or both. Valvulitis results from downward extension of the inflammatory process which starts above the ring; free edges of the cusps become thickened and rolled and their commissures widened (42,44).

Stenosis of the Coronary Ostia

Angina pectoris is a common complication of luetic aortitis. Combination of aortic regurgitation and narrowing of the coronary arteries at their origin are mainly responsible for the vascular insufficiency. Superimposed secondary atherosclerosis may further increase the stenosis, which, if severe enough, may lead to myocardial infarction (34,40). On rare occasions, stenosis of the coronary arteries distal to the ostia (35) or by extrinsic pressure from ventricular gummas (40) have been recorded. Martland cited one case of syphilitic coronary artery aneurysm with rupture into the pericardium (44).

Uncomplicated Aortitis

Syphilitic aortitis is said to be uncomplicated in the absence of the changes described above. However, dilatation of the ascending aorta appears in a significant number of patients with uncomplicated syphilitic aortitis.

Miscellaneous Lesions

Less common cardiovascular lesions due to syphilis are myocarditis (34), gumma of the left ventricle (40,44), aneurysm of pulmonary arteries (10,24), or brachio-cephalic arteries (1,44,67). Ostial stenosis of the latter has also been described (44).

Tuberculous Aortitis

Tuberculosis of the aorta is reported infrequently. In 1965 Silbergleit et al. assembled 110 cases from the literature (64). They were almost equally divided between the thoracic and the abdominal aorta. Only a few additional cases have been added since this review (15,25,28,31,68).

The aorta may be infected with tuberculous bacilli by three mechanisms:

1. *Hematogenous dissemination*: Bacilli circulating in the bloodstream may be implanted in the intima or reach the aortic wall through vasa vasorum, resulting

in diffuse miliary tuberculosis of the intima (33,49), adventitia, and periarterial tissues (49), or they may produce localized tuberculosis of the wall involving all the layers. Tuberculosis of the aortic wall may perforate without aneurysm formation or may remain silent only to be discovered incidentally at autopsy (64). Preexisting aortic aneurysms may be secondarily infected by tuberculous bacilli circulating in the blood (38,41).

2. *Lymphangitic spread*: This route has been shown to be responsible for tuberculosis of the aorta in some cases (32).

3. *Extension by contiguity*: Tuberculosis may involve the aorta by extension from without, i.e., contiguous lymph nodes (15,30–32,57,62,63,66), empyemas (69), pericarditis (29), paraspinal cold abscesses associated with tuberculous spondylitis (31), extensive renal tuberculosis (31), or cavitary pulmonary tuberculosis (28,33).

Aneurysm is a common complication of tuberculous aortitis. It develops in approximately half of the cases of tuberculosis of the aorta (12). The majority of aneurysms are false aneurysms (15,28,69). True and dissecting aneurysms occur rarely (25,33,46). Tuberculous aortic aneurysms are frequently erosive in nature, but they may also be formed as a result of weakening of the aortic wall after hematogenous tuberculosis of the aorta (32).

Tuberculous aortic aneurysms may occur at any age but are more common around the age of 40 (28). Commonly there is coexisting miliary tuberculosis of the lung (15,28,41,62,69), but it is believed that miliary tuberculosis is probably the result rather than the cause of aneurysm in most instances (28).

Constriction and stenosis of the aorta in mediastinal or retroperitoneal fibrosis secondary to tuberculosis is rare (31). However, severe periaortic fibrosis does not prevent formation of aneurysm.

Rupture with fatal hemorrhage is an unavoidable outcome of untreated tuberculous aneurysms (15,32,69). However, bleeding may be slow and intermittent originally, and small openings may be plugged with fibrin (23,63,70). Therefore these slowly bleeding aneurysms can still be treated surgically if the intervention is done without undue delay (69). Hemorrhage may occur into the lung (23), esophagus (69), stomach (63), duodenum (30), jejunum (62), peritoneal and retroperitoneal space (32), trachea and bronchi (70), pericardium (70), and pleura (69).

Clinical presentation is nonspecific and may consist of anorexia, weight loss, fever, chest pain, hemoptysis, dysphagia, abdominal pain, and a palpable mass. If a patient with known or suspected tuberculosis develops an aneurysm, an aortic leak, or both, tuberculous aortitis should be seriously considered and the necessary intervention carried out without delay (64).

The first successful removal of tuberculous aneurysm of the abdominal aorta was performed in 1955 by Rob and Eastcott (57) and was followed by others (11,25,41,64,69,72). However, sudden death resulting from fatal hemorrhage during either the immediate or late postoperative period following uneventful surgery has occurred in some instances (23,69).

Antituberculous therapy must be instituted immediately after surgery (64). Silbergleit et al. suggested that all resected aortic aneurysms be carefully examined microscopically because not all patients with resected tuberculous aortic aneurysm have a preoperative diagnosis of tuberculosis (64).

REFERENCES

1. Avellone, J. C., and Ahmad, M. Y. (1979): Cervical internal carotid aneurysm from syphilis—an alternative to resection. *JAMA*, 241:238–239.
2. Banker, V. P., and Maddison, F. E. (1967): Superior vena cava syndrome secondary to aortic disease: Report of two cases and review of the literature. *Dis. Chest*, 51:656–662.
3. Bardin, J. A., Collins, G. M., Devin, J. B., and Halasz, N. A. (1981): Nonaneurysmal suppurative aortitis. *Arch. Surg.*, 116:954–956.
4. Bennett, D. E. (1967): Primary mycotic aneurysms of the aorta: Report of a case and review of the literature. *Arch. Surg.*, 94:758–765.
5. Bennett, D. E., and Cherry, J. K. (1967): Bacterial infection of aortic aneurysms: A clinicopathologic study. *Am. J. Surg.*, 113:321–326.
6. Blickenstaff, D. E., and Nice, C. M., Jr. (1965): Aortic aneurysm secondary to mediastinal abscess—report of two cases. *Dis. Chest*, 48:534–538.
7. Blum, L., and Keefer, E. B. C. (1962): Cryptogenic mycotic neurysm. *Ann. Surg.*, 155:398–405.
8. Blum, L., and Keefer, E. B. C. (1964): Clinical entity of cryptogenic mycotic aneurysm—report of six cases. *JAMA*, 188:505–508.
9. Bodner, S. J., McGee, Z. A., and Killen, D. A. (1973): Ruptured mycotic aneurysm complicating coarctation of the aorta. *Ann. Thorac. Surg.*, 15:419–426.
10. Boyd, L. J., and McGavack, T. H. (1939): Aneurysm of the pulmonary artery—a review of the literature and report of two new cases. *Am. Heart J.*, 18:562–578.
11. (1960): Case Records of the Masaschusetts General Hospital #46212. *N. Engl. J. Med.*, 262:1084–1089.
12. (1969): Case Records of the Masaschusetts General Hospital #52-1969. *N. Engl. J. Med.*, 281:1414–1419.
13. (1973): Case Records of the Masaschusetts General Hospital #24-1973. *N. Engl. J. Med.*, 288:1290–1296.
14. (1974): Case Records of the Masaschusetts General Hospital #44-1974. *N. Engl. J. Med.*, 291:1021–1027.
15. (1975): Case Records of the Masaschusetts General Hospital #11-1975. *N. Engl. J. Med.*, 292:579–586.
16. Centers for Disease Control: *Sexually Transmitted Disease Fact Sheet*. 34th Ed. U.S. Department of Health, Education and Welfare Publ. 79-8195.
17. Clark, E. G., and Danbolt, N. (1964): The Oslo study of the natural course of untreated syphilis—an epidemiologic investigation based on a re-study of the Boeck-Bruusgaard material. *Med. Clin. North Am.*, 48:613–623.
18. Cliff, M. M., Soulen, R. L., and Finestone, A. J. (1970): Mycotic aneurysms—a challenge and a clue. *Arch. Intern. Med.*, 126:977–982.
19. Collins, G. J., Jr., Rich, N. M., Hobson, R. W., II, et al. (1977): Multiple mycotic aneurysms due to Candida endocarditis. *Ann. Surg.*, 186:136–139.
20. Cornell, H. S. (1973): *The Roentgenographic Diagnosis of the Disease of the Thoracic Aorta*. Charles C Thomas, Springfield, Illinois.
21. Crane, A. R. (1937): Primary multilocular mycotic aneurysm of the aorta. *Arch. Pathol.*, 24:634–641.
22. Crook, B. R. M., Raftery, E. B., and Oram, S. (1973): Mycotic aneurysms of coronary arteries. *Br. Heart J.*, 35:107–109.
23. DeProphetis, N., Armitage, H. V., and Triboletti, E. D. (1959): Rupture of tuberculous aortic aneurysm into lung. *Ann. Surg.*, 150:1046–1051.
24. Deterling, R. A., Jr., and Clagett, O. T. (1947): Aneurysm of the pulmonary artery: Review of the literature and report of a case. *Am. Heart J.*, 34:471–499.
25. Efremidis, S. C., Lakshmanan, S., and Hsu, J. T. (1976): Tuberculous aortitis: A rare cause of mycotic aneurysm of the aorta. *AJR*, 127:859–861.

26. Ernst, C. B., Campbell, H. C., Jr., Daugherty, M. E., Sachatello, C. R., et al. (1977): Incidence and significance of intra-operative bacterial cultures during abdominal aortic aneurysmectomy. *Ann. Surg.*, 185:626–630.
27. Ewart, J. M., Burke, M. L., and Bunt, T. J. (1983): Spontaneous abdominal aortic infections—essentials of diagnosis and management. *Ann. Surg.*, 49:37–50.
28. Felson, B., Akers, P. V., Hall, G. S., Schreiber, J. T., et al. (1977): Mycotic tuberculous aneurysm of the thoracic aorta. *JAMA*, 237:1104–1108.
29. Foley, M. M., Probert, W. R., and Seal, R. M. E. (1956): False aneurysm of ascending thoracic aorta complicating tuberculous pericarditis. *Tubercle*, 37:183–186.
30. Frosch, H. L., and Horowitz, W. (1944): Rupture of abdominal aorta into duodenum (through a sinus tract created by a tuberculous mesenteric lymphadenitis). *Ann. Intern. Med.*, 21:481–485.
31. Gajaraj, A., and Victor, S. (1981): Tuberculous aortitis. *Clin. Radiol.*, 32:461–466.
32. German, J. L., and Green, C. L. (1956): Fatal rupture of a tuberculous aortic aneurysm—a case report. *Ann. Intern. Med.*, 45:698–702.
33. Haythorn, S. R. (1913): Tuberculosis of the large arteries—with a report of a case of tuberculous aneurysm of the right common iliac artery. *JAMA*, 60:1413–1416.
34. Heggtveit, H. A. (1964): Syphilitic aortitis—a clinicopathologic autopsy study of 100 cases, 1950 to 1960. *Circulation*, 29:346–355.
35. Herskowitz, A., Cho, S., and Factor, S. M. (1980): Syphilitic arteritis involving proximal coronary arteries. *N.Y. State J. Med.*, 80:971–974.
36. Jaffe, R. B., and Condon, V. R. (1975): Mycotic aneurysms of the pulmonary artery and aorta. *Radiology*, 116:291–298.
37. Jaffe, R. B., and Koschmann, E. B. (1970): Intravenous drug abuse—pulmonary, cardiac, and vascular complications. *AJR*, 109:107–120.
38. Jarrett, F., Darling, C., Mundth, E. D., and Austen, G. (1975): Experience with infected aneurysms of the abdominal aorta. *Arch. Surg.*, 110:1281–1285.
39. Kampmeier, R. H. (1938): Saccular aneurysm of the thoracic aorta—a clinical study of 633 cases. *Ann. Intern. Med.*, 12:624–631.
40. Kampmeier, R. H. (1964): The late manifestations of syphilis: skeletal, visceral and cardiovascular. *Med. Clin. North Am.*, 48:667–697.
41. Kline, J. L., and Durant, J. (1961): Surgical resection of a tuberculous aneurysm of the ascending aorta. *N. Engl. J. Med.*, 265:1185–1187.
42. Klotz, O. (1918): Some points respecting the localization of syphilis upon the aorta. *Am. J. Med. Sci.*, 155:92–100.
43. Lerner, P. I., and Weinstein, L. (1966): Infective endocarditis in the antibiotic era. *N. Engl. J. Med.*, 274:199–206.
44. Martland, H. S. (1930): Syphilis of the aorta and heart. *Am. Heart J.*, 6:1–29.
45. McNulty, J. S., and Fassett, R. L. (1981): Syphilis: An otolaryngologic perspective. *Laryngoscope*, 91:889–905.
46. Meehan, J. J., Pastor, B. H., and Torre, A. V. (1957): Dissecting aneurysm of the aorta secondary to tuberculous aortitis. *Circulation*, 16:615–620.
47. Miller, B. M., Waterhouse, G., Alford, R. H., Dean, R. H., et al. (1983): Histoplasma infection of abdominal aortic aneurysms. *Ann. Surg.*, 197:57–62.
48. Myerowitz, R. L., Friedman, R., and Grossman, W. L. (1971): Mycotic "mycotic aneurysm" of the aorta due to Aspergillus fumigatus. *Am. J. Clin. Pathol.*, 55:241–246.
49. Neumann, M. A. (1952): Tuberculous lesions of the circulatory system—report of two cases. *Am. J. Pathol.*, 28:919–930.
50. Oldham, H. N., Jr., Phillips, J. F., Jewett, P. H., and Chen, J. T. (1973): Surgical treatment of mycotic aneurysm associated with coarctation of the aorta. *Ann. Thorac. Surg.*, 15:411–418.
51. Pariser, H. (1964): Infectious syphilis. *Med. Clin. North Am.*, 48:625–636.
52. Patel, S., and Johnston, K. W. (1977): Classification and management of mycotic aneurysms. *Surg. Gynecol. Obstet.*, 144:691–694.
53. Phillips, P. L., Amberson, J. B., and Libby, D. M. (1981): Syphilitic aortic aneurysm presenting with the superior vena cava syndrome. *Am. J. Med.*, 71:171–173.
54. Qizilbash, A. H. (1974): Mycotic aneurysm of the sinus of Valsalva with rupture. *Arch. Pathol.*, 98:414–417.
55. Rappaport, B. Z. (1926): Primary acute aortitis. *Arch. Pathol. Lab. Med.*, 2:653–658.
56. Revell, S. T. R., Jr. (1945): Primary mycotic aneurysms. *Ann. Intern. Med.*, 22:431–440.

57. Rob, C. G., and Eastcott, H. H. G. (1955): Aortic aneurysm due to tuberculous lymphadenitis. *Br. Med. J.*, 1:378–379.
58. Rockwell, D. H., Yobs, A. R., and Moore, M. B. (1964): The Tuskegee study of untreated syphilis—the 30th year of observation. *Arch. Intern. Med.*, 114:792–798.
59. Rosahn, P. D. (1947): Autopsy studies in syphilis. *J. Vener. Dis.* (Suppl. 21). U.S. Public Health Service, Venereal Disease Division.
60. Rose, H. D., and Stuart, J. L. (1976): Mycotic aneurysm of the thoracic aorta caused by Aspergillus fumigatus. *Chest*, 70:81–84.
61. Rosenbaum, A. E., Schweppe, H. I., Jr., and Rabin, E. R. (1964): Constrictive pericarditis, pneumopericardium and aortic aneurysm due to Histoplasma capsulatum. *N. Engl. J. Med.*, 270:935–938.
62. Sandrock, R. S., Emerson, G. L., and Emerson, M. S. (1952): A rare complication of tuberculous mesenteric lymphadenitis—a case of fatal hemorrhage from abdominal aorta into jejunum through a tuberculous lymph node. *Am. Rev. Tuberc.*, 65:210–214.
63. Scott, J. W., Maxwell, E. S., and Grimes, A. E. (1949): Tuberculous false aneurysm of the abdominal aorta with rupture into the stomach. *Am. Heart J.*, 37:820–827.
64. Silbergleit, A., Arbulu, A., Defever, B. A., et al. (1965): Tuberculous aortitis—surgical resection of ruptured abdominal false aneurysms. *JAMA*, 193:333–335.
65. Stengel, A., and Wolferth, C. C. (1923): Mycotic (bacterial) aneurysms of intravascular origin. *Arch. Intern. Med.*, 31:527–542.
66. Stiefel, J. W. (1958): Rupture of a tuberculous aneurysm of the aorta—review of the literature and report of a case. *Arch. Pathol.*, 65:506–512.
67. Tadavarthy, S. M., Castenada-Zuniga, W. R., Klugman, J., et al. (1981): Syphilitic aneurysms of the innominate artery. *Radiology*, 139:31–34.
68. Umerah, B. C. (1982): Unfolding of the aorta (aortitis) associated with pulmonary tuberculosis. *Br. J. Radiol.*, 55:201–203.
69. Volini, F. I., Olfield, C., Jr., Thompson, J. R., and Kent, G. (1962): Tuberculosis of the aorta. *JAMA*, 181:78–83.
70. Wetteland, P., and Scott, D. (1956): Tuberculous aortic perforations—review of the literature and report of a case of false aneurysm with rupture into a bronchus. *Tubercle*, 37:177–182.
71. Wilson, S. E., van Wagenen, P., and Passaro, E., Jr. (1978): Arterial infection. *Curr. Probl. Surg.*, 40:6–89.
72. Yeoh, C. B., Ford, J. M., and Garret, R. (1963): Tuberculous pseudoaneurysm of descending thoracic aorta—surgical treatment. *Arch. Surg.*, 86:318–322.
73. Zak, F. G., Strauss, L., and Saphra, I. (1958): Rupture of diseased large arteries in the course of enterobacterial (Salmonella) infections. *N. Engl. J. Med.*, 258:824–828.

Aortitis: Clinical, Pathologic, and Radiographic
Aspects, edited by A. Lande, Y.M. Berkmen, and
H.A. McAllister. Raven Press, New York © 1986.

Takayasu's Arteritis (Nonspecific Aortoarteritis)

Eulo Lupi Herrera and Mario Seoane

National Institute of Cardiology of Mexico, "Ignacio Chávez," Mexico City, Mexico

Nonspecific aortoarteritis was first noted by Savory in 1856 (87). Fifty-two years later the Japanese ophthalmologist Takayasu described in a 21-year-old female a peculiar capillary flush in the ocular fundi, a wreath-like arteriovenous anastomosis around the papillae, and blindness due to cataract (100). Subsequently, in the discussion of this case, Onishi and Kagoshimua called attention to two patients with similar ocular findings who also had absent radial pulses (100). Shimizu and Sano in 1948 detailed the clinical features of this disorder, which in 1954 was termed Takayasu's arteritis by Caccamise and Okuda (94,95). Few entities in the medical literature have been labeled with as many eponyms as has Takayasu's arteritis (TA). It has been known as pulseless disease, aortic arch syndrome, young female arteritis, idiopathic aortitis, reversed coarctation, Martorell syndrome, occlusive thromboaortopathy, and nonspecific aortoarteritis (54,75,94,95,98,100). These eponyms have given rise to confusion because many of the above terms for the condition have been previously considered as separate disease entities; however, this also reflects some of its many features.

GEOGRAPHIC DISTRIBUTION

The majority of cases have been reported from Asia and Africa, and most large series consist of Orientals. However, current reports from western European countries, the United States, and Mexico indicate its worldwide occurrence. The disease is apparently much more common in the United States than was generally suspected (43,44).

The following reasons for the infrequent recognition of this vascular pathology are given: The impression prevails that the disease is mainly confined to the Orient; the full extent of vascular involvement has been recognized only in recent years; symptoms of TA are extremely variable (it has been described as one of the great imitators); and finally the disease is recorded under different names.

Initially, it was thought that the arteritic process was limited to the aortic arch and its branches. Subsequent clinical, angiographic, and pathologic studies have demonstrated that it is not. The process can involve the aortic arch and its branches, the thoracic, descending, and abdominal aorta, and the pulmonary artery.

On the basis of these observations, the disease can be subdivided into four types (107) (Fig. 1): It is called type I, or Shimizu–Sano (94,95) variety, when the

173

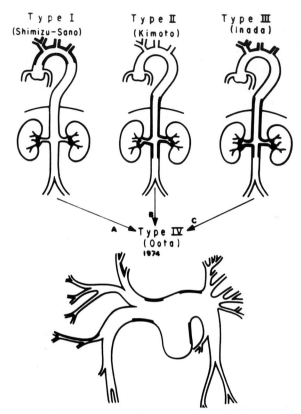

FIG. 1. Clinical and angiographic classification of Takayasu's arteritis as proposed by Ueno and associates and modified by us (50). Thick lines represent areas of involvement. (From Lupi et al., ref. 50, with permission.)

involvement is localized to the aortic arch and its branches. In type II (38), also called atypical coarctation of the aorta or Kimoto variety, the lesions involve the thoracic, descending, and abdominal aorta without involvement of the arch. Type III, Inada (29), or mixed, variety, contains features of both types I and II. We suggested an additional variant (type IV) which may include any of the features of types I, II, and III and, in addition, involves the pulmonary artery (50).

The incidence of the various types is as follows: type I, 8%; type II, 11%; type III, 65%; and type IV, 45% (including several patients in the other groups) (51). Although angiographic classifications are useful for the location of arterial lesions and for diagnostic surgical reasons, no prognostic implications can be determined with such classification.

In one series of TA (31) another classification based on the natural history, prognosis, and clinical features was proposed. The patients were classified into four groups (groups I, IIa, IIb, and III) according to evidence of the four complications attributed to TA at the time the diagnosis was established.

Group I included patients with TA with or without involvement of the pulmonary artery, with narrowing or occlusion in some region of the aorta and/or its main branches but without any of the vascular complications present in group II. In group II were included patients with TA with any one of the following complications: (a) retinopathy; (b) secondary hypertension; (c) aortic regurgitation; or (d) aortic or arterial aneurysm. If TA was mild or moderate it was considered to be in group IIa, and if TA was severe it was in group IIb. Group III patients had two or more of the complications listed for group II.

ETIOLOGY

More than 100 years after its original description (87) and despite voluminous literature on the subject, a specific cause or etiology for TA has not been forthcoming. It has been linked to rheumatic fever, rheumatoid arthritis, collagen vascular diseases (e.g., systemic lupus erythematosus, polymyositis, and scleroderma), parasitic (nematode) infestation, ankylosing spondylitis, giant cell arteritis, syphilis, some patterns of inheritance, an autoimmune etiology, group A streptococcal infection, hormonal imbalance, and tuberculosis.

A possible relationship between TA and rheumatoid arthritis has been suspected by several authors (4,21,27,41,65,84,109) as joint pain, iritis, sclerokeratitis, and positive rheumatoid factor have been found in cases of TA. Aortic lesions histologically similar to those of TA have also been found in cases of rheumatoid arthritis, especially in the presence of rheumatoid nodules, although such nodules are not specific for rheumatoid arthritis and have been observed in lupus erythematosus, granuloma annulare, and diabetes as well. Other authors have related giant cell arteritis to TA. Giant cell arteritis predominantly involves medium-sized muscular arteries but is also known to affect the aorta and may be one of the diverse causes of the aortic arch syndrome. Nevertheless, evidence suggests that this disease is likely to be a separate entity (14,93).

The possible syphilitic nature of TA has been considered for several years, mainly because of the histologic observation that the cicatrization of TA resembles that of syphilitic aortitis (59). On the other hand, it is not usual to find a history of concomitant clinical manifestations of syphilis and positive serologic reactions in TA patients. Furthermore, when aortic calcification is found in TA it usually involves the descending and not the ascending aorta, as in syphilitic aortitis. *Treponema* staining of the lesions in arterial walls has also been shown to be negative. For some authors all these negative features do not rule out a syphilitic origin TA, but we do not believe it to be the case.

Reports from the tropics (57) suggested a possible role of an unidentified nematode with arterial tropism mainly affecting children and young adults. Because nematodes are usually confined to the tropics, this would not explain the worldwide incidence of TA, although nematodes may be a cause of some cases of arteritis observed in the tropics.

The possible role of tuberculosis in TA was pointed out initially by Shimizu and Sano in 1948 (94). They considered this possibility because of the presence of

Langhan's giant cell granulomas morphologically resembling tuberculosis lesions. Others have shown the coexistence of pulmonary or extrapulmonary tuberculosis foci in TA, especially in juxta-arterial and para-aortic lymph nodes (47–49,80–82,89–91,102,103). It had been observed that 48% of the patients had a previous tuberculous infection, e.g., tuberculous adenopathy, pulmonary tuberculosis, and Bazim's erythema induratum. Furthermore, some investigators have reported a strikingly higher incidence of tuberculin skin reactivity to both *Mycobacterium tuberculosis* and atypical mycobacteria in patients with TA when compared with the general population, raising the possibility of a relationship with tuberculosis (49). Others have found that when *M. tuberculosis* is inoculated into the subadventitial layer of the carotid artery of the rabbit changes similar but not identical to those of TA are produced. Also the disease pattern was closer to that of TA when the rabbits were previously sensitized (90).

These pathologic, clinical, and experimental observations suggested that tuberculosis may play a role in TA. On the other hand, they may only be related observations. Humoral antibodies against four mycobacterial products as well as for immune complex which precipitates with human C1q in double diffusion in patients suffering TA in the chronic inactive phase have been investigated (12,73). None showed circulating immune complexes, and only three of the patients had antimycobacterial antibodies. When using an inhibition of cytotoxicity assay, TA patients are found to have circulating immune complexes whose immune reactants could not be characterized in those complexes. The presence of immunopathogenetic mechanisms in chronic TA is partially supported by this work. Immunoregulation studies in TA are now in progress and may offer new insight into this entity.

The role of susceptibility or resistance to disease is controlled by multiple genes including some HLA-linked genes. A susceptible genetic background may play a role in the etiology of the disease (12). The association between TA and HLA, B5, and Bw52 described in Japanese patients was confirmed in Mexican patients, although it was not as marked as in the Oriental population (24,32,60,61). It seems certain that B5 serves only as a marker for the disease-susceptible genes, and this has been the explanation provided for many of HLA–disease associations. At any rate, if an exogenous agent does exist in TA patients, it could develop an unusually strong and continued immune response leading to arterial tissue damage (2,35).

The occurrence of lymphocytotoxic antibodies (LCTA) in human sera has been recognized for many years. An increased frequency of LCTA was noted in sera from patients suffering temporal arteritis. Interestingly, when serum was obtained from patients with chronic TA, it was found that the frequency of LCTA in TA was low and not different from that in the normal population; this is in contrast with the high frequency of LCTA in patients with systemic rheumatic disease (12). All these findings, although negative, have an important significance considering the possible natural occurrence of LCTA in human disease, as both mycobacterial and viral infections, where LCTA are present, have been implicated in the pathogenesis of TA.

The postulated theory that an autoimmune mechanism is in operation is supported by findings such as high gamma globulins, circulating immune complex (anti-aorta antibodies), the failure to detect any etiologic agent in the lesions of the arterial wall, and the systemic arterial nature of the disease (pulmonary and aortic involvement). Although anti-aorta antibodies have been detected in TA patients, there is no definitive evidence at the present supporting that these antibodies are the direct cause of TA. Overall, the bulk of evidence favors an autoimmune etiology (20,27,33,49,56,58,64,66,76,105,110). Most of the difficulties in determining the cause or causes of the disease arise because the pathologic observations are usually made in cicatricial or chronic states and only a few during active arteritis (59). Further experimental work should be encouraged in order to increase our knowledge of the disease. It is possible that the arteritis represents the final common pathologic expression of a number of stimuli.

PATHOLOGY

Takayasu's arteritis is a nonspecific, inflammatory–fibrotic process involving the aorta and its main branches focally and segmentally as well as the pulmonary artery. Histologically, the early stages (acute inflammatory phase) are characterized by an inflammatory infiltrate of plasma cells and lymphocytes in the adventitia and outer layer of the media. Later, all the layers of the wall are involved and its elements destroyed (22,58,59,68). The basic pathologic process is that of marked internal proliferation and fibrosis, fibrous scarring and degeneration of the elastic fibers of the media, and round cell infiltration of variable intensity (6,13,55). The adventitia and the intima become markedly thickened, and the vasa vasorum are destroyed. The proliferation of fibrous tissue starts in the adventitia and extends gradually to all layers of the arterial wall. The lumen narrows and may be obliterated by organizing thrombi. The proliferation process leads to obliterative luminal changes in the aorta and involved arteries (57,59). The end results of the marked fibrosis and thickening of the arterial wall is usually constriction or, as noted before, occlusion and occasionally a saccular aneurysm. In some instances the tissue becomes converted to a thick fibrous cord. In the latter stages of the disease, fibrosis predominates and the cellular exudate is scanty or absent. Shrinkage of the fibrous tissue accounts for the variable degrees of arterial stenosis, and reactive intimal thickening contributes substantially to luminal narrowing. The spectrum of histologic changes is closely related to the activity of the disease (6,13,25,30,55,106). After months or years, the inflammatory activity gradually tapers off and the histology accordingly goes through a cycle of changes. In the old, inactive stage of the disease, the inflammatory process has resolved and the adventitia and media are replaced by fibrous tissue. The presence of periaortic adhesions and fibrosis indicates previous aortitis. In most patients postinflammatory fibrosis is strictly limited to the aortic or pulmonary wall. In advanced stages of the disease there are frequently nondistinguishing signs to permit the crucially important histologic differentiation of nonspecific fibrosis from postinflammatory scar tissue

(19,30,34,104). Histologic examination under this circumstances is liable to be inconclusive.

The degree of secondary atherosclerosis is at times so severe as to totally obscure the underlying intimal changes of arteritis, particularly in older patients. However, in most patients careful microscopic analysis permits distinction of the atheromatous intimal changes from nonatheromatous postinflammatory intimal thickening and the dystrophic changes from atherosclerotic calcifications (6,104). In TA calcification of the aortic and arterial walls is a late complication. Calcification of the arterial walls is a well-known factor for degenerative arterial disease, particularly in atherosclerosis and Monckëberg's calcinosis. Calcifications may also be found in other pathologic processes, e.g., syphilis and metabolic disorders, and in some newborns probably of congenital origin. In TA they seldom receive importance; in fact, their presence, when extensive, has been regarded as a factor against the diagnosis. Studies in this sense have shown that calcifications are not rare and represent a feature of the disease's histopathology. An intentional search for them increases the number of observed cases with TA. The presence of vascular calcifications should not exclude the diagnosis; on the contrary, it should strongly suggest it if found in middle-age females. Calcifications can provide a diagnostic clue when dilated or obstructed areas are seen. Aortic calcifications may resemble aortic dissection images in the angiographic studies (48).

Because of the protean clinical manifestations of TA, the misleading pathologic appearance in some instances, and the difficulty of obtaining tissue material during the clinical course of the disease, arteriography has assumed primary diagnostic importance. The configuration of the diseased aorta as seen by total aortography is highly suggestive of TA. Also, the study can identify the condition even in the presence of secondary atherosclerosis (43,44). Clinicopathologic correlations have shown that minor lesions may be overlooked by angiography. From angiography studies and necropsy findings (51), the arterial lesions most frequently found in TA involve the subclavian arteries (85%), the descending thoracic aorta (67%), the renal arteries (62%), the carotid arteries (44%), and the arch and ascending aorta (27%). Nevertheless, all the main branches of the aorta or the pulmonary artery could be involved. Some authors have noted an unusually high incidence of coronary artery involvement (30%) (37) leading to myocardial infarction in half of the instances with changes that are usually most marked at the points of origin of the arteries from the aorta (8,22,101).

Takayasu's arteritis may present as multisegmental aortic disease with areas of normal wall anatomy between affected sites, diffuse involvement of the aorta, or predominantly disease of individual arteries arising from the aorta. Therefore based on pathologic observations, angiography would reveal one or more of the following images: irregular internal surface of the vessel wall, stenosis, poststenotic dilatation, occlusion of the proximal portions of the branches of the aorta, and saccular aneurysms. Collateral circulation can be demonstrated in most of the aortographic studies and severe coarctation in one-third of the patients. Complications or operative death during aortography are rare.

CLINICAL PICTURE

The disease occurs predominantly in women (female/male ratio 8:1). The age of onset is between 10 and 20 years, although cases beginning during early infancy or late middle age have been reported (11,15,45,52,62,85,88).

The onset of TA is characterized in half of the cases by the sudden appearance of constitutional symptoms suggesting a systemic illness (31,51,58,98). Symptoms such as fever, anorexia, malaise, weight loss, night sweats, and joint pain are present in 78% of the cases. Signs of a local circulatory deficit (86%), high blood pressure (72%), and increased erythrocyte sedimentation rate (ESR) (83%) are the other main clinical findings in TA (51). This clinical picture or first acute clinical inflammatory phase may disappear partly or completely within about 3 months only to reappear in a chronic phase some months later. However, not all the patients proceed (or it is not clinically apparent) through this so-called initial systemic phase, and after a latent period of variable duration they present symptoms and signs referable to the obliterative and inflammatory changes in the vessels. Therefore patients with TA who have advanced arterial obstruction and evidence of collateral circulation can be found when they first develop symptoms (31). These patients, as well as those who go through the above-mentioned initial phase, present the following clinical pictures (5,7,9,10,28,30,36,46,53,71,72,74,78,83,92,99,108,111): diminished or absent pulse, bruits, hypertension, abnormal fundi, and heart failure. The symptomatology of TA is closely related to the presence of aortic coarctations, stenosis, or occlusion of branch vessels. It is important to recognize the four types of TA for diagnostic reasons (50). Among the discriminating clinical features in the four types are the absence of arterial hypertension in type I arteritic patients. Patients with types I and III manifest those findings that are considered to be most typical of this condition, i.e., reversed coarctation of the aorta with absent or diminished upper body pulses and barely detectable blood pressure in the arms, higher pressure in the lower extremities, syncope, and manifestations of ischemia at various affected sites (10,28,83,92).

The cardiovascular and neurologic signs and symptoms are usually present at the same time. In addition to the predominant cardiovascular symptoms previously mentioned, dyspnea on exertion, palpitations, and angina pectoris could be other relevant features (74). Although it has been stated that cardiovascular involvement plays a minor role in the disease process, data demonstrate that the cardiovascular system may be involved at any point in the illness. It should be stressed that, although decreased amplitude of peripheral pulses is a classic finding, normal or even wide pulse amplitude could be found in patients with a mild degree of arteritis, and in those with aortic regurgitation (7% of cases) this complication could mask the disease (31,51). Most of the patients have arterial obstructions, but only a few complain of ischemic pain. This peculiarity is apparently related to the fact that artery obstruction occurs gradually with parallel development of collateral circulation. This can explain why occlusion of the subclavian arteries remains asymptomatic and claudication of the upper limbs is rare. The second most important cardiovascular sign in TA is the systolic vascular bruit resulting from endothelial irregularity, stenosis, and collateral circulation, whose detection and location are described elsewhere (78).

Arterial hypertension is present in more than 70% of the patients with TA (5,28,50,51,92,111), resulting mainly from involvement of the renal arteries, and can be demonstrated in a high percentage of cases by aortography and necropsy studies (Fig. 2). Old and fresh thromboses of the renal arteries are common findings in kidneys obtained at surgery or necropsy. Hypertension also appears to arise from significant coarctation of the aorta; decreased aortic capacitance and reduced baroreceptor reactivity may be contributory factors. Hypertension due to abnormal function of the carotid sinuses and to cerebral ischemia have not been established. The arterial hypertension is generally of moderate degree, and only in a few cases is it severe (diastolic <140 mm Hg, 79%; diastolic >140 mm Hg, 21%) (51). Heart failure, when present in TA, is usually seen in the young and appears to be a consequence of systemic and pulmonary hypertension.

Uncommon causes could result from aortic regurgitation or coronary artery involvement (74), the latter being capable of leading to direct myocardial damage. TA of coronary arteries can give rise to heart failure without the classic symptoms of the disease and be a cause of death. According to most authors, TA of the coronary arteries is rare. In instances in which the diagnosis of Takayasu's coronaritis has been microscopically confirmed, the obstructive process is found to

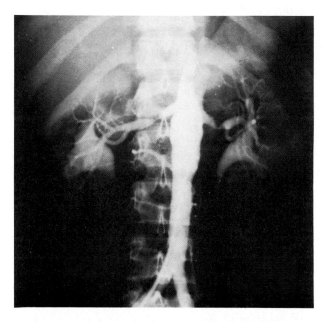

FIG. 2. Abdominal aortogram showing marked narrowing of the abdominal aorta. There are irregularities of the walls of the aorta and bilateral stenosis of the renal arteries. (From Lupi et al., ref. 50, with permission.)

involve the ostia of the coronaries extending from the aorta. However, proximal segments of the coronary arteries can be affected, or distal arteritic lesions can be observed from the coronary ostia, including the formation of saccular aneurysms (47). TA of the coronary arteries can be asymptomatic, giving rise to mild precordial pain or to classic angina pectoris (11% of cases). Symptoms of coronary artery involvement rarely occur in the absence of other manifestations of TA, and coronary involvement is itself a rare complication. It should be stressed that the pathologic findings in the heart are usually nonspecific and are related to heart failure and to systemic and pulmonary arterial hypertension (59,68). There is only one report of TA with granulomatous myocarditis and pericarditis (71).

Aortic regurgitation, when present, is detected by auscultation, echocardiography, and aortography. Pathologically, dilatation of the involved ascending aorta, separation of the aortic commissures, and thickening of the valve cusps themselves are described as the lesions responsible for aortic regurgitation in this disease. It is often difficult to differentiate TA aortic regurgitation from that due to aortitis in giant cell arteritis.

Takayasu's arteritis has been essentially considered one of the occlusive arterial diseases of the aorta, its main branches, and the pulmonary artery. It has been reported, however, that narrowing and/or occlusion are sometimes combined with aneurysm as well as dilatation. In this disease process occlusive lesions may be first produced and in some cases aneurysmal changes follow at any other portion of the aorta and its main branches (1). A clinical differential diagnosis between aneurysm due to this disease and that due to aortitis of giant cell arteritis may also be difficult (14).

Involvement of the vertebral and carotid arteries leads to a variety of cerebral nervous system and ocular manifestations. The neurologic symptoms result from arterial hypertension and cerebral or spinal cord ischemia (46). Variations among neurologic signs and symptoms can be explained on the basis of the irregular distribution of arterial lesions and the development of collateral circulation. Encephalomalacia and cerebral hemorrhage can sometimes be observed and are the cause of both permanent signs and transient neurologic deficits resulting from transient vascular impairment. Headaches are common (57%), and syncope and hemiplegia were observed in less than 15% of the patients in one series (51).

Takayasu's Retinopathy

The stage of retinal arteriovenous anastomosis similar to Takayasu's original finding corresponds to the advanced stage (31,51). Visual disturbances are mainly related to systemic arterial hypertension and can be found in 40% of the cases with grade I abnormal fundi (Keith-Wagner classification). Cataracts and vascular neoformations are rare (31).

Abdominal clinical features in TA can be observed in less than 20%. Occlusion or stenosis of the celiac, superior mesenteric, or inferior mesenteric arteries is observed in 14% of patients, and gastrointestinal symptoms may be related to these

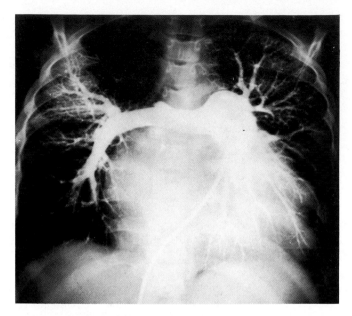

FIG. 3. Pulmonary angiography showing a cutting off of the first anterior trunk to the right upper lobe and asymmetrical arterial flow.

lesions. Perhaps because of abundant collateral circulation, gastrointestinal symptoms are rare (31).

Claudication of the lower limbs (documented in 29%) may be secondary to aortic coarctation or direct involvement of the aortic bifurcation or the iliac or femoral arteries. Most of the patients have arterial obstruction, but only a few complain of ischemic pain. As before, the parallel development of collateral circulation explains this finding.

Pulmonary Arterial Involvement

Oota (62) first described autopsy findings (Fig. 3) in a patient with TA where the pulmonary artery was involved. Since then, pulmonary arterial affection has been confirmed not only by autopsy but also by pulmonary angiography, measurement of pulmonary artery pressure, and lung perfusion scanning (50,59). TA association with pulmonary arterial involvement has been found in 50% or more of patients with the disease (31,51).

There is no relation between pulmonary and systemic arterial systems regarding extent and severity of involvement. In many TA patients lesions in the main pulmonary artery and its main segmental and subsegmental branches are demonstrated (77). As in the systemic territory, the main vessels of the pulmonary circuit are involved. A predilection for involvement of the vessels of the right lung has been observed. When no lesions affecting the main pulmonary artery are observed,

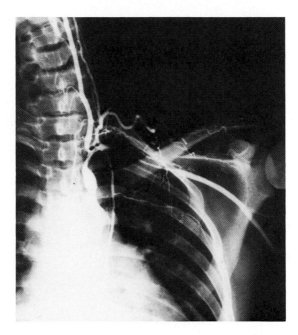

FIG. 4. Arch aortogram showing "flame-shaped" occlusion of the left subclavian artery. Narrowings and irregularity of the vessel walls can be seen.

their existence can be inferred from a pressure gradient between the right ventricle and the pulmonary artery. This gradient may be indistinguishable from that observed in valvular pulmonary stenosis. Pulmonary valve lesions, however, seem to be absent in TA (50). Pressure values are most sensitive in defining lesions in the main pulmonary artery or its branches, whereas angiography provides more clues for detecting the disease in the rest of the pulmonary vasculature. The angiographic pattern of the arteritis lesions closely resembles that observed in pulmonary thromboembolism (18,97,112). Arteritis lesions also produce tortuosity of the vascular wall and stenosis, but these are also seen in atherosclerosis and in congenital stenosis of the pulmonary branches and so cannot be considered pathognomonic (18). Nevertheless, these angiographic findings in patients with TA lesions elsewhere must be interpreted as secondary to pulmonary vascular involvement of the disease itself. It must be emphasized that pulmonary thromboembolism has rarely been documented in these patients.

Pulmonary hypertension, when present, is moderate in most and severe in only a few cases (mean pulmonary arterial pressure = 27 mm Hg; $N = 14$) (50). Although pulmonary hypertension increases the probability of pulmonary vascular involvement, normal pressures do not exclude lesions in the pulmonary vasculature. The lesions in the pulmonary arteries are inflammatory or granulomatous and involve the elastic, medial, and adventitial layers. As in the systemic circulation, the elastic portion seems to be most frequently involved. Most of the pathologic observations of the pulmonary vessels have been made in chronic disease states and not during acute arteritic activity (59).

Clinically, pulmonary manifestations are rare or absent in TA with pulmonary artery involvement. Hemoptysis has rarely been reported as an isolated feature. However, analysis of clinical signs, chest radiographs, and electrocardiograms (ECGs) showed that the majority of the patients with pulmonary involvement had some abnormality.

In more than 50% of the cases the ECG suggests right heart strain, and in some cases a mid-systolic murmur in the pulmonic area may be suggestive of pulmonary arteritis. This last finding, in the absence of an early systolic click, is consistent with the diagnosis (50). Heart failure has generally been regarded as a consequence of systemic arterial hypertension. Most of these patients also have right-sided failure, which may be related to the pulmonary vascular involvement.

Pulmonary artery involvement is an expression of the generalized nature of the disease, and this aspect should also be studied routinely in these patients (43,44). As in other forms of pulmonary artery hypertension, in addition to anatomic lesions on the pulmonary vessels, a passive form from left ventricular origin must be considered.

TAKAYASU'S ARTERITIS IN CHILDREN

Children represent 7% of patients with TA (47). As in the adult type, females predominate (4:1). The first symptoms of TA could be traced to an age of 3 years, but most are seen between 5 and 14 years (3,17,23,26,63,69,70,79,86,96). As has been the experience in adults, type III (mixed variety) is the most prevalent type and is seen in 54% of the studied cases (79). The outstanding clinical features in children are pulse deficit (100%), systemic arterial hypertension (85%), and, in up to two-thirds of the patients, symptoms and signs of congestive heart failure. Arthralgias and arthritis are observed in 65% of the patients (compared with 53% in adults); the large joints are those most frequently involved, and the process usually lasts 1 or 2 weeks without sequelae (79).

The majority of the children are seen during the active phase of the arteritic process, a clinical aspect that produces confusion with such other entities as rheumatic fever (23%), coarctation of the aorta (23%), and glomerulonephritis (8%). TA in children is a serious disease as inferred from the high mortality rate (30–35%) compared to that in the adult population.

LABORATORY, RADIOLOGIC, AND ECG FINDINGS

An increased ESR is the most frequent abnormality among the laboratory studies (83% of the cases). The ESR is considered an excellent index for the activity of this disease (31). It has been demonstrated that the ESR increase during the early and active stages of the disease is generally followed by a gradual return to normal as activity decreases. The accelerated ESR tends to spontaneously decelerate with aging. In young patients the ESR may be normal.

Twenty-five percent of the patients show mild anemia (hypochromic or normochromic/normocytic); a few (10%) have an increase in the leukocyte count (10,000–23,000/mm^3). Urinalysis is abnormal in one-third of the patients, who show albuminuria; cylindruria and hematuria are rare. Creatinine and lipoproteins are usually within normal limits.

C-reactive protein, antistreptolysin O titer, and gamma globulins are abnormal in one-third of the cases. The Mantoux test (2 UT) is positive in a high percentage of the cases (80%). Thoracic or abdominal radiographs are usually abnormal (60%). A moderate increase in heart size (cardiothoracic index of 50 to 55% in 27% of patients; of 56 to 60% in 24%; and of >60% in the very rare patient) (50) is an outstanding feature. An increase in hilar lymph nodes is a feature in half of the cases, and calcifications can be seen in 15% (48) with a few patients showing rib notching. The ECG is abnormal in the majority of the patients with TA (78%); abnormalities include right or left ventricular hypertrophy, myocardial infarction, and left or right bundle branch blocks. Atrial or ventricular arrhythmias as well as auricular-ventricular blocks are rarely documented.

Absolute confirmation of the diagnosis of TA can be made only at necropsy. Arterial biopsy, when feasible, is positive in 35% of the cases. A negative biopsy does not rule out TA.

ARTERIOGRAPHIC FINDINGS

Three basic arteriographic patterns are observed in TA patients: (a) varying degrees of aortic and arterial narrowings (Fig. 4); (b) saccular and fusiform aneurysms; and (c) combinations of the two (25,30,34,43,44) (Fig. 5).

The earliest detectable change at arteriography may be a localized narrowing or irregularity of the aortic wall. Although moderate aortic narrowings may be completely asymptomatic, they represent an important hallmark of TA (43,58). Aortic narrowings may progress to hemodynamically significant coarctations and occasionally total occlusion. Coarctation and complete aortic blocks have been described at various levels from the distal aortic arch to the aortic bifurcation. An excellent collateral circulation usually reconstitutes the distal vessel. Aortic constrictions can be short and segmental or long and diffuse. Elongate coarctations of the thoracic aorta frequently originate distal to the left subclavian artery and gradually taper toward the diaphragm. The appearance is quite characteristic and has been described as the "rat-tail" thoracic aorta (44). Infradiaphragmatic narrowing (atypical abdominal coarctation) can be supra-, inter-, or infrarenal in location. Supra- and interrenal coarctations are usually associated with severe diastolic hypertension. Abdominal narrowings are frequently long and diffuse, extending downward to the bifurcation. Branch vessels are usually involved, with occlusion and stenosis of the visceral and mainly the renal arteries. Aneurysm is not rare in TA; and when destruction of the aortic walls is extensive and the production of supporting fibrous tissue is deficient, the weakened aortic wall balloons out forming fusiform or saccular aneurysms. The dilatation may involve long, continuous segments of the

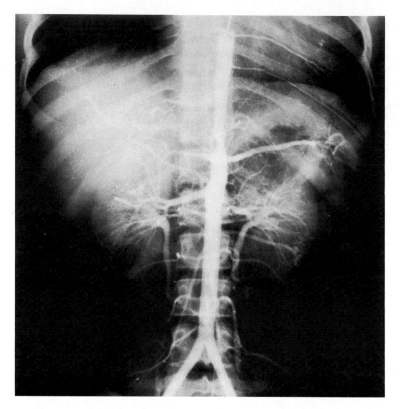

FIG. 5. Abdominal aortography showing diffuse, irregular narrowing of the vessels with a short area of segmental coarctation. There is also stenosis of the left renal artery.

aorta; and in some instances the entire aorta may be irregularly dilated. When this happens and the contours of the vessels remain smooth and symmetrical, the appearance is that of simple aortic ectasia. This appearance is usually an expression of extensive patchy involvement of contiguous segments of the vessels. Mild to moderate intimal irregularity often escapes arteriographic detection, and the contour of the vessels remains smooth. In some patients a saccular aneurysm is superimposed on diffuse aortic dilatation. Skipped areas of aortic involvement in which aneurysms and narrowing alternate with normal segments are the most characteristic aortographic findings of TA (29,31,38,43,44,51,58).

MEDICAL TREATMENT

It has been stated that a delay in diagnosis and commencement of medical treatment means a poor prognosis, except for a few patients with spontaneous healing and mild circulatory sequelae. It should be stressed, however, that at present there is no specific therapy for TA. The response to treatment for heart failure and systemic arterial hypertension is usually good (50). Some authors have obtained remarkable clinical remissions with corticosteroids, and in isolated cases an impressive amelioration of stenotic lesions affecting the abdominal aorta and renal arteries with reversal of hypertension has been claimed (42). In adults we have obtained only remission of systemic symptoms. In children with TA who receive corticosteroids there was an improvement in such parameters as the sense of well-being, arthritis, and erythema nodosum, but there was no restoration in pulse deficits (79). Some patients showed worsening of the systemic hypertension. At the present time this therapy needs further evaluation, and we believe there are not enough clinical and experimental data to justify the routine use of corticosteroids.

Medical treatment for tuberculosis is indicated only when active tuberculosis is found; it should not be used routinely until the exact role of tuberculosis in TA has been established. When treatment for tuberculosis was applied in the early and acute stages of TA no significant effects were noted (51,79). Anticoagulant treatment, chloroquine vasodilators, and salicylic acid do not seem to have any place in TA therapy.

Surgical treatment of many types may be needed to deal with late complications of TA. However, their precise efficacy is not established. Surgical procedures include endarterectomy, bypass of obstructed arteries, and resection of localized coarctations. Surgery is performed preferably during the chronic phase. It should be carefully evaluated in each case and utilized only when medical treatment has failed to control severe arterial hypertension or vascular insufficiency, or when the possibility of a ruptured aneurysm ensues.

PROGNOSIS

The nature of TA gives rise to complications (39,50,51,58) that influence the subsequent course of TA. The course of the disease can be unpredictable; however, in the majority of cases slow progression over a period of months to years is frequent. In a recent series 5-year survival after diagnosis was established at 83% (31), whereas for children the 5-year survival was 64% (79). Heart failure and cerebrovascular accidents are common causes of death. Death can also be related to surgery, renal failure, myocardial infarction, or rupture of an aneurysm; and in children sudden death can occur. As is the case in most diseases, the sooner the diagnosis is established and adequate therapy initiated, the better is the prognosis.

REFERENCES

1. Abrahamns, D. G., and Cockshott, W. P. (1962): Multiple non-luetic aneurysms in young Nigerians. *Br. Heart J.*, 24:83–91.
2. Albert, E. D., Mickey, M. R., and Terasaki, P. I. (1972): Genetics of the HLA system in four populations: American Caucasians, Japanese Americans, American Negroes and Mexican Americans. In: *Histocompatibility Testing*, p. 233. Munksgaard, Copenhagen.
3. Ansell, B. M., Bywaters, E. G. L., and Doniack, I. (1958): The aortic lesion of ankylosing spondylitis. *Br. Heart J.*, 20:507.
4. Ask-Upmark, E. (1954): On the pulseless disease outside of Japan. *Acta Med. Scand.*, 149:161.
5. Ask-Upmark, E. (1961): On the pathogenesis of hypertension in Takayasu's syndrome. *Acta Med. Scand.*, 169:467.

6. Ask-Upmark, E., and Fajers, C-M. (1956): Further observations on Takayasu's syndrome. *Acta Med. Scand.*, 155:275–291.

7. Austen, G. N., and Shaw, R. S. (1964): Surgical treatment of pulseless disease. *N. Engl. J. Med.*, 270:1228.

8. Barker, N. W., and Edwards, J. E. (1955): Primary arteritis of the aortic arch. *Circulation*, 11:486–492.

9. Birke, G., Ejrup, B., and Olhagen, B. (1957): Pulseless disease: Clinical analysis of ten cases. *Angiology*, 8:433.

10. Brownnel, W. H. (1963): The many faces of pulseless disease. *Dis. Chest*, 43:433.

11. Caccamise, W. C., and Okuda, K. (1954): Takayasu's or pulseless disease: An unusual syndrome with ocular manifestations. *Am. J. Ophthalmol.*, 37:784.

12. Castro, G., Chávez-Peón, F., Sánchez, T. G., and Reyes, P. (1982): HLA A and B antigens in Takayasu's arteritis. *Rev. Invest. Clin.*, 34:15.

13. Césarman, E., Cárdenas, M., Escudero, J., Zajarías, S., and Contreras, R. (1963): Arteritis de Takayasu: Observaciones clínicas y anatomopatológicas, *Arch. Inst. Cardiol. Mex.*, 33:690.

14. Contreras, R., Castañeda, H. I., and Quijano Pitman, F. (1965): Aneurisma aórtico por arteritis de celulas gigantes. *Arch. Inst. Cardiol. Mex.*, 35:818.

15. Correa, P., and Araujo, J. (1958): Arteritis of the aorta in young women. *Am. J. Clin. Pathol.*, 29:560.

16. Danaraj, T. J., and Ong, W. H. (1959): Primary arteritis of the abdominal aorta in children causing bilateral stenosis of renal arteries and hypertension. *Circulation*, 20:856–863.

17. Danaraj, T. J., and Wong, H. O. (1959): Primary arteritis of abdominal aorta in children causing bilateral stenosis of renal arteries and hypertension. *Circulation*, 20:856.

18. Delaney, T. B., and Nadas, A. S. (1964): Peripheral pulmonic stenosis. *Am. J. Cardiol.*, 13:451.

19. Esclavissat, M., Ginefra, P., and Espino-Vela, J. (1957): Enfermedad sin pulso: A propósito de dos casos en mujeres jóvenes. *Arch. Inst. Cardiol Mex.*, 27:645.

20. Fabius, A. J. M. (1959): Failure to demonstrate precipitating antibodies against vessel extracts in patients with vascular disorders. *Vox Sang.*, 4:247.

21. Falicov, R. E., and Cooney, D. F. (1954): Takayasu's arteritis and rheumatoid arthritis. *Arch. Intern. Med.*, 114:594.

22. Frovig, A. G., and Loken, A. C. (1951): Syndrome of obliteration of the arterial branches of the aortic arch due to arteritis. *Acta Psychiatr. Neurol. Scand.*, 26:313.

23. González, C. J., Villavicencio, L., Molina, B., and Bessudo, J. (1967): Nonspecific obliterative aortitis in children. *Ann. Thorac. Surg.*, 4:193.

24. Gorodezky, C., Terán, L., and Escobar-Gutiérrez, A. (1979): HLA frequencies in a Mexican Mecstizo population. *Tissue Antigens*, 14:347.

25. Harrell, J. E., and Manion, W. C. (1970): Sclerosing aortitis and arteritis. *Semin. Roentgenol.*, 5:260–266.

26. Hirsch, M. S., Aikat, B. K., and Basu, A. K. (1964): Takayasu's arteritis: Report of five cases with immunologic studies. *Johns Hopkins Med. J.*, 115:29.

27. Ikeda, M. (1966): Immunologic studies on Takayasu's arteritis. *Jpn. Circ. J.*, 30:87.

28. Inada, K., and Kawahara, T. (1963): Atypical coarctation of the aorta: Its genesis and mechanism of hypertension. *Jpn. Circ. J.*, 27:729.

29. Inada, K., Shimizu, H., and Yokoyama, T. (1962): Pulseless disease and atypical coarctation of the aorta with special reference to their genesis. *Surgery*, 52:433.

30. Isaacson, C. (1961): An idiopathic aortitis in young Africans. *J. Pathol. Bacteriol.*, 81:69–79.

31. Ishikawa, K. (1978): Natural history and classification of occlusive thromboaortopathy (Takayasu's disease). *Circulation*, 57:27.

32. Isohisa, I., Numano, F., Maezawa, H., and Sasazuki, T. (1978): HLA-Bw52 in Takayasu's disease. *Tissue Antigens*, 12:246.

33. Ito, I. (1966): Aortitis syndrome, with reference to detection of antiaorta antibody from patients sera. *Jpn. Circ. J.*, 30:75.

34. Joffe, N. (1965): Aortitis of obscure origin in the African. *Clin. Radiol.*, 16:130–140.

35. Joysey, V. C. (1978): HLA-A-B and C antigens, their serology and cross reaction. *Br. Med. Bull.*, 34:217.

36. Judge, R. D., Currier, R. D., Gracie, W. A., and Figley, M. M. (1962): Takayasu's arteritis and the aortic arch syndrome. *Am. J. Med.*, 32:379.

37. Juzi, U. (1967): Takayasusche Arteritis mit Herzinfarkt. *Schweiz. Med. Wochenschr.*, 13:397–405.
38. Kimoto, S. (1960): Surgical treatment of coarctation of the aorta, with special reference to atypical coarctation. *Clin. Surg.*, 15:5 [in Japanese].
39. Kozuka, T., and Nosaki, T. (1969): Aortic insufficiency as a complication of the aortitis syndrome. *Acta Radiol. [Diagn.] (Stockh.)*, 8:49.
40. Kozuka, T., Nosaki, T., Sato, K., et al. (1968): Aortitis syndrome with special reference to pulmonary vascular changes. *Acta Radiol. (Stockh.)*, 7:25.
41. Kulka, J. P. (1959): The pathogenesis of rheumatoid arthritis. *J. Chronic Dis.*, 10:388.
42. Kulkarni, T. P., D' Cruz, I. A., Gandhi, M. J., and Dadhich, D. S. (1974): Reversal of renovascular hypertension caused by non-specific aortitis after corticosteroid therapy. *Br. Heart J.*, 36:114.
43. Lande, A., and Gross, A. (1972): Total aortography in the diagnosis of Takayasu's arteritis. *AJR*, 116:165.
44. Lande, A., and Rossi, P. (1975): The value of total aortography in the diagnosis of Takayasu's arteritis. *Radiology*, 114:287.
45. Lobato, O. (1956): Enfermedad de Takayasu: A propósito de un caso. *Arq. Bras. Cardiol.*, 9:277.
46. Lupi, H. E., and Sánchez Torres, G. (1972): Arteritis inespecífica y paraplejia intermitente. *Arch. Inst. Cardiol. Mex.*, 42:131.
47. Lupi, H. E., Contreras, R., Espino-Vela, J., Sánchez Torres, G., and Horwitz, S. (1972): Arteritis inespecífica en la niñez: Observaciones clínicas y anatomopatologicas. *Arch. Inst. Cardiol. Mex.*, 42:477.
48. Lupi, H. E., Horwitz, S., and Sánchez Torres, G. (1973): Calcifications in Takayasu's arteritis. *Vasc. Surg.*, 7:259.
49. Lupi, H. E., Sánchez Torres, G., and Castillo, P. U. (1972): Reactividad cutánea al PPD a los antígenos de myocobacterias atípicas (Kansasii, avium y fortuitum) en pacientes con arteritis inespecífica. *Arch. Inst. Cardiol. Mex.*, 42:717.
50. Lupi, H. E., Sánchez, T. G., Horwitz, S., and Gutiérrez, F. E. (1975): Pulmonary artery involvement in Takayasu's arteritis. *Chest*, 67:69.
51. Lupi, H. E., Sánchez, T. G., Marcuschamer, J., Mispireta, J., Horwitz, S., and Vela, J. E. (1977): Takayasu's arteritis: Clinical study of 107 cases. *Am. Heart J.*, 93:94.
52. Marquis, Y., Richardson, J. B., Ritchie, A. C., and Wigle, D. (1968): Idiopathic medial aortopathy and arteriopathy. *Am. J. Med.*, 44:939.
53. Martorell, F. (1972): Maladie de Takayasu et syndrome de Martorell. *Folia Angiol.*, 20:124.
54. Martorell, F., and Fabré, J. (1944): El síndrome de obliteración de los troncos supraaórticos. *Med. Clin. (Barc.)*, 2:26.
55. McKusick, V. A. (1962): Form of vascular disease relatively frequent in the Orient. *Am. Heart J.*, 63:57.
56. Miller, G. A. H., Thomas, M. L., and Medd, W. Z. (1962): Aortic arch syndrome and polymyositis with L. E. cells in peripheral blood. *Br. Med. J.*, 1:771.
57. Muñoz, N., and Correa, P. (1970): Arteritis of the aorta and its major branches. *Am. Heart J.*, 80:319.
58. Nakao, K., Ikeda, M., Kimato, S., Nhtani, H., Miyahara, M., Ishimi, Z., Hashiba, K., Takeda, Y., Ozawa, T., Matsushita S., and Kuromochi, M. (1967): Takayasu's arteritis: Clinical report of eighty-four cases and immunological studies of seven cases. *Circulation*, 35:1141.
59. Nasu, T. (1962): Pathology of pulseless disease: Systematic study and critical review of twenty-one autopsy cases reported in Japan. *Angiology*, 14:225.
60. Numano, F., Isohisa, I., Kishi, U., Arita, M., and Maezawa, H. (1978): Takayasu's disease in twin sisters. *Circulation*, 58:173.
61. Numano, F., Isohisa, I., and Maezawa, H. (1978): HLA antigens in Takayasu's disease. *J. Jpn. Soc. Intern. Med.*, 67:258.
62. Oota, K. (1940): Ein seltener Fall von veiderseitigem carotis Subclaviaerchluss (ein Beitrag zur Pathologie du anasto-Mosis peripapillaires des Anges mit fehlendem Radioalpuls). *Trans. Soc. Pathol. Jpn.*, 30:680.
63. Paton, B. C., Charttkanij, K., Buri, P. T., and Jumbala, B. (1965): Obliterative aortic disease in children in the tropics. *Circulation [Suppl.]*, 31:197.
64. Piomelli, S., Stefanini, M., and Mele, R. H. (1959): Antigenicity of human vascular endothelium: Lack of relationship to the pathogenesis of vasculitis. *J. Lab. Clin. Med.*, 54:241.

65. Planchecka, M., Kopec, M., and Kowalska, M. (1966): Rheumatoid factor in Takayasu syndrome. *Acta Rheum. Scand.*, 12:29.
66. Pokoruny, J., and Jezková, Z. (1962): Significance of immunological studies in peripheral obliterating vascular disease. *Circ. Res.*, 11:961.
67. Rao, G. R., and Krishnamurti, M. (1969): Idiopathic arteritis of aorta and pulmonary artery. *J. Assoc. Physicians India*, 17:443.
68. Rentería, V. G., and Contreras, M. (1978): Aorto-arteritis inespecífica: Estudio anatomopatológico de 18 casos. *Arch. Inst. Cardiol. Mex.*, 481:104.
69. Riehl, J., and Brown, W. J. (1965): Takayasu's arteritis: An auto-immune disease. *Arch. Neurol.*, 12:92.
70. Rivera de Reyes, A. Ma., Pérez-Treviño, C., and Pérez-Alvarez, J. J. (1969): Arteritis inespecífica en la niñez. *Arch. Inst. Cardiol. Mex.*, 39:1.
71. Roberts, W. C., and Wibin, E. A. (1966): Idiopathic panaortitis, supraaortic arteritis, granulomatous myocarditis and pericarditis. *Am. J. Med.*, 41:453.
72. Robicsek, F., Sanger, P. W., and Daugherty, H. K. (1965): Coarctation of the abdominal aorta diagnosed by aortography. *Ann. Surg.*, 162:227.
73. Rojas, E., Sánchez, T., and Reyes, P. A. (1981): Estudios inmunológicos en la arteritis de Takayasu. I. Anticuerpos circulantes a productos de microbacterias y complejos inmunes circulantes. *Arch. Inst. Cardiol. Mex.*, 51:185.
74. Rosen, N., and Gaton, E. (1972): Takayasu's arteritis of coronary arteries. *Arch. Pathol.*, 94:225.
75. Ross, R. S., and McKusick, V. A. (1953): Diminished or absent pulses in arteries arising from the arch of the aorta: Aortic arch syndrome. *Arch. Intern. Med.*, 92:701.
76. Roth, L. M., and Kissane, J. M. (1964): Panaortitis and aortic valvulitis in progressive systemic sclerosis (scleroderma). *Am. J. Clin. Pathol.*, 41:287.
77. Saito, Y., Hirota, K., Ito, I., et al. (1972): Clinical and pathological studies of five autopsied cases of aortitis syndrome. Part I. Findings of the aorta and its branches, peripheral arteries and pulmonary arteries. *Jpn. Heart J.*, 13:20.
78. Sánchez, T. G. (1971): Compresión arterial: Una maniobra clínica para localizar algunos soplos vasculares. *Arch. Inst. Cardiol. Mex.*, 41:531.
79. Sánchez, T. G., Pineda, C., Morales, E., and Martínez- Lavín, M. (1983): Takayasu's arteritis in children. *Arthritis Rheum.*, 26:535.
80. Sánchez Torres, G. (1972): Arteritis inespecífica y enfermedad tuberculosa: Aspectos clínicos. *Arch. Inst. Cardiol. Mex.*, 42:717.
81. Sánchez Torres, G., and Barroso, M. R. (1971): Eritema nodoso, y eritema indurado de Bazin, su relación con las arteritis inespecíficas. *Arch. Inst. Cardiol. Mex.*, 41:414.
82. Sánchez Torres, G., Contreras, R., Barroso, M. B., Zajarías, S., Dávila, R., and Lupi, H. E. (1972): Adenitis tuberculosa y arteritis de Takayasu. *Arch. Inst. Cardiol. Mex.*, 42:663.
83. Sánchez Torres, G., Zamora, C., Melcom, G., and Alvarez, A. (1970): Coartacion atípica de la aorta por arteritis inespecífica. *Arch. Inst. Cardiol. Mex.*, 40:602.
84. Sanching, H., and Welin, G. (1961): Aortic arch syndrome with special reference to rheumatoid arthritis. *Acta Med. Scand.*, 170:1.
85. Santos-Botello, O. E. (1956): Enfermedad sin pulso o síndrome de obstrucción de los troncos arteriales que nacen del cayado aórtico. *Rev. Hosp. Univ. Monterrey*, 3:83.
86. Saveleva, L. A., and Sivkovas, J. (1963): Pulseless disease in childhood. *Pediatriia*, 42:67 [in Russian].
87. Savory, W. S. (1856): Case of a young woman in whom the main arteries of both upper extremities and of the left side of the neck were throughout completely obliterated. *Med. Chir. Trans. Lond.*, 39:205.
88. Schire, V., and Asherson, R. A. (1964): Arteritis of the aorta and its major branches. *Q. J. Med.*, 33:439.
89. Sen, P. K., Kinare, S. G., Engineer, S. D., and Parulkar, G. B. (1963): Middle aortic syndrome. *Br. Heart J.*, 25:610.
90. Sen, P. K., Kinare, S. G., Kelkar, M. D., and Nanivadkar, S. A. (1972): Nonspecific stenosing arteritis of the aorta and its branches: A study of a possible etiology. *Mt. Sinai J. Med.*, 39:221.
91. Sen, P. K., Kinare, S. G., Kulkarni, T. P., and Parulkar, G. B. (1962): Stenosing aortitis of unknown etiology. *Surgery*, 51:317.
92. Shapiro, M. J. (1959): Coarctation of the abdominal aorta. *Am. J. Cardiol.*, 4:547.

93. Shimada, S., Sugiyama, Y., and Ogawa, I. (1956): Giant cell arteritis: Report of a case. *Acta Med. Biol.*, 4:67.
94. Shimizu, K., and Sano, K. (1948): Pulseless disease. *Clin. Surg (Tokyo)*, 3:377 [in Japanese].
95. Shimizu, K., and Sano, K. (1951): Pulseless disease. *J. Neuropathol. Clin. Neurol.*, 1:37.
96. Steeger, A., and Vargas, L. (1960): Enfermedad de Takayasu. *Rev. Chil. Pediatr.*, 31:377.
97. Stein, P. D., O'Connor, J. F., Dalen, J. E., et al. (1967): The angiographic diagnosis of acute pulmonary embolism: Evaluation of criteria. *Am. Heart J.*, 73:730.
98. Strachnan, R. W. (1964): The natural history of Takayasu's arteriopathy. *Q. J. Med.*, 33:57.
99. Sunada, T., and Inada, K. (1966): Atypical coarctation with a special reference to the genesis. *Jpn. Circ. J.*, 30:72.
100. Takayasu, M. (1908): Case with unusual changes of the central vessels in the retina. *Acta Soc. Ophthalmol. Jpn.*, 12:554.
101. Takeda, R., Oneda, G., Suto, K., et al. (1961): Pulseless disease: Report of an autopsy case, with special reference to the morphogenesis of the arterial lesions. *Gunma J. Med. Sci.*, 1:27–45.
102. Takezawa, H., Sakakura, M., Kokan, Y., and Hamaguchi, Y. (1966): Report of two cases of Takayasu's disease complicated with tuberculoid exanthemas. *Jpn. Circ. J.*, 30:1045.
103. Thiffault, C. R., and Smith, S. P. (1966): Extrapulmonary tuberculosis with erythema nodosum and occlusive arterial disease. *Can. Med. Assoc. J.*, 95:275.
104. Thurlberck, W. M., and Currens, J. H. (1959): Aortic arch syndrome (pulseless disease): Report of ten cases with three autopsies. *Circulation*, 19:499.
105. Ueda, H., Ito, I., and Saito, Y. (1964): Auto-antibody in the cardiovascular disease. *Jpn. J. Clin. Med.*, 22:1271.
106. Ueda, H., Morooka, S., Ito, I., et al. (1969): Clinical observation of 52 cases of aortitis syndrome. *Jpn. Heart J.*, 10:277–288.
107. Ueno, A., Awane, Y., Wakabayachi, A., and Shimizu, K. (1967): Successfully operated obliterative brachiocephalic arteritis (Takayasu) associated with the elongated coarctation. *Jpn. Heart J.*, 8:538.
108. Vinijchaikul, K. (1967): Primary arteritis of the aorta and its main branches (Takayasu's arteriopathy). *Am. J. Med.*, 43:15.
109. Waaler, E., and Milde, E. J. (1968): Is there a relationship between "giant cell" arteritis with "polymyalgia rheumatica" and rheumatoid arthritis? *Acta Pathol. Microbiol. Scand.*, 72:347.
110. Willoughby, W. F. (1972): Pulmonary arteritis induced by cationic proteins. *Am. Rev. Respir. Dis.*, 105:50.
111. Zajarías, S., Rotberg, T., Stevens, H., and Durán, P. (1969): Arteriopatía tipo Takayasu con localización renovascular. *Arch. Inst. Cardiol. Mex.*, 39:499.
112. Zimerman, H. A. (1972): *Intravascular Catheterization*, p. 311. Charles C Thomas, Springfield, Illinois.

Aortitis: Clinical, Pathologic, and Radiographic Aspects, edited by A. Lande, Y. M. Berkmen, and H. A. McAllister. Raven Press, New York © 1986.

Giant Cell Arteritis and Giant Cell Aortitis

Gene G. Hunder

Department of Medicine, Mayo Medical School, Rochester, Minnesota 55905

Giant cell arteritis, also referred to as temporal arteritis, cranial arteritis, or granulomatous arteritis, is a form of vasculitis which affects persons over the age of 50 years (11). The inflammatory processes tend to involve the aorta and branches of the arteries originating from the arch of the aorta most prominently, but lesions may be found in almost any artery of the body and occasionally in some veins (16). The relationship of giant cell arteritis to other forms of vasculitis is unclear, but the combination of clinical and pathologic features is sufficiently distinctive to suggest that it is a specific disease. Hutchinson described a case in 1890, but the condition was not generally recognized until the report of Horton and associates in 1932 (8,12).

The etiology of giant cell arteritis is unknown. A variety of causative agents and infectious organisms have been implicated, but none is proved. The occurrence of giant cell arteritis in older individuals has implied a relationship to aging. One hypothesis proposes that certain protein structures of the artery wall may become biochemically and antigenically altered with advancing years, and in giant cell arteritis an autoimmune reaction develops against an altered constituent of the artery wall. Several workers have noted that the inflammatory infiltrations are most prominent in the regions of elastic fibers in the artery wall and have raised the idea that a cell-mediated autoimmune reaction develops against aged elastin (14,23). There are no experimental data to support this concept. In this chapter a general review of giant cell arteritis is provided, and the clinical aspects of cases with involvement of larger arteries are emphasized.

GIANT CELL ARTERITIS

Giant cell arteritis is a relatively common disorder in the United States and Europe (2,11). Less is known about the incidence elsewhere. Familial aggregations have been observed occasionally. An epidemiologic study in Minnesota showed an average annual incidence during the 25-year period 1950 through 1974 of 11.7 cases per 100,000 persons aged 50 years and older, and a prevalence of active and resolved cases of 133 per 100,000 persons 50 years of age and older (11). Somewhat similar figures have been found in Europe (2). Study of pathologic material suggests that giant cell arteritis is even more common. Östberg found histologic evidence of giant cell arteritis in 1.7% of 899 unselected postmortem cases in which sections of the aorta and temporal arteries were prepared (21).

193

Women are affected twice as commonly as men. The mean age at onset is about 70 years; 90% of the patients are over age 60 at onset. The illness may begin abruptly or insidiously (Tables 1 and 2). Constitutional symptoms such as fatigue, malaise, and weight loss are frequent. Confusion or apparent mental depression may occur and be misinterpreted as senility. A low-grade fever is present in somewhat fewer than one-half of cases, and in 15% the clinical picture of "fever of unknown origin" is the presenting manifestation (3).

Headache is the most common symptom and is present in 60 to 90% of cases in different series. The headaches may be severe or mild, transient or persistent. Giant

TABLE 1. *Initial manifestations of giant cell arteritis in 100 patients[a]*

Finding	No. of patients
Headache	32
Polymyalgia rheumatica	25
Fever of undetermined origin	15
Visual symptoms without loss	7
Weakness/malaise/fatigue	5
Myalgias	4
Tenderness over arteries	3
Weight loss/anorexia	2
Jaw claudication	2
Permanent loss of vision	1
Tongue claudication	1
Sore throat	1
Vasculitis on angiogram	1
Stiffness of hands and wrists	1

[a]After Calamia and Hunder (3).

TABLE 2. *Clinical findings in 100 patients with giant cell arteritis[a]*

Finding	No. of patients
Fever	42
Polymyalgia rheumatica	39
Symptoms related to arteritis	83
Jaw claudication	45
Headache	68
Visual loss	14
Limb claudication	4
Signs related to arteries	66
Artery tenderness	27
Decreased temporal artery pulse	46
Erythematous/nodular/swollen temporal arteries	23
Large artery bruit	21
Decreased large artery pulse	7

[a]After Calamia and Hunder (3).

cell arteritis should be considered in any patient over the age of 50 years with a new type of headache.

Abnormalities of the extracranial arteries are the most helpful physical findings in recognizing giant cell arteritis. The temporal or occipital arteries may be tender or enlarged and nodular or thrombosed. However, arteritis may be present on biopsy even when the temporal arteries are normal on physical examination. Jaw claudication nearly always indicates the presence of giant cell arteritis. It occurs in approximately one-half of the cases. With this symptom the patient develops a sensation of fatigue or discomfort in one or more groups of muscles of mastication when chewing food, especially meat. The discomfort is relieved by rest. Claudication also may occur in the muscles of the tongue or deglutition or the extremities.

Permanent loss of vision is the most common serious complication of giant cell arteritis. Visual symptoms of any type are found in about one-third of cases. They are usually secondary to ischemia of ocular structures supplied by the ophthalmic and posterior ciliary arteries. Transient visual blurring and diplopia should alert the physician to the possible presence of giant cell arteritis. Partial or complete unilateral or bilateral visual loss occurs in 10 to 20% of cases. Once fixed, visual loss is permanent (3).

Polymyalgia rheumatica is a clinical syndrome characterized by the presence of aching and stiffness located in the neck and torso, shoulder girdle muscles, and hip girdle muscles along with evidence of a systemic reaction which is usually documented by an erythrocyte sedimentation rate (ESR) of 40 mm in 1 hr or more, according to the Westergren method (4). Polymyalgia rheumatica is closely related to giant cell arteritis. About 40 to 50% of patients with giant cell arteritis have polymyalgia rheumatica (3,11). However, only 15 to 20% of patients with polymyalgia rheumatica can be shown to have giant cell arteritis (4). The aching and stiffness in polymyalgia rheumatica appear related to inflammation in the proximal joints, ligaments, or tendons (19).

Laboratory Findings

The ESR is the most useful laboratory test in the diagnosis of giant cell arteritis. It is markedly elevated in nearly all patients with active disease (Table 3). A mild to moderate normochromic or normocytic anemia is present in most cases, but the leukocyte count is usually normal. The alpha-2-globulin fraction of serum proteins and platelet counts are frequently elevated (3). In about one-third of cases mild elevation of the liver enzymes has been noted (3). All laboratory tests revert to normal with corticosteroid therapy.

Diagnosis

The diagnosis of giant cell arteritis may be difficult because the findings and presentations are diverse (Tables 1 and 2). Giant cell arteritis should be considered in any older patient who has developed transient or sudden visual changes, prolonged fever, polymyalgia rheumatica, or headaches. The manifestations may vary

TABLE 3. *Findings in patients with giant cell arteritis*[a]

Parameter	Large artery involvement	No large artery involvement
Patients (No.)	23	52
Age at onset (years)	65 (51–83)[b]	69 (54–82)
Sex (M/F)	4/19	11/41
With polymyalgia rheumatica (No.)	7	28
With permanent visual loss (No.)	1	3
Hemoglobin (g/dl)	12.1 (9.1–14.4)	11.3 (7.4–14.3)
ESR (mm in 1 hr)	80 (46–116)	97 (58–144)
Alpha-2-globulin (g/dl)	1.29 (0.75–2.19)	1.25 (0.48–2.06)
Albumin (g/dl)	3.12 (2.27–4.28)	2.83 (1.32–3.47)

[a]After Klein et al. (16).
[b]Mean (range).

over a week or two and even subside spontaneously. Thus it is important to inquire thoroughly about the presence of symptoms the patient has currently or has had in the recent past. The arteries of the head, neck, and extremities should be examined carefully for tenderness, enlargement, or alterations in pulses, as well as auscultated for bruits.

A temporal or occipital artery biopsy is recommended in all patients suspected of having this disease. When the artery is clearly abnormal, a short segment is usually sufficient to establish the diagnosis. If the artery is not obviously altered, a 4- to 6-cm temporal biopsy is suggested. The specimen should be examined at multiple levels for arteritis (15). If the first temporal artery is normal, the opposite side should be biopsied. In 15 to 20% of cases histologic evidence of giant cell arteritis is obtained only on the second biopsy (3).

Histologically, a chronic, granulomatous-type inflammatory reaction is present marked by the infiltration of lymphocytes, plasma cells, and histiocytes. Multinucleated giant cells are seen in most cases and tend to be located about disrupted elastic laminae. The inflammatory processes may involve portions or quadrants of the vessel wall, or a panarteritis may develop and result in occlusion of the vessel lumen.

Treatment/Course

Nearly all patients respond rapidly to corticosteroid therapy. These drugs should be started as soon as the diagnosis is made in order to prevent vascular complications, e.g., blindness. The initial dose should be 40 to 60 mg of prednisone per day or the equivalent dose of a similar corticosteroid. This dose should be continued for about 1 month. After that, if all reversible symptoms have resolved and laboratory tests are normal, the dose can be gradually tapered by a maximum of 10% of the daily dose per week using the patient's clinical course, the ESR, the alpha-2-globulin levels, and the hemoglobin concentrations as guidelines.

The duration of giant cell arteritis is variable and ranges from several months to several years or more (11). The average length is approximately 1 year. Relapses may occur and may need to be treated by increasing the prednisone dose to higher levels again temporarily.

Large Artery Involvement

Jennings was one of the first to call attention to large artery involvement in temporal arteritis (13). He described a patient with headache, jaw claudication, polymyalgia rheumatica, tender temporal arteries, and narrowing of the left brachial artery and arteries of the right foot. Subsequently other cases were reported, and it has become apparent that inflammation in the aorta and its branches is not a rare finding in giant cell arteritis. Clinically, large artery involvement has been detected in 10 to 15% of patients with giant cell arteritis. Hamrin found aortic arch symptoms in 14 of 93 patients, and Klein and co-workers found 23 patients with definite evidence for large vessel involvement and 11 others with possible large artery involvement in a total of 254 patients (7,16). However, actual inflammatory lesions in the aorta and large proximal vessels are likely to be much more frequent as suggested by the fact that findings on history and physical examination are detected only when inflammatory changes are extensive enough to cause significant alteration of the lumen of the affected arteries (21).

Findings that suggest large artery involvement include tenderness over the arteries, reduced pulses, bruits, intermittent claudication of the extremities, and cerebrovascular ischemia. In occasional instances a vessel may appear enlarged as a result of mural or periarterial inflammation or dilation. Aortic dilation and rupture and aortic valve insufficiency have been reported also (7,9,16). Reduced pulses, bruits, and claudication should develop at the time of active arteritis in order to differentiate it from arteriosclerosis, which commonly develops in this age group.

Clinical Features

The clinical and laboratory features in patients with giant cell arteritis who have large artery involvement are similar to those without such findings. In Table 3 the clinical and laboratory findings in a group of 23 patients with large artery involvement are compared with 52 randomly selected patients with giant cell arteritis without large artery symptoms or findings (16). Systemic manifestations were present in all 23 patients and were similar to those without large artery involvement. In this group of 23 patients with definite large artery involvement, the duration of illness when large vessel findings were noted ranged from 0 to 84 months with a mean of 8.8 months and a median of 3.5 months. Clinical manifestations were related to both the upper and lower extremities in 7 patients, to the upper extremities alone in 11, and to the lower extremities alone in 3. Intermittent claudication of an extremity was the most common symptom and was present in 17 of the 23 patients (Table 4). Raynaud's phenomenon occurred in 5 patients and was unilateral at times, affecting only the extremity overtly involved with arteritis. In 2 patients paresthesias in the extremities were suggestive of neuropathy, but a nerve deficit was not documented in these cases. Neuropathy occurs only occasionally in giant

TABLE 4. *Clinical features in 23 patients with definite large artery involvement[a]*

Symptom or sign	No. of patients
Intermittent claudication	17
Upper extremity	9
Lower extremity	3
Both	5
Raynaud's phenomenon	5
Paresthesias	2
Decreased or absent pulses	21
Upper extremity	14
Lower extremity	4
Both extremities	3

[a]After Klein et al. (16).

cell arteritis. Physical examination in the 23 patients revealed bruits over large arteries or decreased pulses in all but two subjects, one of whom was not examined before death. Bruits often were noted over a long segment of vessel, e.g., along a subclavian artery and distally in the axilla and arm to the elbow. Hamrin's earlier experience was similar (7). Hamrin pointed out the predilection for the left brachial artery over the right (7). Wilkinson and Russell reviewed the autopsy findings in 12 patients whose deaths were related to giant cell arteritis (23). All patients had died with cerebral infarctions secondary to narrowing or thrombosis of the vertebral or carotid arteries.

The findings in the above studies suggest that subclavian, axillary, and brachial arteries are the most common larger vessels affected symptomatically in giant cell arteritis. Although ischemic symptoms occur in the limbs, gangrene is uncommon. When death occurs as a result of this disease, ih is likely to be the result of occlusion of the cervical arteries, especially the vertebral arteries, or rupture of the aorta.

Symptoms related to large arteries may be the initial manifestation or occur late in the disease. In 4 of Klein and co-workers' 23 patients, intermittent claudication of the arms and absence of pulses in the upper extremities were the initial manifestations of arteritis (Table 5). None of these 4 had polymyalgia rheumatica, scalp tenderness, or headaches at any time during the illness, and in each a diagnosis was determined by biopsy of a temporal artery which felt normal on physical examination. The presenting complaints of eight other patients were due to large artery involvement, but careful questioning revealed that scalp pain or polymyalgia rheumatica also had been present during the months preceding the initial examination. Large artery disease in 6 of the 23 patients first became evident an average of 6.8 months after corticosteroid therapy had been initiated and while these drugs were being withdrawn after initial control of the disease. The ESR had risen again and exceeded 60 mm in 1 hr in all 6 patients at the time large artery symptoms were diagnosed. Three final patients in this group of 23 developed evidence of large artery involvement after corticosteroid therapy had been discontinued. In 2

TABLE 5. *Initial presentation of large artery involvement[a]*

Condition	No. of patients
Without symptoms of polymyalgia rheumatica or giant cell arteritis	4
With symptoms of polymyalgia rheumatica or giant cell arteritis	8
During corticosteroid reductions	6
After corticosteroid discontinued	3
Postmortem	2
Total	23

[a]After Klein et al. (16).

patients the diagnosis was made at autopsy; one of these died of a ruptured aorta secondary to giant cell arteritis, and the second died from a cardiac arrest but also had an aortic aneurysm. A third patient in this series died from rupture of the aorta during corticosteroid withdrawal.

Diagnosis

Careful examination of the arteries for tenderness, decreased pulses, and bruits help determine the presence of large artery involvement. Angiographic studies should be carried out to define the extent of the vessel changes when clinical evidence for large vessel lesions is found (22). Arteriographic features most suggestive of arteritis are (a) long segments of smooth arterial stenoses alternating with areas of normal or increased caliber; (b) smooth, tapered occlusions of affected large arteries; (c) absence of irregular plaques and ulcerations; and (d) anatomic distribution of these changes with major involvement of subclavian, axillary, and brachial arteries (Figs. 1 and 2). Dilation of the ascending aorta is also seen frequently, although it is of limited differential value in this age group. A temporal artery biopsy is recommended even when typical arteriographic changes are present.

Pathology

In 16 autopsy cases with large artery involvement studied by Östberg, lesions were found in the aorta in 12 (20). In 6 the entire aorta was involved, in 1 the proximal thoracic and distal abdominal aorta were affected, in 2 the thoracic aorta was inflamed, and in 3 inflammation was found in the distal two-thirds of the aorta. Changes were found in the arm arteries in 13 of the 16 cases. The extent of the lesions varied, the proximal subclavian arteries being involved in 10, whereas in 3 the first portions of these arteries were normal. In 11 cases typical lesions were found in the carotid arteries. In 10 cases changes were found in leg arteries. The lesions in the large arteries were fairly symmetrical on both sides of the body and disseminated with normal areas between.

Common changes described in the intima of the aorta are diffuse thickening and fine wrinkling which produces cushion-like projections into the arterial lumen. The

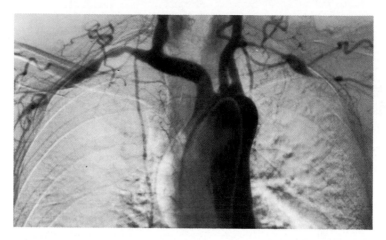

FIG. 1.   Giant cell arteritis proved by temporal artery biopsy. This subtraction print of an arch aortogram shows alternating segments of stenosis and dilation of the subclavian arteries and axillary arteries. (From Klein et al., ref. 16, with permission.)

projections may be oriented longitudinally or transversely (16,20). As noted, aortic dilation and rupture may be found.

The histologic appearance depends on the extent and age of the lesion. Active foci have the appearance of a chronic granulomatous inflammatory process marked by the presence of lymphocytes, plasma cells, multinucleated giant cells, and histiocytes. In old lesions fibrosis predominates. Necrosis in the media is present in varying amounts surrounded by inflammatory cells (Fig. 3). The elastic fibers are frayed and decreased in number. The intima contains loose connective tissue with fibroblasts or smooth muscle cells and thin bundles of collagen and metachromatic ground substance but generally few inflammatory cells. The adventitia may be infiltrated with chronic inflammatory cells. Diffuse fibrous thickening of the adventitia may develop.

Treatment/Course

In general, the symptoms and findings related to the large arteries respond favorably to corticosteroids when given in doses that are adequate to cause ESR to return to normal. In Klein and co-workers' series, 14 of the 23 patients showed improvement in intermittent claudication, pulses, and blood pressure in the affected extremities (16). In 3 other patients claudication improved, but pulses remained the same. Follow-up information was not available for 3 other patients, and 3 patients died.

In some patients with severe deficits, improvement may be noted only after 2 to 4 months of corticosteroid treatment. If an artery has become completely occluded before the initiation of treatment, return of pulses or blood pressure generally is not found, even though improvement in the use of the extremity may be noted. If

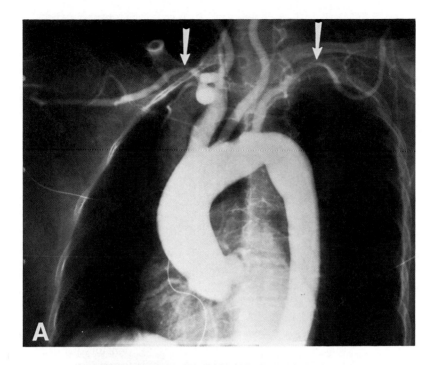

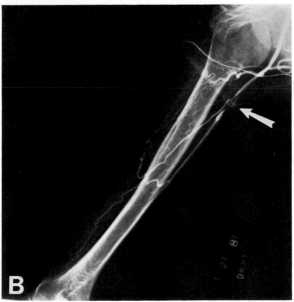

FIG. 2. Giant cell arteritis proved by temporal artery biopsy. **A:** Arch aortogram with smooth-walled stenoses of segments of both subclavian arteries *(arrows).* **B:** Right brachial arteriogram of the same patient showing marked narrowing of a segment of the proximal brachial artery *(arrow)* and collateral circulation.

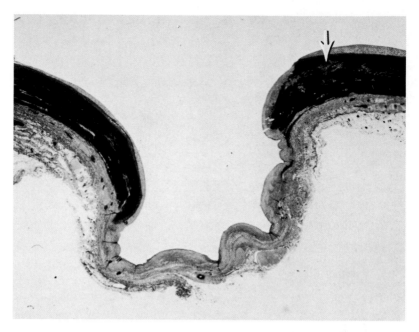

FIG. 3.   Giant cell arteritis of the aorta. Cross section at the edge of a saccular aneurysm. Intima is at top. Elastic tissue stain shows areas of disruption of elastic laminae at the edges of the section *(arrow)* and complete separation of elastic fibers in the aneurysmal portion at the center of the figure. (Lawson's elastic stain, × 16.)

circulation is marginal at the onset of treatment, ischemic symptoms may continue or worsen.

Relationship of Giant Cell Arteritis to Takayasu's Disease

Determining the relationship of the various forms of vasculitis to each other has been difficult because little is known about the causes and important pathophysiological mechanisms in this group of diseases (10). Some authors classify Takayasu's disease (aortic arch arteritis) with giant cell arteritis (1,5). Similarities between the two are present, as is apparent from the data in this book. The distribution of arterial lesions in giant cell arteritis may be identical with those found in Takayasu's disease. Similarly, the histopathologic appearances may be indistinguishable. However, Fiessinger and colleagues, as well as others, have suggested that in giant cell arteritis the most intense inflammation tends to be located at the region of the internal elastic lamina and inner media, whereas in Takayasu's disease the lesions tend to be more prominent in the adventitia and outer part of the arterial wall (6). Intimal thickening and narrowing of the arterial lumen occurs in both conditions, but only Takayasu's disease is capable of producing aortic arch narrowing or coarctation (18). Aortic dilation is seen in both diseases.

A number of other findings also suggest that these conditions are separate disease entities. Takayasu's disease generally begins during the first three decades of life, but the onset of giant cell arteritis is rare before the age of 50 years. Giant cell arteritis appears more commonly in Caucasians, whereas Takayasu's disease has been reported more frequently in persons of Oriental and Indian ancestry and in Mexican mestizos. In the population of Olmsted County, Minnesota, a preliminary survey showed the average annual incidence of Takayasu's disease to be 0.4 cases per year per 100,000 population, whereas the incidence of giant cell arteritis in the same population was 2.4 cases per year per 100,000 population (17). Large artery involvement is clinically evident in essentially all patients with Takayasu's disease, whereas this is true in only a minority of patients with giant cell arteritis. Although blindness occurs in both conditions, in giant cell arteritis lesions in the ophthalmic and posterior ciliary arteries are responsible for ocular ischemia, whereas in Takayasu's disease visual impairment is generally caused by obstructive lesions in the carotid and vertebral arteries. Both conditions respond favorably to corticosteroids early in the course of the disease. Little is known regarding the pathophysiology of either disease.

REFERENCES

1. Alarcón-Segovia, D. (1980): Classification of the necrotizing vasculitides in man. *Clin. Rheum. Dis.*, 6:223–231.
2. Bengtsson, B-A., and Malmvall, B-E. (1981): The epidemiology of giant cell arteritis including temporal arteritis and polymyalgia rheumatica. *Arthritis Rheum.*, 24:899–904.
3. Calamia, K. T., and Hunder, G. G. (1980): Clinical manifestations of giant cell (temporal) arteritis. *Clin. Rheum. Dis.*, 6:389–403.
4. Chuang, T-Y., Hunder, G. G., Ilstrup, D. M., and Kurland, L. T. (1982): Polymyalgia rheumatica: A ten-year epidemiologic and clinical study. *Intern. Med.*, 97:672–680.
5. Cupps, T. R., and Fauci, A. S. (1981): *Major Problems in Internal Medicine, Vol. 21: The Vasculitides*. Saunders, Philadelphia.
6. Fiessinger, J-N., Camilleri, J-P., Chousterman, M., Cormier, J-M., and Housset, E. (1978): Maladie de Horton et maladie de Takayasu: Criteres anatomopathologiques. *Nouv. Presse Med.*, 7:639–642.
7. Hamrin, B. (1972): Polymyalgia arteritica. *Acta Med. Scand. [Suppl.]*, 533:1–133.
8. Horton, B. T., Magath, T. B., and Brown, G. E. (1932): An undescribed form of arteritis of the temporal vessels. *Proc. Staff Meet. Mayo Clin.*, 7:700–701.
9. How, J., and Strachan, R. W. (1978): Aortic regurgitation as a manifestation of giant cell arteritis. *Br. Heart J.*, 40:1052–1054.
10. Hunder, G. G., and Lie, J. T. (1983): The vasculitides. *Cardiovasc. Clin.*, 12:261–291.
11. Huston, K. A., Hunder, G. G., Lie, J. T., Kennedy, R. H., and Elveback, L. R. (1978): Temporal arteritis: A 25-year epidemiologic, clinical, and pathologic study. *Ann. Intern. Med.*, 88:162–167.
12. Hutchinson, J. (1889–1890): Diseases of the arteries: On a peculiar form of thrombotic arteritis of the aged which is sometimes productive of gangrene. *Arch. Surg.*, 1:323–329.
13. Jennings, G. H. (1938): Arteritis of the temporal vessels. *Lancet*, 1:424–428.
14. Kimmelstiel, P., Gilmour, M. T., and Hodges, H. H. (1952): Degeneration of elastic fibers in granulomatous giant cell arteritis (temporal arteritis). *Arch. Pathol.*, 54:157–168.
15. Klein, R. G., Campbell, R. J., Hunder, G. G., and Carney, J. A. (1976): Skip lesion in temporal arteritis. *Mayo Clin. Proc.*, 51:504–510.
16. Klein, R. G., Hunder, G. G., Stanson, A. W., and Sheps, S. G. (1975): Large artery involvement in giant cell (temporal) arteritis. *Ann. Intern. Med.*, 83:806–812.
17. Kurland, L. T., Chuang, T-Y., and Hunder, G. G. (1984): Epidemiology of systemic arteritis. In: *Epidemiology of the Rheumatic Diseases*, edited by R. C. Lawrence and L. E. Shulman, pp. 196–205. Grower Medical Publishing Limited, New York.

18. Lande, A., and Berkman, Y. M. (1976): Aortitis: Pathologic, clinical and arteriographic review. *Radiol. Clin. North Am.*, 14:219–240.
19. O'Duffy, J. D., Hunder, G. G., and Wahner, H. W. (1981): A follow-up study of polymyalgia rheumatica: Evidence of chronic axial synovitis. *J. Rheumatol.*, 7:685–693.
20. Östberg, G. (1972): Morphologic changes in large arteries in polymyalgia arteritica. *Acta Med. Scand. [Suppl.]*, 533:135–164.
21. Östberg, G. (1973): On arteritis with special references to polymyalgia arteritica. *Acta Pathol. Microbiol. Scand. [A] [Suppl.]*, 237:1–59.
22. Stanson, A. W., Klein, R. G., and Hunder, G. G. (1976): Extracranial angiographic findings in giant cell (temporal) arteritis. *AJR*, 127:957–963.
23. Wilkinson, I. M. S., and Russell, R. W. R. (1972): Arteries of the head and neck in giant cell arteritis: A pathological study to show the pattern of arterial involvement. *Arch. Neurol.*, 27:378–391.

Aortitis: Clinical, Pathologic, and Radiographic Aspects, edited by A. Lande, Y. M. Berkmen, and H. A. McAllister. Raven Press, New York © 1986.

Takayasu's Arteritis in Children

John Baum

Departments of Pediatrics and Medicine, University of Rochester School of Medicine and Dentistry, Rochester, New York 14620; and Arthritis and Clinical Immunology Unit, Monroe Community Hospital, Rochester, New York 14603

Takayasu's arteritis is an inflammatory process which can often present during childhood but is more usually seen in young women (13). Lupi-Herrera et al. (14), in a review of 107 cases of Takayasu's disease, noted a characteristic appearance in the young with the sudden onset of constitutional symptoms noted above but also including such symptoms and signs of a local circulatory defect and high blood pressure. They stated that this clinical picture represented the initial inflammation, which could disappear partly or completely over an approximate 3-month period and then reappear several months later in a chronic phase. Sixty-seven percent of their patients under age 15 presented initially in heart failure. In 77% of the group the onset occurred between the ages of 10 and 20.

In the discussion of their eight patients, Wiggelinkhuizen et al. (27) reported other types of early symptoms in children: palpitations, dyspnea, epistaxis, and headache. Lee and his colleagues (13), also looking at the disease only in children, found dyspnea to be the most common manifestation followed by edema or a puffy face. However, these patients may have reached the chronic stage as all of them had cardiomegaly. Eight of the 10 had hypertension, and 7 of the 10 had a bruit heard over the abdomen.

Fever, fatigue, weight loss, and anemia are nonspecific manifestations of inflammatory disease, especially when accompanied by an elevated erythrocyte sedimentation rate (ESR). It is clear that it would require a high index of suspicion to make the diagnosis in these cases. Accompaniment of these symptoms by any symptom referable to the cardiovascular system, e.g., palpitation, edema, or cardiomegaly, are more definitive pointers toward a correct diagnosis.

Lande et al. (12) reemphasized that this disease shows early and late stages as originally pointed out in Japan. When the disease appears early, it presents as a generalized systemic disease with "fever, arthritis, cough, chest pain, hemoptysis, abdominal pain, skin rashes, and so forth." The subsequent disease is characterized by symptom complexes that result from the reduction in the circulatory system (arterial occlusions and regional ischemia). The latter symptoms, the late phase of the disease, is apparently being seen more often as the presenting phase.

It might seem that because the symptoms seen in the initial systemic phase appear in a number of acute and chronic childhood illnesses that it is much more difficult to diagnosis the disease in children. However, in Ishikawa's series (9) the

younger patients (under age 20) had significantly higher ESRs, and in these patients
the diagnosis was made sooner. There was an interval from onset to diagnosis of
4 years, which was less than half the time it took to make the diagnosis in those
patients who had ESRs under 40 mm/hr. It appears that a child with an elevated
ESR is more likely to be diagnosed in the systemic phase of the disease if a high
ESR is kept in mind as providing a high index of suspicion for arteritis.

Some authors (15,24) pointed out that in the younger children there is a higher
frequency of thoracic and abdominal aorta involvement than the aortic arch type
or combined type. Table 1 shows the frequencies in two Japanese studies. Ueda et
al. (24) and Nakao et al. (16) showed larger numbers of children with thoracic and
abdominal aorta involvement compared to involvement of the aortic arch, ranging
anywhere from 2.5 to 3.0 times as much. Children presenting with combined
disease or lesions, including all of the areas, ranged from one-third to one-half of
the patients.

The distribution of the lesion in Takayasu's syndrome can extend from involvement of the whole aorta and its major branches to the pulmonary arteries. It can
go on to dilatations or narrowing, even to occlusion of affected vessels. When the
aortic arch is involved, there is reduction of or even absent pulses in the arms and
neck and narrowing of those vessels which come out of the aortic arch. With those
lesions involving only the arch, aortography would not show any involvement of
the thoracic aorta or abdominal aorta. There is another group in which the whole
aorta is involved as well as its branches. Another type shows involvement of the
descending thoracic and abdominal aortas and their branches. Involvement of the
aorta and vessels is often described as coarctation.

Thoracic and abdominal aorta involvement, i.e., those cases with lesions below
the arch, are more often seen in younger patients (6,15,24). With involvement of
these areas the children present with clinical manifestations of coarctation rather
than the more classical syndromes that are seen with aortic arch involvement.
Hypertension is prominent because of involvement of the abdominal aorta and
blockage of renal vessels. Involvement here might be more conducive to surgical
intervention and replacement with prosthetic material.

Schrire and Asherson (22) reported a series of cases from Cape Town. Eighteen
patients had been seen during the 12-year period. Of these 18 cases, 12 were 18
years old or younger. The only three males were in this younger age group with

TABLE 1. *Distribution of aortitis sites in children (under age 19)*

Measurement	Aortic Arch		Thoracic and abdominal aorta		Combined	
	Ueda	Nakao	Ueda	Nakao	Ueda	Nakao
Total cases (No.)	24	47	9	10	19	27
Percent	25	26	78	40	37	52

one male age 4. The nine females who were 10 to 19 years old represented the largest single group.

These authors categorized their patients by the dominant symptomatology. The largest group are those who presented with cardiac symptoms and signs (8 patients). Two had cerebral vascular insufficiency, 5 intermittent claudication, 2 thoracic aneurysm, and 1 constitutional symptoms. Five of the 8 patients with the onset of cardiac symptoms were in the younger age group, 1 of the 2 with cerebral vascular insufficiency, 3 of the 5 with intermittent claudication, 1 of the 2 with thoracic aneurysms, and the single case with constitutional symptoms. It is quite clear, then, that in this series the children did not show a single type of presentation that was exclusive to this younger age group but, rather, distributed themselves through all the various types of presentation. However, all 4 of the 19 patients who presented with congestive heart failure were in the younger age group. Aortic incompetence was not restricted to the younger group but was found throughout the series. There were three cases of mitral incompetence, all in the younger age group.

In studies of the ocular lesions it was reported that ocular lesions were more important in the "young female" group of patients (25). Ocular symptoms are produced by involvement of the aortic arch, particularly the internal carotid artery. Cataract formation, which is a late change, results from chronic circulatory insufficiency.

Although central nervous system (CNS) symptoms have been reported frequently in patients with Takayasu's disease, a review by Currier and his colleagues (2) of 41 cases showed only three with the onset at age 18 or younger in whom they reported manifestations of this type. One patient had headache and two were described as having syncope and loss of consciousness at onset. Dizziness has been reported frequently in several series, but it appears that CNS manifestations are a rarer feature of the disease in children.

EPIDEMIOLOGY

A number of reports have noted the varying age distribution of the patients with Takayasu's syndrome. In Table 2 it can be seen that the larger the series reported

TABLE 2. *Age distribution of Takayasu's disease (under age 20)*

Investigator	Country	Under age 20/ total		Females/total	
		No.	%	No.	%
Ueda	Japan	17/52	33	6/7	86
Ueda	Japan	65/321	20	61/64	95
Ishikawa	Japan	10/43	23	50/54	93
Kinare	India	9/20	45	8/9	89
Lupi-Herrera	Mexico	82/107	77	—	~80
Fraga	Mexico	1/20	5	—	~90
Lande	USA	3/30	10	3/3	100

the higher is the frequency of patients under 20 years of age. In Ueda and co-workers two series in Japan (23,24) these young patients comprised one-third to one-fifth of the total. The larger single series (321 patients) was that of Ueda wherein 20% of the patients were under age 20 (23). It is of interest that Ishikawa's series, also from Japan (9), had approximately the same frequency. The study of Lupi-Herrera et al. (14) from Mexico showed the highest frequency of young patients, with 77% in the younger age group. This is in marked contradistinction to the series with the smallest percentage of young patients, that of Fraga et al. (5), also from Mexico. However, this was one of the smallest groups reported. In the United States Lande et al. (12) reported a 10% frequency in children.

When a breakdown was made of the percentage of female patients in all of the series, it ranged from 80 to 95%, so that the high frequency of Takayasu's disease in females was seen as consistently in the children as it was in older age groups.

DIFFERENTIAL DIAGNOSIS

The differential diagnosis of this disease can be a problem, especially in children. Owing to its rarity the disease is virtually never considered because its features of systemic onset, e.g., fatigue, fever, cough, pleurisy, anemia, and polyarthralgias, suggest a number of systemic diseases. Its manner of presentation is similar to that of systemic lupus erythematosus (SLE). In both diseases the patients can present with fever, fatigue, weight loss, joint pains, cardiomegaly, anemia, and an elevated ESR. The differences between them are those related directly to the cardiovascular system so that congestive heart failure, cerebral symptoms (e.g., headache, syncope), and ocular findings are rarely if ever seen in the children with SLE. Systemic juvenile-onset arthritis can present in this way, but here lymphadenopathy is prominent as well as a characteristic high spiking fever. Marked elevation of the ESR is a feature of juvenile arthritis so there is no clear-cut laboratory feature which would point to either disease. The appearance of congestive heart failure, more particularly hypertension, is the strongest indication in a child that one might be dealing with aortitis. If there is aortic arch involvement, cerebral symptoms or the ocular symptoms originally described by Takayasu also lead to consideration of this diagnosis. Absence of pulses might be considered pathognomonic, especially if there have been generalized systemic symptoms.

SURVIVAL AND MORBIDITY

Ishikawa (10) studied the survival and morbidity of patients with Takayasu's disease. Eighty-one patients had been followed prospectively for a mean of 7.4 years. Of this group 11 patients died during the follow-up period. Although the author made no note of the age of onset as a predictor, dividing the data still further produced interesting results. The four younger patients died an average of 7.8 years after the onset of their disease, whereas the seven patients in the age group beyond 18 lived an average of 18.3 years after diagnosis. This seems to indicate that there is an increased mortality with a younger age of onset. The age of onset in the older patients was almost twice that of the younger patients, with the average in the seven older patients being 29 and that of the younger patients 15 years.

An indication of the frequency of Takayasu's arteritis has been provided by Restrepo et al. (20) and Rose and Sinclair-Smith (21). Restrepo et al. found a frequency of 0.61%, and Rose and Sinclair-Smith found 16 cases of Takayasu's disease among more than 17,000 autopsies, giving an autopsy incidence of 0.09%. The marked frequency of young patients was again noted, with 9 of the 16 patients age 16 or under. Tuberculosis was frequently seen, although not as often as had been reported in the past. It was found in 6 of the 16 cases for a frequency of 37.5%. The significance of the finding in this particular series is the fact that all of the patients with tuberculosis were age 16 or under. Thus tuberculosis seems to be a strong etiological agent in the younger patient in this South African population. Their series also had a high frequency of male patients. Nine of the 16 were male, with 4 in the younger age group.

ETIOLOGICAL FACTORS

A frequently associated factor in aortitis has been its appearance against a background of tuberculosis. This has been seen with active disease or with a high frequency of positive tuberculin tests. These findings have led to the consideration that tuberculosis might be an etiological factor.

In a report from Thailand describing seven cases found in children in that country, the authors reported that though active tuberculosis was noted in several of their patients, they believed there was no association between the two diseases. The background frequency for tuberculosis is high in the population they studied, and so the authors are probably correct in not trying to make the association (19).

A study from Korea (13) of 10 children reported with pulseless disease showed that 9 had a positive Mantoux test. Again, because of a high frequency of tuberculosis in the population, the significance of this finding related to the etiology of the disease is questionable.

However, Kinare (11) believed on the basis of studies in Indian children that there was a correlation. His population of 20 individuals included 9 under age 20. Tuberculosis was present in 14 cases; 9 had clinically active disease, and 5 showed active disease. The 70% frequency he thought far exceeded the frequency of tuberculosis in their general population, which he claimed was only 10%. This report, however, runs into the problem of Berkson's fallacy (1). Berkson pointed out that the association of two diseases especially when found in a hospital population, either one of which would be enough to cause hospitalization of the patient and especially necropsy, can lead to a falsely high picture of association. This consideration probably reduces the importance of the association claimed by the author in his paper.

A number of cases reported from Japan by Nakao and his colleagues (16) reported a positive Mantoux test in 55 of 64 patients, but the authors did not believe that this was significantly higher than the average positive rate in Japan. In this series 36% of the patients studied were age 19 or under. Although the authors reported on the intensity of the test with 25 of the 55 patients showing strong reactions with papules, induration, and even ulceration it was not possible to determine if the frequency of strong reactions was any higher in the children in his cases.

The relationship between aortitis and tuberculosis has been extensively studied in Mexico. Lupi-Herrera and his colleagues (14) looked at a group of 107 patients. In 77% the age of onset was between 10 and 20. In these patients, 14% had tuberculous adenopathy, 7% had a history of tuberculous adenopathy, one had pulmonary tuberculosis, and one had tuberculosis of the hip. Erythema induratum was found in 26%, so that 48% of the patients had either active or previous tuberculosis infection. The PPD reaction was positive in 81% compared to 66% in the normal Mexican population. These authors also reported that some of their patients had a strong reaction. In previous studies this group found that intradermal reactions to *Mycobacterium kansasii* antigens was found in 84% and to *Mycobacterium avium* antigens in 78% of the Takayasu population. In their control population positivity to these antigens was only 11 to 15%. These authors thus believed that tuberculosis does play an important role in the etiology of Takayasu's aortitis.

From South Africa (27) a study of 8 children found all to have strongly positive Mantoux tests. These investigators thought that the strong reaction in all of their patients, although tuberculosis was common in the population, was unusual in its severity. They further reported that 5 of their 8 patients showed evidence of tuberculosis on x-ray film examination or at autopsy. However, they were unable to isolate the organism from the aorta.

Another study from Mexico reporting 6 children with aortitis (11) found a strongly positive tuberculin reaction in 5 of the 6. They also reported that there was no history of tuberculosis in the families of these children, who ranged in age from 5 to 12 years. They noted that the 5 patients with tuberculosis were females, the 1 male patient not showing a positive tuberculin test. These authors also claimed that this disease is related to tuberculosis.

A report in the United States has again strongly revived the association between Takayasu's arteritis and tuberculosis in children. Pantell and Goodman (18) reported a case of a 12-year-old child from South Carolina who showed arteritis within a month of the appearance of tuberculous cervical adenitis. There was a strong history of tuberculosis in the family; her father had cavitary tuberculosis when the patient was age 2, and she herself was treated for active pulmonary tuberculosis when she was 26 months of age with a year of isoniazid therapy. These authors reviewed the association of tuberculosis with Takayasu's arteritis and showed in their review, which included most of the reports noted above, that the frequency of active tuberculosis in the individuals with Takayasu's aortitis exceeded the frequency of active tuberculosis in the general population. However, again data to prove the association of two diseases when each disease alone has symptomatology that would bring the patient to a hospital and thus lead to extensive investigation is suspect. For example, in an earlier report of a case of aortitis reported from North

Carolina (26), a 7-year-old girl showed a negative skin test for tuberculosis. These authors further pointed out that all attempts to identify or isolate the organism from aortic lesions had been unsuccessful. This author concurs with their statement that the finding of positive tuberculin reactions seem to be related to the frequency of tuberculosis in the countries where the disease has been reported most often.

In general, in reports where treatment for tuberculosis was instituted because of either the presence of active disease in the patients or the thought that tuberculosis might be an etiological factor in this disease, no improvement related to anti-tuberculosis therapy has been noted.

The markedly elevated ESR frequently noted in this condition certainly goes along with a granulomatous or inflammatory lesion and in this way shows a similarity to the findings in tuberculosis where the induction of multiple granu-lomatous lesions in the body usually leads to a markedly high ESR.

A large-scale study from several hospitals in Paris has renewed the question of the role of tuberculosis in Takayasu's disease (4). These investigators found in a study of 86 patients that 31% had had prior tuberculosis. Patients with positive Mantoux tests were significantly higher from nonmetropolitan areas than among city dwellers. Thirty-four of the group originally came from North Africa. This geographic distribution may account for the increased presence of tuberculosis.

Surgery has been done in a number of patients, and immunofluorescence studies were performed in six cases in one report. Using appropriate antiserum, there was no evidence of a deposition of any of the immunoglobulins (IgA, IgG, or IgM) or of complement factors C3 and C1q. This seemed to decrease the importance of an immunological mechanism (at least in the late stage). The authors claimed that this finding increases the possibility that tuberculosis does play a role in this disease. This series was also unusual in that there were only 55% females. The average age of their patients was 32, but the age breakdown was not given except that a child of five was the youngest patient in this series.

Gupta (7) also studied a small group of patients for immunological features. There was a 45% frequency of positive Mantoux tests, a high serum IgG level in 55% (5 of 9 patients), but only 3 had substantially elevated levels (33%). There were normal values for other immunoglobulins and low-normal values for C3 and C4. Circulating complexes were not found in any of the 9 patients studied.

Another etiological factor that has been proposed for Takayasu's disease is a genetic feature. The availability of transplantation antigens has stimulated a study in Japan by Numano et al. (17), who studied a group of patients looking for any disease-associated haplotypes. Their study was based on a review of the Japanese literature looking at the family incidence of this condition. Ten occurrences linking family members have been noted in Japan. There were three mother and daughter combinations, four sisters including one twin sister, two brothers and sisters, and one aunt and niece. Five of these groups had their HLA antigens studied. The investigators found a statistically significant high level of a haplotype composed of A9, A10, B5, or Bw40 in patients with Takayasu's disease. In a further study of 65 patients with the disease, a significantly high frequency of A10 and B5 were noted. On this basis they believed that genetic factors are strong in this disease. It is interesting to note that the appearance of the disease in most of these cases was while the patients were in their childhood. Although the information is not available, it would be interesting to find out whether the appearance of the disease is earlier in those patients having these particular haplotypes.

THERAPY

Fraga and his colleagues (5) treated a number of patients with corticosteroids and showed a favorable response to maintenance steroid therapy. Although only 1 of the 22 patients they treated was in the childhood years, the general response when the treatment was given early was good. It appears that if treatment can be given during the initial inflammatory stages of this disease a favorable response can be obtained with standard anti-inflammatory therapy. Late therapy, as indicated by several other reports, is surgery.

A case report of Takayasu's arteritis in an 11-year-old boy (3) reported that this young boy had had a strongly positive Mantoux test 3 years before being seen. At the time of admission his blood pressure was 180/80 and he showed irregularity and stenosis of the descending aorta. He was treated by surgery with correction of the first coarctation with a plastic graft. The result of the therapy was a decrease in the hypertension, with the final blood pressure being 120/70. This case again seems to show that surgery can be effective in the treatment of children with this syndrome.

Gupta and his colleagues (8) described two cases in children: one an 11-year-old girl and one a 9-year-old girl, each of whom presented with cardiac failure. Both children had an elevated ESR; the first had a value of 50 and the second of 35. Both had hypertension, and both had a positive Mantoux test. An aortogram on the first child showed diffuse narrowing of the descending thoracic and upper abdominal aorta. In the second the aortogram showed a diffuse stricture of the descending thoracic aorta with maximum constriction just above the diaphragm. The second child was operated and had a Dacron prothesis inserted. The child did well. The first child, who was not operated on, died.

The authors in this case beleived that the main cause of heart failure in these children was the hypertension caused by the stricture of the descending aorta. The aortoplasty procedure was devised for use in a child as the child would be likely to outgrow a long bypass graft.

CONCLUSION

It thus appears that Takayasu's aortitis, though a rare disease in general and more particularly regarded as a disease of young women, looms large in this limited framework as a disease of the childhood years. In countries such as Mexico, Japan, and South Africa where the disease is well recognized, there is reported high frequency in children. Its apparent rarity in other countries may be due to a lack of recognition. There might also be different etiological factors present in these countries. Aortitis will remain an unknown threat during the childhood years unless it is considered in the differential diagnosis of a child with a number of nonspecific complaints.

REFERENCES

1. Berkson, J. (1946): Limitations of the application of fourfold table analysis to hospital data. *Biomet. Bull.*, 2:47–53.
2. Currier, R. D., Dejong, R. N., and Bole, G. C. (1954): Pulseless disease: Central nervous system manifestation. *Neurology (NY)*, 4:818–830.
3. Dedios, R. M., Pey, J., Cazzaniga, M., Villaran, E. S., Espino, R. F., Brito, J. M., and Cerezo, L. (1980): Coronary arterial stenosis and subclavian steel in Takayasu's arteritis. *Eur. J. Cardiol.*, 12:229–234.
4. Fiessinger, J. N., Tawfik-Taher, S., Capron, L., Laurian, C., Cormier, J. M., Camilleri, J. P., and Housset, E. (1982): Maladie de Takayasu: Criteres diagnostiques. *Nouve. Presse Med.*, 20:583–586.
5. Fraga, A., Mintz, G., Valle, L., and Flores-Izquierdo, G. 1972): Takayasu's arteritis: Frequency of systemic manifestations (study of 22 patients) and favorable response to maintenance steroid therapy with adrenocorticosteroids (12 patients). *Arthritis Rheum.*, 15:617–624.
6. Gonzalez-Cerna, J. L., Villavicencio, L., Molina, B., and Bessudo, L. (1967): Nonspecific obliterative aortitis in children. *Ann. Thorac. Surg.*, 4:193–204.
7. Gupta, S. (1981): Surgical and immunological aspects of Takayasu's disease. *Ann. R. Coll. Surg. Engl.*, 63:325–332.
8. Gupta, S., Goswani, B, Ghosh, D. C., and Sen Gupta, A. N. (1981): Middle aortic syndrome as a cause of heart failure in children and its management. *Thorax*, 36:63–65.
9. Ishikawa, K. (1978): Natural history and classification of occlusive thromboaortopathy (Takayasu's disease). *Circulation*, 57:27–35.
10. Ishikawa, K. (1981): Survival and morbidity after diagnosis of occlusive thromboaortopathy (Takayasu's disease). *Am. J. Cardiol.*, 47:1026–1032.
11. Kinare, S. G. (1969): Aortitis in early life in India and its association with tuberculosis. *J. Pathol.*, 100:69–76.
12. Lande, A., Bard, R., Rossi, P., Passariello, R., and Castrucci, A. (1976): Takayasu's arteritis: A worldwide entity. *N.Y. State J. Med.*, 76;1477–1482.
13. Lee, K., Sohn, K., Hong, C., Kang, S., and Berg, K. (1967): Primary arteritis (pulseless disease) in Korean children. *Acta Paediatr. Scand.*, 56:526–536.
14. Lupi-Herrera, E., Sanchez-Torres, G., Marcushamer, J., Mispireta, J., Horwitz, S., and Vela, J. (1977): Takayasu's arteritis: Clinical study of 107 cases. *Am Heart J.*, 93:94–103.
15. Munoz, N., and Correa, P. (1970): Arteritis of the aorta and its major branches. *Am. Heart J.*, 80:319–328.
16. Nakao, K., Ikeda, M., Kimata, S., Niitani, H., Miyahara, M., Ishimi, Z., Hashiba, K., Takeda, Y., Ozawa, T., Matsushita, S., and Kuramochi, M. (1967): Takayasu's arteritis: Clinical report of eighty-four cases and immunological studies of seven cases. *Circulation*, 35:1141–1155.
17. Numano, F., Isohisa, I., Maezawa, H., and Juji, T. (1979): HLA-A antigens in Takayasu's disease. *Am. Heart J.*, 98:153–159.
18. Pantell, R. H., and Goodman, B. W., Jr. (1981): Takayasu's arteritis: The relationship with tuberculosis. *Pediatrics*, 67:84–88.
19. Paton, B. C., Chartikavanij, K., Buri, P., Prachuabmoh, K., and Jumbala, M. R. B. (1965): Obliterative aortic disease in children in the tropics. *Circulation [Suppl. 1]*, 31/32:I197–I202.
20. Restrepo, C., Tejeda, C., and Correa, P. (1969): Nonsyphilitic aortitis. *Arch. Pathol.*, 87:1–12.
21. Rose, A., and Sinclair-Smith, C. C. (1980): Takayasu's arteritis. *Arch. Pathol. Lab. Med.*, 104:231–237.
22. Schrire, V., and Asherson, R. A. (1964): Arteritis of the aorta and its major branches. *Q. J. Med.*, 33:439–463.
23. Ueda, H., Ito, I., and Saito, Y. (1965): Studies on arteritis with special reference to pulseless disease and its diagnosis. *Naika*, 15:239–256.
24. Ueda, H., Morooka, S., Ito, I., Yamaguchi, H., Takeda, T., and Saito, Y. (1969): Clinical observation of 52 cases of aortitis syndrome. *Jpn. Heart J.*, 10:277–288.

25. Wagener, H. P. (1958): The ocular lesions of pulseless disease. *Am. J. Med. Sci.*, 235:220–234.
26. Warshaw, J. B., and Spach, M. S. (1965): Takayasu's disease (primary aortitis) in childhood: Case report with review of literature. *Pediatrics*, 35:620–626.
27. Wiggelinkhuizen, J., and Cremin, B. J. (1978): Takayasu arteritis and renovascular hypertension in childhood. *Pediatrics*, 62:209–217.

Aortitis: Clinical, Pathologic, and Radiographic
Aspects, edited by A. Lande, Y. M. Berkmen, and
H. A. McAllister. Raven Press, New York © 1986.

Neurologic Aspects of Aortitis

John C. M. Brust

*Department of Clinical Neurology, Columbia University College of Physicians and
Surgeons, New York, New York 10027; and Department of Neurology, Harlem Hospital,
New York, New York 10037*

The frequency of neurologic symptoms and signs in aortitis (particularly in Takayasu's disease) is not really known, for many case reports and clinical series of "aortic arch syndrome" or "pulseless disease" have presumed a diagnosis without pathologic verification (39,40,97,114). The converse—determining the incidence of aortitis within a stroke population—is also uncertain (2). The first autopsy case of neurologic symptoms and marked stenosis of aortic arch vessels was reported by Yelloly in 1823 (186); the patient was a 58-year-old man with syncopal attacks and probably both syphilis and atherosclerosis. Davy (33) described two patients, aged 55 and 36, who had syncope and decreased arm and neck pulses for several years before death. In one, postmortem examination revealed a dissecting aortic aneurysm and occlusion of the three great vessels off the aortic arch; the diagnosis was probable syphilis, although the patient had been severely wounded at the Battle of Waterloo 24 years before. The second patient had only a cursory autopsy, and no diagnosis was reached.

Focal cerebral symptoms with absent arm and neck pulses were first described in 1855 by Gull (50) in a 41-year-old woman with right hemiplegia but in whom autopsy similarly failed to determine a cause. Perhaps the first description of Takayasu's arteritis was by Savory (151) in 1856: A 22-year-old woman had dyspnea, left limb fatigue, orthostatic visual dimming, and eventually left blindness. Prior to death she developed a gangrenous area over the left parietal calvarium which extended through the bone to the cerebral cortex. At gross pathologic examination, the author noted, "the main arteries of both upper extremities and the left side of the neck were throughout completely obliterated." Syphilis, although unlikely in this patient, could not be excluded.

The descriptions half a century later by Takayasu, Onishi, and Kagoshima (169) were strictly clinical and did not mention other than visual symptoms. Although "Takayasu's arteritis" has since been recognized as a disease entity (6,20,72,142), the terms "aortic arch syndrome," "pulseless disease," and "Takayasu's arteritis" have not always been rigorously defined, and have sometimes been used synonymously. Currier et al. (29) in 1954 culled from the literature 40 patients who had either completely absent arm and neck pulses or, at most, a patent radial pulse or a "doubtfully pulsatile" or only "minimally patent" common carotid artery, and in whom clinical descriptions were reasonably extensive. By these criteria the patients of Savory and of Takayasu were excluded. Of the 40 patients, 12 were considered to have had probable arteritis, but in none was that diagnosis certain. The authors' own patient was a 32-year-old woman with multiple strokes and syphilis.

Nine years later Judge et al. (72) stressed the need to distinguish between the broad terms "pulseless disease," "aortic arch syndrome," and Takayasu's arteritis and, observing that more than 140 patients with the latter had by then been reported, described four of their own, one of whom had left hemiparesis, bulbar palsy, and optic atrophy. Only one of their patients had an autopsy, and another, who had neither an aortogram nor a postmortem examination, was 61 years old. The diagnosis of Takayasu's arteritis was apparently based on hyperglobulinemia and an eythrocyte sedimentation rate (ESR) of 38 mm/hr.

The same year Riehl (140), addressing the "neurological implications" of "the idiopathic arteritis of Takayasu," described six patients, none with postmortem examinations. One, a 46-year-old man with sudden left hemiparesis, had positive serologic tests for syphilis, which, because the *Treponema* immobilizing test was negative, were considered to represent biologic false positivity. Another, a 22-year-old woman with sudden right hemiparesis and aphasia, had narrowed left common and internal carotid arteries with "segmental constrictions (beading)"; the aortic arch and other major vessels were normal, and so although such proximal location would be unusual this woman may in fact have had fibromuscular dysplasia (123).

The predisposition of the inflamed aorta to develop premature atherosclerosis is another reason for occasional diagnostic ambiguity, even when autopsy is performed (139). Thus diagnostic certainty is not always present even in reports purportedly focusing on aortitis of Takayasu's type. The significance of such vagary to a neurologist is that although the "aortic arch syndrome" is stereotypical enough the underlying disease, e.g., Takayasu's arteritis, syphilis, atherosclerosis, giant cell arteritis, other connective tissue diseases, or radiation injury (88,175), might cause neurologic symptoms and signs of its own.

NEUROLOGIC MANIFESTATIONS OF AORTIC ARCH SYNDROME

What, then, are the neurologic manifestations of the "syndrome of obliteration of the supra-aortic branches" (107) regardless of cause? Ischemia of the brain or eye may begin as transient ischemic attacks (TIAs) or as fixed occlusive strokes. Headache, vertigo, dizziness, amaurosis fugax, and transient focal deficts (e.g., hemiparesis, hemisensory loss or paresthesias, aphasia, homonymous hemianopia, unilateral or bilateral blindness, or bulbar signs) depend on the vascular territory affected, and there is nothing about these TIAs or brain infarcts that points specifically to aortic arch diease (94). Symptoms may, however, be strikingly precipitated by neck turning or extension, standing up, walking, or exercise. Headache may be severe and dominate the clinical picture (21). Syncope has been reported in 6 to 62% of patients (153) and seizures in 6 to 23% (142,152), an unexpectedly high frequency for intermittent focal cerebral ischemia and attributed in some cases to hypersensitivity of the carotid sinus baroreceptor (11,20,70,73,82,83,92,

105,122,142,146–148,158,159,179). Internal carotid artery compression often pre-cipitates such symptoms, and relief reportedly follows denervation of the carotid sinus and removal of the carotid body (158). In another report (1) elevated plasma renin activity disappeared after carotid sinus denervation. However, reduced bar-oreceptor sensitivity has been reported in atherosclerotic rabbits (5) as well as in patients with Takayasu's arteritis (170), and so it seems likely that dizziness, syncope, or seizures occurring with neck compression are caused in many instances not by baroreceptor-mediated bradycardia or hypotension but by a critical decrease in already borderline cerebral perfusion.

Other frequently encountered neurologic symptoms include gait ataxia, tinnitus or deafness, diplopia, dysphagia, and facial weakness (54,105,115,155). Vertigo may, like syncope, be precipitated by standing or head-turning (174). Dysarthria occurs either on a central basis or secondary to direct lingual ischemia (14,158). Jaw muscle claudication is common (6,21,44,73,137); in one report (73) an affected middle-aged woman had to give up chewing gum. Paraplegia has followed spinal cord ischemia (100).

Mental abnormalities are not unusual (10,109,147,156); in one series 38% of patients had decreased concentration or memory (153). Reported mental changes also include depression (175), irritability or "bad temper" (6), anxiety (166), and emotional incontinence including a vague "neurasthenic reaction" (18,173). Pro-gressive mental deterioration has been described (142), but most reports of "low IQ" have lacked premorbid baselines (42,82).

Ischemic ophthalmologic symptoms and signs, described in detail elsewhere (see Baum, *this volume*), include eye pain, photophobia, and blurred vision or blindness. Amaurosis fugax sometimes occurs with exercise, resembling Uthoff's syndrome in multiple sclerosis (134), or with neck extension (6,42), accounting for a char-acteristic "head flexion" posture (6,19,42,100,124,150,154). A 19-year-old girl had difficulty seeing on arising in the morning (44). Such symptoms might lead to neurologic rather than ophthalmologic referral, as may hyperemic or atrophic optic discs (92,177), retinal hemorrhages, mydriatic poorly reactive pupils, orbital pain, or a peculiar sensation of "the eyes being drawn into the head" (54). Keratitis, iris atrophy, cataracts, peripapillary arterial anastomoses, vitreous hemorrhage, and glaucoma are more obviously nonneurologic.

The subclavian steal syndrome (130,183), frequently diagnosed angiographically or ultrasonically in aortic arch disease, may produce brainstem ischemia (143,185) but usually is asymptomatic, especially in slowly progressive arteritides with ade-quate brainstem and upper extremity collaterals (121,187). An 11-year-old boy with Takayasu's arteritis and a subclavian steal variant—subclavian artery occlusion distal to the vertebral artery origin but significant vertebral artery stenosis, with steal from the thyrocervical trunk—was similarly asymptomatic neurologically (106).

For the same reason, symptoms of intermittent claudication of the arms, although common among patients with aortic arch disease, are less frequent than might be expected for the degree of large vessel compromise. Upper extremity pain, fatigue, weakness, or paresthesias rarely occur at rest but may be precipitated by exercise or elevation of the arms (6,42,64,72,105,107) and if a careful history is not obtained may be mistaken for transient cerebral ischemia. Pain in the arms (and nipples) has also been precipitated by cold (12). Disease of the descending aorta can cause lower extremity claudication with pain suggesting lumbosacral radiculopathy; there may even be impotence (19). Except for Raynaud's phenomenon and hyperpigmentation of the skin of the hands (125), upper extremity trophic changes such as atrophy, ulcerated fingertips, or slow nail growth occur infrequently (18,27,31,45,55,105,107). In the head, however, ischemic trophic changes are common and include: facial muscle atrophy; decalcification of cranial or jaw bones; perforation of the nasal septum; saddle nose; ulceration or gangrene of the face, tongue, ears, or palate; accelerated dental caries; loss of teeth or hair; and bleeding gums (3,17,18,20,42,55,63,70,73,105,107,108,120,122,127,154). The face may appear prematurely aged.

Involvement of other organs by aortic disease may indirectly produce neurologic symptoms. Renal artery stenosis, carotid sinus hyposensitivity, and decreased aortic distensibility may lead to systolic or diastolic hypertension (100,156), which in turn causes intracranial atherothrombotic disease, lacunar infarcts of the diencephalon or brainstem, intracerebral hemorrhage (14,181), and hypertensive encephalopathy (100). Hypertension may also contribute to visual disturbance and fundal changes (100). Paroxysmal hypertension and tachycardia with decreased vision, headache, dizziness, sweating, palpitations, and flushing suggest pheochromocytoma; in one report such symptoms occurred with micturation, mimicking pheochromocytoma of the bladder (171).

Cardiac disease may be secondary to hypertension or to involvement of the coronary arteries or cardiac valves (72). Congestive heart failure lowers cardiac output, raises intracranial pressure, and further reduces an already precarious cerebral blood flow. Cardiac arrhythmias cause syncope or seizures. Myocardial infarction sets the stage for embolic strokes via collateral circulation. Aortitis of any cause can damage the aortic valve (88) with consequent systemic or cerebral emboli, including septic emboli; brain abscess, ruptured mycotic aneurysm, or meningitis may follow.

Collateral circulation to the head in aortic arch syndrome is discussed in detail elsewhere (see Lande and Berkman, *this volume*). Except when they are affected by atherosclerosis, the vertebral arteries are usually the major suppliers of blood to the brain (13,89,127,149,175). Anastomoses are seen between internal and external carotid arteries, which probably account for the frequently encountered hyperemia of the perilimbic bulbar conjunctiva (14), between vertebral and internal carotid arteries, and between carotid arteries and the thyrocervical trunks (11), the subclavian and innominate arteries, and the aorta itself (96,136,149). The pattern of collaterals of course depends on eccentricities of the underlying disease. For example, in Takayasu's arteritis inflammation sometimes extends into the internal carotid artery all the way to the base of the skull (6,42,112), with a "characteristic filiform narrowing" (90). Single internal carotid occlusion as the only manifestation of brachiocephalic involvement has also been reported. When internal carotid artery involvement is bilateral, the vertebral arteries assume even greater importance as suppliers of blood to the entire brain, and when the vertebral arteries arise directly from the aortic arch they may be directly affected by the underlying disease process (16,51,54,152). Collaterals from the thyrocervical trunk, internal mammary arteries, or upper intercostal arteries may then provide the entire intracranial circulation (51).

Supraclavicular and cervical bruits are often prominent, including a systolic–diastolic murmur suggesting patent ductus arteriosus (100). A woman with transitory visual obscuration, dizziness, tinnitus, and arm and jaw claudication had, when lying supine, a rightward rotation of her head with each beat of her pulse (6).

SPECIFIC AORTITIDES: TAKAYASU'S ARTERITIS

Clues that a patient with aortic arch syndrome has Takayasu's arteritis include clinical and laboratory findings discussed by Spiera and Kerr *(this volume)*, especially age, sex, and in many subjects early constitutional or systemic symptoms such as fever, sweating, malaise, myalgia, arthralgia, anorexia, nausea, vomiting, weight loss, night sweats, irregular menses, skin rash (e.g., erythema nodosum), pleurisy, abdominal pain, scleritis, choroiditis, arthritis, pericarditis, and hemoptysis (3,6,12,15,23,36,46,100,119,145,164). Such symptoms may precede signs of vascular insufficiency, and during this phase of illness a neurologist is unlikely to be consulted. When a patient presents with a stroke, however, systemic symptoms can point to the nature of the underlying disease. Their nonspecificity should nonetheless be stressed: A young woman with such symptoms and a stroke could also have systemic lupus erythematosus; and temporomandibular joint arthralgia or arthritis (85) could suggest rheumatoid arthritis or lead to neurologic consultation for "atypical facial pain." Moreover, although it has been claimed that systemic symptoms occur at the outset in over 70% of cases of Takayasu's arteritis (14,119) and that such symptoms can persist for months or years before arterial compromise supervenes (164), others maintain that they occur in only a small minority (88). A young person with only neurologic symptoms raises the possibility of multiple sclerosis (164) or, if seizures occur in the presence of a normal neurologic examination, idiopathic epilepsy (146,164). Neurologic disease in otherwise healthy young children can be particularly perplexing. Autopsy reports include a documented example of Takayasu's arteritis with severe cerebral and circulatory disturbance in a 9-month-old infant (182).

In some patients the problem is initially considered emotional (45). A 16-year-old girl had easy fatigability, palpitations, and "progressively less satisfactory scholastic performance" prior to a stroke with right hemiparesis (158). For several months before an aphasic TIA a 26-year-old woman had headache, dizzy spells, frequent drowsiness, and cramps in the shoulders and arms on doing housework (63). A 28-year-old woman had headache, attacks of lightheadedness, "generalized paresthesias," and attacks of weeping (21); and a 26-year-old woman had insomnia, headaches, blurred vision, and dizziness (86). A 34-year-old woman was considered to have anorexia nervosa: Epigastric pain aggravated by food led to anorexia, nausea, vomiting, and a 40-pound weight loss; there was also, however, angina pectoris and upper extremity intermittent claudication. Autopsy revealed aortitis (41).

In some patients with Takayasu's arteritis, during the stage of systemic symptoms there is tenderness over the subclavian or carotid arteries (11,14,82,119), mimicking carotidynia, a migraine variant (138). Severe neck pain or pain beneath the chin or in the tongue (125,126) may occur only on swallowing, with radiation to the head, shoulders, arms, fingers, or back (63,165).

Vessels affected by Takayasu's arteritis tend to be spared distally (54), and intracranial involvement has been reported so rarely as to invite skepticism (141); in some cases hypertensive cerebrovascular disease is the likelier culprit.

Like other aortitides, Takayasu's arteritis can affect the distal aorta preferentially, leading to leg pain or other symptoms of vascular insufficiency (168). Spinal cord ischemia has produced myelopathy suggesting multiple sclerosis (34).

Neurologic symptoms in Takayasu's arteritis can be mild or severe (81,118). Patients may live for decades, but the appearance of recurrent neurologic deficits is a grave prognostic sign: Such patients do not usually survive more than 5 years (14), although some do develop adequate collaterals and their symptoms plateau or even improve (14). In Lupi-Herrera et al.'s (100) series of 107 patients seen over 19 years (diagnostic criteria were clinical and angiographic; only 28% had histologic confirmation, and patients over age 35 were excluded), 14 died but only one from a stroke, said to be a cerebral hemorrhage. Neurologic symptoms were common, however: 61 patients had headache, 14 syncope, 8 hemiplegia, 1 paraplegia, and 4 "hypertensive encephalopathy" [an oft-overdiagnosed entity (58)]. Neurologic (and cardiovascular) symptoms were especially prominent in patients with advanced arterial obstruction and collaterals when they first became symptomatic.

The 84 patients of Nakao et al. (119) were diagnosed on the basis of symptoms and signs; only 30 had aortograms, and onset began from age 11 to 48. Some therefore probably had arteriosclerosis. Neurologic symptoms such as dizziness, syncope, headache, or decreased vision were mentioned but not quantitated. Six patients died, three from acute heart failure, one from massive ovarian bleeding, and two from unexplained sudden death. Apparently no patient had a stroke.

The diagnosis of Takayasu's arteritis in Ishikawa's (68) series of 54 patients, seen during an 18-year period, was based variably on clinical manifestations, angiography, or autopsy. Onset was from age 9 to 43. Of eight deaths, three followed a stroke (one "cerebral thrombosis," one cerebral embolus, and one cerebral hemorrhage). Of surviving patients, one had a cerebral hemorrhage during the second stage of delivery, one had subarachnoid hemorrhage, and one had unilateral blindness. All three stroke deaths occurred in patients with hypertension (which was present in 59% of the total).

Fraga et al. (40) followed 22 patients over 6 years; diagnosis was based on clinical signs, arteriography, and in four instances histology. Five died of congestive heart failure, cardiac arrest with surgery, uremia, "multiple thromboses of systemic arteries," and "obliteration of the innominate and left renal artery stenosis." Although none died of stroke, neurologic symptoms were common: 19 had headache, 15 limb paresthesias, 10 dizziness, 1 tinnitus, and 1 hemiplegia. The authors, reviewing 306 cases from the literature they thought met criteria for Takayasu's arteritis, stated that three-fourths of all patients had died within 2 years of symptomatic onset.

Sano and Saito's (148) 77 patients were diagnosed on the basis of absent radial pulses; not all had aortography, and histology, mentioned in only a few instances, concerned immunologic studies. Inasmuch as 74 patients were female with age of onset 8 to 40, the great majority probably did have Takayasu's arteritis. During follow-up of 1 to 21 years, 17 died, 2 as a result of corrective surgery, 5 from "cardiovascular insufficiency," 1 from nephrosis, 3 incidentally, 3 of unknown cause, and 3 from "cerebral embolism." Neurologic symptoms were common. Fifty-one percent of patients presented with dizziness or syncope, 40% with upper extremity coldness, paresthesias, or fatigability, and 14% with decreased visual acuity or restricted visual fields. Completed stroke with hemiplegia or hemiparesis occurred in 6.2%, "worsening stroke" in 2.5%, and TIA in 28.6%. (It was not stated if any of these patients were the same as those who died of "cerebral embolism.")

The 64 patients of Morooka et al. (116) were followed 3 months to 15 years. Criteria for diagnosis were not given. Thirteen died, 4 of congestive heart failure, 3 of cerebral hemorrhage, 2 of cerebral infarct, 2 operatively, 1 of respiratory paralysis, and 1 from suicide. The authors noted that hypertension predisposed patients to stroke but did not say how many survivors were so afflicted.

SYPHILITIC AORTITIS

Syphilis was so prevalent in the nineteenth century (9,33,50,186) that syphilitic aortitis was undoubtedly overdiagnosed, and series probably contain patients with Takayasu's arteritis (103,120). Although syphilitic aortitis has become less common, as recently as 1964 it was considered to account for "the largest single group of aortic inflammatory lesions" (59). As the following patient demonstrates, syphilitic aortitis can present neurologically.

Case Report

A 56-year-old nurse in 1978 developed diffuse continuous headache and, 3 weeks later, diplopia. Hospitalized, she had normal vital signs and pulses, and the only abnormality on examination was a complete left oculomotor palsy. Abnormal laboratory values included 10,400 white blood cells/ml (78% polymorphonuclears, 14% lymphocytes, 4% monocytes, and 3% eosinophils), ESR 73 mm/hr, and reactive serum FTA. Serum VDRL, however, was negative. Cerebrospinal fluid (CSF) was normal, including serology, as were computed tomography (CT) scans, edrophonium test, chest radiograph, blood glucose level, and temporal artery biopsy. She received prednisone with immediate clearing of headache and gradual resolution of ophthalmoparesis. A year later, however, she was readmitted with sudden left hemiparesis, facial weakness, and sensory loss. The ESR and CSF were normal. Initially improving, she was found unresponsive 4 days later, with electro-cardiographic (ECG) evidence of myocardial infarction. She died the same day. At autopsy there was syphilitic arteritis involving the thoracic and abdominal aorta and the right brachiocephalic, left common carotid, and left subclavian arteries. Multiple mural thrombi were seen on the ascending aorta, and there was recent infarction of the right frontoparietal cerebrum. Atherosclerosis was minimal except for a plaque in the left anterior descending coronary artery. Myocardial fibrosis was present in the left ventricle.

Syphilitic aortitis can cause neurologic symptoms indistinguishable from those encountered in other diseases affecting the aortic arch (9,16,25,49,75,87,129, 150,159,172,176,178). Cerebral emboli can be either from mural thrombi, as in this patient, or from thrombi forming within an aneurysmal sac (156). Cerebral infarction can also follow occlusion of the great vessels themselves from either scarring, aneurysm formation and secondary thrombosis, or compression of the great vessels by giant syphilitic aneurysms (16,25,27,75,156). Aneurysms of the ascending aorta can obstruct the superior vena cava, causing a superior vena caval syndrome with increased intracranial pressure. Aneurysms of the transverse aorta produce dysphagia by compressing the esophagus or dysarthria by compressing the trachea or the recurrent laryngeal nerve (74).

How often syphilitic aortitis causes neurologic disease is difficult to estimate, for in many older patients hypertensive or atherosclerotic cerebrovascular disease exists independently. For example, of 100 autopsy cases of syphilitic aortitis re-ported by Heggvett (59) (the diagnosis was suspected during life in only 17), stroke was considered the cause of death in 16, two of whom had been receiving antico-agulation therapy for "thromboembolic disease," but neither clinical nor pathologic details of these patients were offered (e.g., their ages, whether their strokes were considered clinically to be embolic, or whether at autopsy mural thrombi were present on the luetic aortas).

In an analysis of 1,330 patients with syphilis, 202 were found to have cardio-vascular disease (101). The majority of these had no symptoms; some had dyspnea, angina pectoris, or palpitations; none had neurologic symptoms except for 4 with aneurysms and hoarseness. In a further study of 61 patients with "uncomplicated syphilitic aortitis" (66) (no aortic regurgitation or aneurysm), 10 died, 4 from stroke, but it was unclear if the strokes had anything to do with the syphilitic aortitis.

Because 10 to 30% of patients with luetic aortitis have negative serology (59,74), the diagnosis is not usually considered when focal neurologic symptoms occur without radiographic aortic abnormalities. Kampmeier (74) stressed, "the diagnosis of cardiovascular syphilis in the absence of aortic regurgitation, aneurysm, or narrowing of the coronary artery is for all practical purposes impossible." Yet treatment must be given before such complications develop to prevent catastrophes.

Syphilitic aortitis may coexist with neurosyphilis, including general paresis, tabes dorsalis, or meningovascular syphilis. General paresis causes mental changes rarely encountered in aortic arch syndrome, and tabes dorsalis is a sensory radiculopathy unrelated to spinal cord vascular insufficiency. Meningovascular syphilis infrequently affects large cerebral vessels (113), and therefore major strokes are unusual. Either aortic arch syndrome or meningovascular lues can cause headache, optic atrophy, or dementia, however.

GIANT CELL (TEMPORAL) ARTERITIS

Giant cell arteritis often presents neurologically, but infrequently from involvement of the aortic arch. Although weakness is not a feature of polymyalgia rheumatica, such patients are sometimes referred to neurologists for consideration of polymyositis. Headache occurs in 60% of patients, jaw claudication in 36%, and unilateral or bilateral blindness in one-third (48). Visual loss may be sudden, with both eyes affected days or weeks apart, or there may first be amaurosis fugax. Other neurologic symptoms include vertigo, diplopia, facial neuralgia, tongue claudication, depression, and confusional states. Synovitis at the wrist has led to carpal tunnel syndrome (57). There may be tenderness over the carotid as well as the temporal arteries (53).

Strokes are well documented in giant cell arteritis and include infarction in the territories of the middle and anterior cerebral arteries (22,28,38,43,60–62,77,111,132,167) or the vertebral-basilar system (26,32,60,111,132,135). In such patients the arteritic process most often involves the internal carotid arteries in their petrous or intracavernous portions and the vertebral arteries cervically, without affecting the cerebral vessels themselves. Strokes are often embolic.

When, as occurred in 34 of 248 patients in one series (78), giant cell arteritis affects primarily the aortic arch (4,46,52,56,76,98,161,162) or its major branches (163), a syndrome indistinguishable from Takayasu's arteritis may ensue (35,52,65,69) including systemic symptoms and elevated ESR. Reported series of either giant cell arteritis or Takayasu's arteritis lacking autopsies are each probably contaminated by inclusion of the other disease, and sometimes even postmortem examination fails to relieve diagnostic uncertainty (7,8,82). Giant cell arteritis is rare in patients under age 50, and Takayasu's arteritis is predominantly a disease of young adults, although an individual patient can be an exception to a general rule (52). Giant cell arteritis with aortic arch syndrome causes strokes either by thrombotic occlusion of the great vessels or by emboli from mural thrombi. Dissecting aneurysms, which can acutely occlude vessels supplying the brain, are not unusual in giant cell arteritis (98,110), in contrast to their great rarity in aortitis from Takayasu's disease or syphilis (88).

THROMBOANGIITIS OBLITERANS (BUERGER'S DISEASE)

Although the nosologic status of Buerger's disease remains unclear, it is believed to represent a disease entity (37). Reports of its association with aortic arch syndrome have mostly been unsubstantiated by autopsy (20,42,49,84,85,104,105, 107,122,142), but a few well-documented cases do exist, some with neurologic presentation. For example (11), a 54-year-old man had 2 weeks of progressive confusion and then decreased alertness, dysphagia, and "speech disturbances." Pulses were absent in arms and neck, but he was hypertensive in his legs. Five years earlier he had had a stroke with hemiplegia and 2 years afterward gait disturbance, vertigo, and hand paresthesias. Autopsy revealed thromboangiitis obliterans with occlusion of the subclavian and carotid arteries. Buerger's disease probably can also affect intracranial vessels, although early reports describing such effects predated current sophistication regarding the arteritides (93,95,99).

IDIOPATHIC AORTITIS IN CHILDREN

Isaacson (67) in 1961 described six African children, aged 7 to 16, with hypertension secondary to aortitis. In three there were seizures, coma, and death, considered hypertensive encephalopathy, although the only brain examined was normal and fibrinoid arteriolitis was not seen in organs of any patient. "Panaortitis" was histologically indistinguishable from Takayasu's arteritis, yet the author, on the basis of the young ages of the patients and the propensity for the disease to affect the descending aorta, with hypertension and a fulminating course, believed it represented "a different as yet unnamed disease entity." Similar patients have been described in Africa (71), India (157), Singapore (30), and Thailand (131) in reports emphasizing the absence of aortic arch syndrome and the frequency of hypertension and its cerebral complications, including seizures. More typical Takayasu's arteritis also occurs in Africa (155), but that does not answer the question of whether a similar but distinct disease affecting children exists there as well.

TRANSIENT EMBOLIGENIC AORTOARTERITIS

A report from Sri Lanka (184) described 10 patients, aged 16 to 36, with strokes (hemiparesis or hemiplegia in 8, quadriparesis in 1, and cerebellar and brainstem signs in 1) secondary to emboli from disease of the aorta or its major branches. Patchy active or healed inflammatory lesions with fragmented elastic lamellae were seen in vessel walls beneath mural thrombi. The lesions were more focal and transient than those of Takayasu's arteritis, and "transient emboligenic aortoarteritis" was therefore considered a "new disease entity," possibly accounting for some previously unexplained cases of stroke in the young, including moyamoya disease (160). Further studies are needed to test the validity of the notion that transient emboligenic aortoarteritis is separate from Takayasu's arteritis.

MISCELLANEOUS AND PROBLEMATIC AORTITIDES

Aortitis in association with other connective tissue or immunologic diseases such as acute rheumatic fever (80), rheumatoid arthritis (24,36,119,180,188), ankylosing spondylitis (24,125), Reiter's syndrome (47,133), systemic lupus erythematosus

(91,125), polyarteritis nodosa (12), scleroderma (144), and relapsing polychondritis (88) is discussed by Spiera and Kerr *(this volume)*. These diseases can affect the nervous system independently of aortitis, causing, for example, chorea or behavioral disturbance in acute rheumatic fever, seizures or psychosis in systemic lupus erythematosus, or mononeuritis multiplex in polyarteritis nodosa.

Mycotic aneurysms of the aorta (88,128) are usually the result of bacterial endocarditis, which can otherwise cause cerebral infarction, brain abscess, meningitis, or cerebral mycotic aneurysms. Infectious granulomatous aortitis [e.g., tuberculosis or nematode infestation (79,117,128,131,158)] is rare, although, as discussed by Virmani and McAllister *(this volume)*, these organisms have been invoked etiologically in Takayasu's arteritis (100,102). When it occurs, the nervous system may be independently involved (e.g., tuberculous meningitis, brain tuberculomas, or Pott's disease).

Pseudoxanthoma elasticum can cause aortic arch syndrome (12), but strokes are more often the result of hypertension or of direct cardiac or cerebrovascular involvement.

REFERENCES

1. Abe, K., Miyazaki, S., Kusaka, T., Irokawa, N., and Aoyagi, H. (1976): Elevated plasma renin activity in aortitis syndrome. *Jpn. Heart J.*, 17:1–11.
2. Abraham, J., Shetty, G., and Jose, C. J. (1971): Strokes in the young. *Stroke*, 2:258–267.
3. Aggeler, P. M., Lucia, S. P., and Thompson, J. H. (1941): A syndrome due to the occlusion of all the arteries arising from the aortic arch: Report of a case featured by primary thrombocytosis and autohemagglutination. *Am. Heart J.*, 22:825–834.
4. Alestig, K., and Barr, J. (1963): Giant cell arteritis: A biopsy study of polymyalgia rheumatica, including one case of Takayasu's disease. *Lancet*, 1:1228–1230.
5. Angell-James, J. E. (1974): Arterial baroreceptor activity in rabbits with experimental atherosclerosis. *Circ. Res.*, 34:27–39.
6. Ask-Upmark, E. (1954): On the pulseless disease outside of Japan. *Acta Med. Scand.*, 149:161–178.
7. Austen, W. G., and Blennerhassett, J. B. (1965): Giant cell aortitis causing an aneurysm of the ascending aorta and aortic regurgitation. *N. Engl. J. Med.*, 272:80–83.
8. Barker, N. W., and Edwards, J. E. (1955): Primary arteritis of the aortic arch. *Circulation*, 11:486–492.
9. Barker, W. F. (1949): Syphilitic aortitis with obstruction of multiple aortic ostia. *N. Engl. J. Med.*, 241:524–527.
10. Benchimol, A. B., Schlesinger, P., Anache, M., and Carneiro, R. D. (1962): Pulseless disease: A clinical, hemodynamic and angiographic study of 6 cases. *Mal. Cardiovasc.*, 3:489–519.
11. Bernsmeier, A., and Held, K. (1972): The aortic arch syndrome. In: *Handbook of Clinical Neurology*, Vol. 12, edited by P. Vinken and G. W. Bruyn, pp. 398–421. North Holland, Amsterdam.
12. Birke, G., Ejrup, B., and Olhagen, B. (1957): Pulseless disease: A clinical analysis of ten cases. *Angiology*, 8:433–455.
13. Bloss, R. S., Duncan, J. M., Cooley, D. A., Leatherman, L. L., and Schnee, M. J. (1978): Takayasu's arteritis: Surgical considerations. *Ann. Thorac. Surg.*, 27:574–579.
14. Bonventre, M. V. (1974): Takayasu's disease, revisited. *N.Y. State J. Med.*, 74:1960–1967.
15. Breutsch, W. L. (1971): Aortic arch syndrome (Takayasu's arteritis, pulseless disease). In: *Pathology of the Nervous System*, Vol. 2, edited by Minekler, J., pp. 1488–1499. McGraw-Hill, New York.
16. Broadbent, W. A. (1875): Absence of pulsation in both radial arteries, the vessels being full of blood. *Trans. Clin. Soc. Lond.*, 8:165.
17. Brown, C. F. (1929): Absence of pulse: Case of absence of pulse in both axillary, radial and

carotid arteries, while normal in femoralis and dorsalis pedis arteries. *Chin. Med. J.*, 43:269–274.

18. Burstein, J., Lindström, B., and Wasastjerna, C. (1957): Aortic arch syndromes: A survey of five cases. *Acta Med. Scand.*, 157:365–378.

19. Bustamante, R. A., Milanes, B., Casas, R., and de la Torre, A. (1954): The chronic subclavian-carotid obstruction syndrome (pulseless disease). *Angiology*, 5:479–485.

20. Caccamise, W. C., and Whitman, J. F. (1952): Pulseless disease: A preliminary case report. *Am. Heart J.*, 44:629–633.

21. Caldwell, R. A., and Skipper, E. W. (1961): Pulseless disease: A report of 5 cases. *Br. Heart J.*, 23:53–65.

22. Castleman, B., and Towne, V. (1976): Case records of the Massachusetts General Hospital. *N. Engl. J. Med.*, 295:944–950.

23. Christian, C. L., and Sargeant, J. S. (1976): Vasculitis syndromes: Clinical and experimental models. *Am. J. Med.*, 61:385–392.

24. Clark, S. W., Kulka, J. P., and Bauer, W. (1957): Rheumatoid aortitis with aortic regurgitation. *Am. J. Med.*, 22:580–592.

25. Cohen, H., and Davie, T. B. (1933): Bilateral obliteration of radial and carotid pulses in aortic aneurysm. *Lancet*, 1:852–855.

26. Cooke, W. T., Cloake, P. C. P., Govan, A. D. T., and Colbeck, J. C. (1946): Temporal arteritis: A generalized vascular disease. *Q. J. Med.*, 15:47–75.

27. Crawford, I. R. (1921): Bilateral pulse obliteration in thoracic aneurysm. *JAMA*, 76:1395–1396.

28. Crompton, M. R. (1959): The visual changes in temporal (giant-cell) arteritis. *Brain*, 82:377–390.

29. Currier, R. D., DeJong, R. N., and Bole, G. G. (1954): Pulseless disease: Central nervous system manifestations. *Neurology (NY)*, 4:818–830.

30. Damaraj, T. J., Wang, H. O., and Thomas, M. A. (1963): Primary arteritis of aorta causing renal artery stenosis and hypertension. *Br. Heart J.*, 25:153–165.

31. Darling, S. T., and Clark, H. C. (1915): Arteritis syphilitica obliterans. *J. Med. Res.*, 32:1–26.

32. Das, A. K., and Laskin, D. M. (1966): Temporal arteritis of the facial artery. *J. Oral Surg.*, 24:226–232.

33. Davy, J. (1839): Notice of a case in which the arteria innominata and the left subclavian and carotid arteries were closed without loss of life. *Res. Physiol. Anat.* Cited by A. Bernsmeier and K. Held, ref. 11.

34. Ederli, A., Lo-Russo, F., Natali, G., and Carratelli, D. (1978): Pulseless disease (clinical case with unusual neurologic manifestations). *Riv. Neurobiol.*, 24:115–120.

35. Editorial (1965): Arteritis of the aorta and its branches. *Lancet*, 1:642–643.

36. Falicov, R. E., and Cooney, D. F. (1964): Takayasu's arteritis and rheumatoid arthritis: A case report. *Arch. Intern. Med.*, 114:594–600.

37. Fauci, A. S., Haynes, B. F., and Katz, P. (1978): The spectrum of vasculitis: Clinical, pathologic, immunologic, and therapeutic considerations. *Ann. Intern. Med.*, 89:660–676.

38. Ferris, E. J., and Levine, H. L. (1973): Cerebral arteritis: Classification. *Radiology*, 109:327–341.

39. Follmann, P., Littman, J., Heszberger, I., Ura, I. L., and Kali, A. (1970): Ophthalmodynamography and ophthalmodynamometry in the aortic arch and the subclavian steal syndromes. *Acta Chir. Acad. Sci. Hung.*, 11:149–161.

40. Fraga, A., Mintz, G., Valle, L., and Flores-Izquierdo, G. (1972): Takayasu's arteritis: Frequency of systemic manifestations (study of 22 patients) and favorable response to maintenance steroid therapy with adrenocorticosteroids. *Arthritis Rheum.*, 15:617–624.

41. Frank, N., and Frank, M. J. (1973): Pulseless disease producing abdominal angina and simulating anorexia nervosa. *J. Med. Soc. N.J.*, 70:830–833.

42. Frövig, A. G., and Löken, A. C. (1951): The syndrome of obliteration of the arterial branches of the aortic arch due to arteritis: A post-mortem angiographic and pathologic study. *Acta Psychiatr. Neurol. Scand.*, 26:313–337.

43. Fulton, A. B., Lee, R. V., Jampol, L. M., Keltner, J. L., and Albert, D. M. (1976): Active giant cell arteritis with cerebral involvement. *Arch. Ophthalmol.*, 94:2068–2071.

44. Giffin, H. M. (1939): Reversed coarctation and vasomotor gradient; report of a cardiovascular anomaly with symptoms of brain tumor. *Proc. Staff Meet. Mayo Clin.*, 14:561–565.

45. Gillanders, L. A., and Strachan, R. W. (1965): The role of radiology in the diagnosis of Takayasu's arteriopathy ("pulseless disease"). *Clin. Radiol.*, 16:119–129.
46. Gilmour, J. R. (1941): Giant-cell arteritis. *J. Pathol. Bacteriol.*, 53:263–277.
47. Good, E. A. (1973): Reiter's disease: A review with special attention to cardiovascular and neurologic sequelae. *Semin. Arthritis Rheum.*, 3:253–286.
48. Goodman, B. W. (1979): Temporal arteritis. *Am. J. Med.*, 67:839–852.
49. Gremmel, H., and Schulte-Brinkmann, W. (1963): Das Aortenbogensyndrom. *Fortschr. Roentgenstr.*, 99:144–167.
50. Gull, W. (1855): Thickening and dilation of the arch of the aorta with occlusion of the innominata and left carotid: Atrophic softening of the brain. *Guys Hosp. Rep.*, 16:12.
51. Hachiya, J. (1970): Current concepts of Takayasu's arteritis. *Semin. Roentgenol.*, 5:345–359.
52. Hamilton, C. R., Shelley, W. M., and Tumulty, P. A. (1971): Giant cell arteritis: Including temporal arteritis and polymyalgia rheumatica. *Medicine (Baltimore)*, 50:1–27.
53. Hamrin, B., Jousson, N., and Landberg, T. (1965): Involvement of large vessels in polymyalgia arteritica. *Lancet*, 1:1193–1196.
54. Harbitz, F. (1926): Bilateral carotid arteritis. *Arch. Pathol. Lab. Med.*, 1:499–510.
55. Harders, H., and Wenderoth, H. (1955): Das "aortenbogensyndrom" mit Hypotonie der oberen und Hypertonie der unteren Körperhälfte. *Dtsch. Arch. Klin. Med.*, 202:194–213.
56. Harris, M. (1968): Dissecting aneurysm of the aorta due to giant cell arteritis. *Br. Heart J.*, 30:840–844.
57. Healey, L. A., and Wilskie, K. R. (1977): Manifestations of giant cell arteritis. *Med. Clin. North Am.*, 61:261–271.
58. Healton, E. B., Brust, J. C. M., Feinfeld, D. A., and Thomson, G. E. (1982): Hypertensive encephalopathy and the neurologic manifestations of malignant hypertension. *Neurology (NY)*, 32:127–132.
59. Heggvett, H. A. (1964): Syphilitic aortitis: A clinicopathologic autopsy study of 100 cases, 1950–1960. *Circulation*, 29:346–355.
60. Hepinstall, R. H., Porter, K. A., and Barkley, H. (1954): Giant cell (temporal) arteritis. *J. Pathol. Bacteriol.*, 67:507–519.
61. Hinck, V. C., Carter, C. C., and Rippey, I. G. (1964): Giant cell (cranial) arteritis: A case with angiographic abnormalities. *AJR*, 92:769–775.
62. Hirsch, M., Mayersdorf, A., and Lehmann, E. (1974): Cranial giant-cell arteritis. *Br. J. Radiol.*, 47:503–506.
63. Hirsch, M. S., Aikat, B. K., and Basu, A. K. (1964): Takayasu's arteritis: Report of five cases with immunologic studies. *Bull. Hopkins Hosp.*, 115:29–64.
64. Högerstedt, A., and Nemser, M. (1897): Über die krankhafte Verengerung und Verschliessung vom Aortenbogen ausgehender grosser Gefasse. *Z. Klin. Med.*, 31:130–147.
65. Hunder, G. G., Ward, L. E., and Burbank, M. D. (1967): Giant cell arteritis producing an aortic arch syndrome. *Ann. Intern. Med.*, 66:578–582.
66. Irvine, R. E. (1956): Outcome of uncomplicated syphilitic aortitis. *Br. Med. J.*, 1:832–834.
67. Isaacson, C. (1961): An idiopathic aortitis in young Africans. *J. Pathol. Bacteriol.*, 81:69–79.
68. Ishikawa, K. (1978): Natural history and classification of occlusive thromboaortopathy (Takayasu's disease). *Circulation*, 57:27–35.
69. Jennings, G. H. (1938): Arteritis of temporal arteries. *Lancet*, 1:424–428.
70. Jervell, A. (1954): Pulseless disease. *Am. Heart J.*, 47:780–784.
71. Joffe, N. (1965): Aortitis of obscure origin in the African. *Clin. Radiol.*, 16:130–140.
72. Judge, R. D., Currier, R. D., Gracie, W. A., and Figley, M. M. (1963): Takayasu's arteritis and the aortic arch syndrome. *Am. J. Med.*, 32:379–392.
73. Kalmansohn, R. B., and Kalmansohn, R. W. (1957): Thrombotic obliteration of the branches of the aortic arch. *Circulation*, 15:237–244.
74. Kampmeier, R. H. (1964): The late manifestations of syphilis: Skeletal, visceral, and cardiovascular. *Med. Clin. North Am.*, 48:667–698.
75. Kampmeier, R. H., and Neumann, V. F. (1930): Bilateral absence of pulse in the arms and neck in aortic aneurysm. *Arch. Intern. Med.*, 45:513–522.
76. Kent, D. C., and Arnold, H. (1967): Aneurysm of the aorta due to giant cell aortitis. *J. Thorac. Cardiovasc. Surg.*, 53:572–577.
77. Kjeldsen, M., and Reske-Nielsen, E. (1968): Pathological changes of the central nervous system in giant cell arteritis. *Acta Ophthalmol. (Copenh.)*, 46:49–56.

78. Klein, R. G., Hunder, G. G., Stanson, A. W., and Sheps, S. G. (1975): Large artery involvement in giant cell (temporal) arteritis. *Ann. Intern. Med.*, 83:806–812.
79. Kline, J. I., and Durant, J. (1961): Surgical resection of a tuberculous aneurysm of the ascending aorta: Report of a case. *N. Eng. J. Med.*, 265:1185–1187.
80. Klinge, F. (1933): Die rheumatische Narbe. *Ergebn. Allg. Pathol.*, 27:106–136.
81. Komarnicki, M., and Zawilska, K. (1978): A case of aorto-arteritis with widespread vascular changes from immunological causes. *Mat. Med. Pol.*, 10:320–321.
82. Koszewski, B. J., and Hubbard, T. F. (1957): Pulseless disease due to branchial arteritis. *Circulation*, 16:406–410.
83. Kouretas, D., and Djacas, C. (1941): Réflectivité exagerée du sinus carotidien avec accès épileptique et spasme des artères rétiniennes, dans un cas d'oblitération lente des carotides et des sousclavieres. *Ann. Oculist (Paris)*, 177:161–178.
84. Krayenbuhl, H., and Weber, G. (1944): Die thrombose der Arteria carotis interna und ihre Beziehung zur Endangiitis obliterans (v. Winiwarter-Buerger). *Helv. Med. Acta*, 11:289–333.
85. Kremer, K. (1959): Klinik und operative Behandlung des Aortenbogensyndroms (Takayasu-Krankheit). *Thoraxchirurgie*, 7:334–339.
86. Kucukcakirlar, T., Guven, I., Ozsaruhan, O., Ozkan, E., and Buyukozturk, K. (1974): Obstructive arteritis of Takayasu's type complicated by acute myocardial infarction. *Acta Cardiol. (Brux.)*, 29:485–493.
87. Lampen, H., and Wadulla, H. (1950): Stenosierende Aortenlues unter dem klinischen Bild einer "umgekehrten Isthmusstenose." *Dtsch. Med. Wochenschr.*, 75:144–147.
88. Lande, A., and Berkman, Y. M. (1976): Aortitis: Pathologic, clinical and angiographic review. *Med. Clin. North Am.*, 14:219–240.
89. Lande, A., and La Porta, A. (1976): Takayasu's arteritis: An arteriographic-pathologic correlation. *Arch. Pathol. Lab. Med.*, 100:437–440.
90. Lande, A., Bard, R., Bole, P., and Guarnarcia, M. (1978): Aortic arch syndrome (Takayasu's arteritis): Arteriographic and surgical considerations. *J. Cardiovasc. Surg.*, 19:507–513.
91. Lessof, M. H., and Glynn, L. E. (1959): The pulseless syndrome. *Lancet*, 1:799–801.
92. Lewis, T., and Stokes, J. (1942): A curious syndrome with signs suggesting cervical arterio-venous fistula, and the pulses of neck and arm lost. *Br. Heart J.*, 4:57–65.
93. Lindenburg, R., and Spatz, H. (1939): Über die Thromboendarteritis obliterans der Hirugefasse (Cerebrale Form der v. Winiwarter-Buergerschen Krankheit). *Virchows Arch. [Pathol. Anat.]*, 305:531–557.
94. Linnemann, M. P., and Johnson, V. W. (1975): Pulseless disease with optic atrophy, aortic incompetence, and recurrent peptic ulceration. *Proc. R. Soc. Med.*, 68:806–808.
95. Llavero, F. (1946): Thromboendangiitis obliterans des Gehirns. *Schweiz. Arch. Neurol. Psychiatr.*, 57:290–319.
96. Lovisetto, P., and Marfisi, F. (1968): La Sindrome dell'arco aortico. *Edizioni Minerva Medica*.
97. Lovisetto, P., Marfisi, F., and Pochettino, G. (1973): Syndrome de la crosse de l'aorte, maladie de Takayasu-Onishi, syndrome aortique: Considerations clinico-nosographiques. *Nouv. Presse Med.*, 2:33–37.
98. Ludin, H., Fernex, M., and Schleidegger, S. (1963): Aortographic demonstration of aortic dissection in a case of generalized giant cell arteritis. *Der Radiol.*, 3:411–418.
99. Lüers, T. (1943): Weitere Mitteilungen zur Klinik und Anatomie der cerebralon Form der Thromboangiitis obliterans (v. Winiwarter-Buergersche Krankheit). *Arch. Psychiatr. Nervenkr.*, 115:319–348.
100. Lupi-Herrera, E., Sanchez-Torres, G., Marcushamer, J., Mispireta, J., Horwitz, S., and Espina Vela, J. (1977): Takaysu's arteritis: Clinical study of 107 cases. *Am. Heart J.*, 93:94–103.
101. MacFarlane, W. V., Swan, W. G. A., and Irvine, R. E. (1956): Cardiovascular disease in syphilis: A review of 1330 patients. *Br. Med. J.*, 1:827–832.
102. Mahapatra, R. K., and Krasnow, N. (1981): Takayasu's arteritis associated with panhypopituitarism: A case report. *Angiology*, 32:653–655.
103. Mallory, T. B. (1936): Case records of the Massachusetts General Hospital. *N. Engl. J. Med.*, 214:690–698.
104. Mangold, R., and Roth, F. (1954): Zur Kenntnis des Aortenbogensyndroms (Maladie san pouls). *Schweiz. Med. Wochenschr.*, 84:1192–1194.
105. Marinesco, G., and Kreindler, A. (1936): Oblitération progressive et complète des deux carotides

primitives; accès épileptiques: Considérations sur le rôle des sinus carotidiens dans la pathologénie de l'accès épileptique. *Presse Med.*, 44:833–836.

106. Martin, D. E., Dios, R., Pey, J., Cazzaniga, M., Villaran, E. S., Espino, R. F., Brito, J. M., and Cerezo, L. (1981): Coronary arterial stenosis and subclavian steal in Takayasu's arteritis. *Eur. J. Cardiol.*, 12:229–234.

107. Martorell, F., and Fabre, I. (1954): The syndrome of obliteration of the supraaortic branches. *Angiology*, 5:39–42.

108. Maspetiol, R., and Taptas, I. N. (1948): Thrombose des gros troncs de la crosse l'aorte chez une jeune femme; ses rapports avec les diverses arterites thrombosantes. *Sem. Hop. Paris*, 24:2705–2710.

109. McKusick, V. A. (1962): A form of vascular disease relatively frequent in the Orient. *Am. Heart J.*, 63:57–64.

110. McMillan, C. G. (1950): Diffuse granulomatous aortitis with giant cells *Arch. Pathol*, 49:63–69.

111. Meadows, S. P. (1966): Temporal or giant cell arteritis. *Proc. R. Soc. Med.*, 59:329–333.

112. Mengis, C. L., Dubilier, V., and Barry, K. G. (1958): The aortic arch syndrome of Takayasu. *Am. Heart J.*, 55:435–442.

113. Merritt, H. H., Adams, R. D., and Solomon, H. C. (1946): *Neurosyphilis*. Oxford University Press, New York.

114. Mohanta, K. D., Mahakur, A. C., Panda, T. N., and Misra, D. (1971): Takayasu's disease in a child. *Indian Pediatr.*, 8:125–126.

115. Morl, C., and Morl, H. (1976): Otological symptoms due to disturbances of the major extracranial arteries. *Laryngol. Rhinol. Otol.*, 55:989–994.

116. Morooka, S., Ito, I., Yamaguchi, H., Takeda, T., and Saito, Y. (1972): Follow-up observations of aortitis syndrome. *Jpn. Heart J.*, 13:201–213.

117. Munoz, N., and Correa, P. (1970): Arteritis of the aorta and its major branches. *Am. Heart J.*, 80:319–328.

118. Naceur, M. B., Houissa, D., Maamouri, T., Hafsia, M., and Dite, B. (1972): Non-atherosclerous truncal arteriopathies: Evolution of the angiographic clinical signs (so-called Takayasu's disease: apropos of 5 cases). *Arch. Mal. Coeur*, 65:607–622.

119. Nakao, K., Ikeda, M., Kimata, S., Nhtani, H., Miyahara, M., Ishimi, Z., Hashiba, K., Takeda, Y., Ozawa, T., Matsushita, S., and Kuramochi, M. (1967): Takayasu's arteritis: Clinical report of eighty-four cases and immunological studies of seven cases. *Circulation*, 35:1141–1155.

120. Nasu, T. (1963): Pathology of pulseless disease: A systematic study and critical review of 21 autopsy cases reported in Japan. *Angiology*, 14:225–242.

121. Newton, T. H., and Wylie, E. J. (1964): Collateral circulation associated with occlusion of the proximal subclavian and innominate arteries. *AJR*, 91:394–405.

122. Oata, K. (1940): Ein seltener Fall von beiderseitigem Carotis-Subclaviaverschluss: Ein Beitrag zur Pathologie der Anastomosis peripapillaris des Augen mit fehlendem Radialpuls. *Trans. Soc. Pathol. Jpn.*, 30:680–690.

123. Osborn, A. G., and Anderson, R. E. (1977): Angiographic spectrum of cervical and intracranial fibromuscular dysplasia. *Stroke*, 8:617–626.

124. Pahwa, J. M., Pandey, M. P., and Gypha, D. P. (1959): Pulseless disease or Takayasu's disease. *Br. Med. J.*, 1:1439–1442.

125. Paloheimo, J. A. (1967): Obstructive arteritis of Takayasu's type: Clinical, roentgenological and laboratory studies on 36 patients. *Acta Med. Scand. [Suppl.]*, 488:1–45.

126. Paloheimo, J. A., Julkunen, H., Siltanen, P., and Kajander, A. (1966): Takayasu's arteritis and ankylosing spondylitis. *Acta Med. Scand.*, 179:77–85.

127. Panter, K., and Ueberberg, H. (1959): Klinische und pathologisch-anatomische Untersuchungser-gebnisse zum Aortenbogensyndrom (pulseless disease, maladie sans pouls). *Dtsch. Z. Nerven-heilk.*, 179:285–297.

128. Parkhurst, G. F., and Decker, J. P. (1955): Bacterial aortitis and mycotic aneurysm of the aorta: A report of twelve cases. *Am. J. Pathol.*, 31:821–835.

129. Parsons, C. (1872): Case of occlusion of the arteries arising from the arch of the aorta: With aortic degeneration and aneurysms. *Boston Med. Surg. J.*, 86:400.

130. Patel, A., and Toole, J. F. (1965): Subclavian steal syndrome—reversal of cephalic blood flow. *Medicine (Baltimore)*, 44:289–303.

131. Paton, B. C., Charikavanij, K., Buri, P., Prachuabmah, K., and Jumbala, M. R. B. (1965): Obliterative aortic disease in children in the tropics. *Circulation [Suppl. 1]*, 31:197–202.

132. Paulley, J. W., and Hughes, J. P. (1960): Giant-cell arteritis, or arteritis of the aged. *Br. Med. J.*, 2:1562–1567.
133. Paulus, E. H., Pearson, M. C., and Pitts, H. (1972): Aortic insufficiency in five patients with Reiter's syndrome. *Am. J. Med.*, 53:464–472.
134. Persson, H. E., and Sachs, C. (1981): Visual evoked potentials elicited by pattern reversal during provoked visual impairment in multiple sclerosis. *Brain*, 104:369–382.
135. Pollock, M., Blennerhassett, J. B., and Clarke, A. M. (1973): Giant cell arteritis and the subclavian steal syndrome. *Neurology (NY)*, 23:653–657.
136. Porstmann, W. (1960): Die gezielte Angiographie der supraaortischen Äste als notwendige präoperative Massnahme beim Aortenbogensyndrom. *Fortschr. Roentgenstr.*, 93:735–745.
137. Raeder, J. G. (1927): Ein Fall von symmetrischer Karotisaffektion mit präseniler Katarakt und "Glaukom" sowie Gesichtatrophie. *Klin. Monotsbl. Augenheilkd.*, 63(Suppl. 78):63–78.
138. Raskin, N. H., and Prusiner, S. (1977): Carotidynia. *Neurology (NY)*, 27:43–46.
139. Reaves, L. E., and Wasserman, A. J. (1964): The Takayasu aortic arch syndrome: Report of a case with associated hypoplasia of the aorta and review of the literature. *Angiology*, 15:280–282.
140. Riehl, J-L. (1963): The idiopathic arteritis of Takayasu: A re-evaluation of its anatomical distribution and neurological implications. *Neurology (NY)*, 13:873–884.
141. Riehl, J-L., and Brown, W. J. (1965): Takayasu's arteritis: An auto-immune disease. *Arch. Neurol.*, 12:92–97.
142. Ross, R. S., and McKusick, V. (1953): Aortic arch syndromes: Diminished or absent pulses in arteries arising from arch of aorta. *Arch. Intern. Med.*, 92:701–740.
143. Rostad, H., and Hall, K. V. (1980): Arterial occlusive disease of the upper extremity. *Scand. J. Thorac. Cardiovasc. Surg.*, 14:223–226.
144. Roth, M. L., and Kissane, M. J. (1964): Panaortitis and aortic valvulitis in progressive systemic sclerosis (scleroderma). *Am. J. Clin. Pathol.*, 41:287–296.
145. Sandring, H., and Welin, G. (1961): Aortic arch syndrome with special reference to rheumatoid arthritis. *Acta Med. Scand.*, 170:1–19.
146. Sano, K. (1961): Obstructive diseases of the carotid artery. *Igaku No Ayumi*, 37:236. Cited by R. J. Schwartzman and J. C. Parker, ref. 156.
147. Sano, K., and Aiba, T. (1966): Pulseless disease: Summary of our 62 cases. *Jpn. Circ. J.*, 30:63–67.
148. Sano, K., and Saito, I. (1972): Pulseless disease: Summary of our experiences and studies. *Schweiz. Arch. Neurol. Neurochir. Psychiatr.*, 111:417–433.
149. Sano, K., Aiba, T., and Saito, I. (1970): Angiography in pulseless disease. *Radiology*, 94:69–74.
150. Sato, T. (1938): Ein seltener Fall von Arterien Obliteration. *Klin. Wochenschr.*, 17:1154–1157.
151. Savory, W. S. (1856): Case of a young woman in whom the main arteries of both upper extremities and of the left side of the neck were throughout completely obliterated. *Trans. Med. Chir. Soc. Lond.*, 39:205.
152. Schliack, H., and Dahl, V. P. (1963): Hirndurchblutungsstörungen beim Aortenbogensyndrom (Takayasu). *Dtsch. Med. Wochenschr.*, 88:41–46.
153. Schmidt, H., Heine, H., and Rascovic, M. (1967): Klinik und Prognose des Aortenbogensyndrom. *Munch. Med. Wochenschr.*, 109:777–783.
154. Schneider, G., Amthor, K. J., and Piskorz, R. (1964): Uber das Aortenbogensyndrom. *Bruns Beitr. Klin. Chir.*, 209:70–79.
155. Schrire, V., and Asherson, R. A. (1964): Arteritis of the aorta and its major branches. *Q. J. Med.*, 33:439–463.
156. Schwartzman, R. J., and Parker, J. C. (1979): The aortic arch syndrome. In: *Handbook of Clinical Neurology*, Vol. 39, edited by P. Vinken and G. W. Bruyn, pp. 213–238. North Holland, Amsterdam.
157. Sen, P. K., Kinare, S. G., Kulkarni, T. P., and Panulkar, G. B. (1961): Stenosing aortitis of unknown etiology. *Surgery*, 51:317–325.
158. Shimuzu, K., and Sano, K. (1951): Pulseless disease. *J. Neuropathol. Clin. Neurol.*, 1:37–47.
159. Skipper, E., and Flint, F. J. (1952): Symmetrical arterial occlusion of upper extremities, head and neck: A rare syndrome. *Br. Med. J.*, 2:9–14.
160. Solomon, G. E., Hilal, S. K., Gold, A. P., and Carter, S. (1970): Natural history of acute hemiplegia of childhood. *Brain*, 93:107–120.
161. Sproul, E. E. (1942): A case of temporal arteritis. *N.Y. State J. Med.*, 42:345–346.

162. Sproul, E. E., and Hawthorne, J. J. (1937): Chronic diffuse mesaortitis: Report of 2 cases of unusual type. *Am. J. Pathol.*, 13:311–324.
163. Stanson, A. W., Klein, R. G., and Hunder, G. G. (1976): Extracranial angiographic findings in giant cell (temporal) arteritis. *AJR*, 127:957–963.
164. Strachan, R. W. (1964): The natural history of Takayasu's arteriopathy. *Q. J. Med.*, 33:57–69.
165. Strachan, R. W., Wigzell, F. W., and Anderson, J. R. (1966): Locomotor manifestations and serum studies in Takayasu's arteriopathy. *Am. J. Med.*, 40:560–568.
166. Suwaki, H., Nishii, Y., Hosokawa, K., and Otsuki, S. (1978): Anxiety symptoms of the patients with aortic arch syndrome. *Folia Psychiatr. Neurol. Jpn.*, 32:517–523.
167. Symonds, C., and MacKenzie, I. (1957): Bilateral loss of vision from cerebral infarction. *Brain*, 80:415–455.
168. Szczeklik, A., Gryglewski, R. J., Nizankowski, R., Skawinski, S., Guszko, P., and Korbut, R. (1980): Prostacyclin therapy in peripheral arterial disease. *Thromb. Res.*, 19:191–199.
169. Takayasu, M. (1908): A case with peculiar changes of the central retinal vessels. *Acta Soc. Ophthal. Jpn.*, 12:554.
170. Takeshita, A., Tanaka, S., Orita, Y., Kanaide, H., and Nakamura, M. (1977): Baroreflex sensitivity in patients with Takayasu's aortitis. *Circulation*, 55:803–806.
171. Tanaka, N., Tanaka, H., Toyama, Y., Kashima, T., Niimura, T., and Kanehisa, T. (1975): Paroxysmal hypertension in aortitis syndrome. *Am. Heart J.*, 90:369–375.
172. Tanret, P., Rykner, G., and Solignac, H. (1962): La fonction du sinus carotidien au cours du syndrome de Takayasu. *Presse Med.*, 70:2403–2404.
173. Tardif, L., Mignault, J. de L., Derome, L., and Roy, P. (1965): Maladie de Takayasu: Démonstration d'un cas par l'angiographie. *Un. Med. Can.*, 94:703–709.
174. Tazekawa, H., Sakakura, T., Komada, M., Kotani, Y., and Hamaguchi, T. (1966): Report on two cases of Takayasu's disease, complicated by tuberculide- or tuberculoma-like exanthemas. *Jpn. Circ. J.*, 30:1045–1053.
175. Thurlbeck, W. M., and Currens, J. H. (1959): The aortic arch syndrome (pulseless disease): A report of ten cases with three autopsies. *Circulation*, 19:499–510.
176. Töppich, G. (1921): Über nichtthrombotischen Verschluss der grossen Gefässostien des Aortenbogens, insbesondere des Ostiums der Carotis. *Frankfurt Z. Pathol.*, 25:236–260.
177. Trias de Bes, L., Sanchez Lucas, J. G., and Ballesta Barrens, F. (1955): A case of Takayasu's syndrome: The pulseless disease. *Br. Heart J.*, 17:484–488.
178. Turk, W. (1901): Arterieller Collateralkreislaufbei Verschluss der grossen Gefasse am Aortenbogen durch deformierende Aortitis. *Wien Klin. Wochenschr.*, 14:757–763.
179. Ueda, H. (1968): Clinical and pathological studies of aortitis syndrome: Committee report. *Jpn. Heart J.*, 9:76–87.
180. Valaitis, J., Pilz, G. C., and Montgomery, M. M. (1957): Aortitis with aortic valve insufficiency in rheumatoid arthritis. *Arch. Pathol.*, 63:207–212.
181. Vinijchaikul, K. (1967): Primary arteritis of the aorta and its main branches (Takayasu's arteriopathy): A clinicopathologic autopsy study of eight cases. *Am. J. Med.*, 43:15–27.
182. Westphal, J., Lobbecke, F., and Mietens, C. (1976): Arteritis of the large vessels originating at the aorta (Takayasu arteritis) in childhood. *Klin. Paediatr.*, 188:570–577.
183. Wheeler, H. B. (1967): Surgical treatment of subclavian artery occlusions. *N. Engl. J. Med.*, 276:711–717.
184. Wickremasinghe, H. R., Peiris, J. B., Thenabadu, P. N., and Sheriffdeen, A. H. (1978): Transient emboligenic aortoarteritis: Noteworthy new entity in young stroke patients. *Arch. Neurol.*, 35:416–422.
185. Wood, C. P., and Meire, H. B. (1980): Intermittent bilateral subclavian steal detected by ultrasound angiography. *Br. J. Radiol.*, 53:727–730.
186. Yelloly, J. (1823): Case of preternatural growth in the lining membrane covering the trunks of the vessels proceeding from the arch of the aorta. *Med. Clin. Tr.*, 12:565.
187. Yoneda, S., Nukada, T., Tada, K., Imaizumi, M., Takano, T., and Abe, H. (1977): Subclavian steal in Takayasu's arteritis: A hemodynamic study by means of ultrasonic doppler flowmetry. *Stroke*, 8:264–268.
188. Zvaifler, N. J., and Weintraub, A. M. (1963): Aortitis and aortic insufficiency in chronic rheumatic disorders: A re-appraisal. *Arthritis Rheum.*, 6:241–245.

Aortitis: Clinical, Pathologic, and Radiographic
Aspects, edited by A. Lande, Y. M. Berkmen, and
H. A. McAllister. Raven Press, New York © 1986.

Ocular Manifestations of Takayasu's Disease

Murk-Hein Heinemann and Jesse Sigelman

*Department of Ophthalmology, Cornell University Medical College, and New York
Hospital, New York, New York 10021*

Takayasu's disease is a chronic inflammatory condition that causes widespread obliterative endarteritis of the aorta and its larger branches. Although of worldwide distribution, the disease characteristically manifests in young women of Japanese extraction (2,6). In addition to symptomatic hypertension, delayed or absent extremity pulsations, fatigue, and exertional dyspnea, ocular signs and symptoms are among the most frequent findings in affected patients. Arteritis, in which pulselessness of the brachiocephalic circulation is apparent, was initially described in 1865 by Savory, who reported the case of a young woman with absent radial and left carotid pulsations (17). Takayasu, a Japanese ophthalmologist, noted peculiar retinal vascular changes in a 1908 clinical report (15) of the case of a 21-year-old woman. In a discussion of the case, Ohnishi and Kagoshima commented on two additional cases in which retinal vascular changes were accompanied by absent radial pulses in young women. Since the observations by Takayasu, Ohnishi, and Kagoshima, attempts have been made to classify the disease on a pathophysiological basis (14,16).

By convention, type I (Shimizu–Sano) disease is characterized by involvement of the ascending aorta and its branches, resulting in upper extremity and cephalic hypotension (14). In this form of the disease, cerebral and retinal ischemia plays a prominent role in the clinical course. Disease in which the descending aorta is primarily involved and segmental stenosis is common is classified as type II (Kimoto) (10). In this form of the disease, the eye can be involved as a result of secondary hypertension in the face of normal brachiocephalic circulation. The most common form of the disease is type III in which both the ascending and descending thoracoabdominal aorta are involved (10). Type IV disease is characterized by pulmonary artery as well as aortal involvement.

Transient complete or partial visual loss in one or both eyes is one of the most consistent complaints of patients with Takayasu's disease (17). In a review of 107 cases, however, Lupi-Herrera and co-workers noted that only 8% of patients complained of visual disturbances (12). Shimizu and Sano reported that amaurosis was often precipitated by postural changes, with many of their patients preferring a position in which the head was flexed (14). In addition, the exacerbation of visual disturbances by exercise in cases of carotid occlusion has been well documented (17). Because of the complexity of the brachiocephalic and vertebral circulations, there is no consistent pattern to the visual loss experienced by many patients.

Monocular visual loss is most commonly the result of retinal or optic nerve ischemia; bilateral symptoms can be caused by either retinal or cerebral ischemia. In the latter case, transient homonymous visual field defects can be elicited. In some cases of carotid vascular insufficiency secondary to arteritis, light flashes (photopsia) have been described (3,7,17).

SIGNS

Chronic impairment of the cephalic circulation can cause characteristic signs evident on external ophthalmologic examination. Most dramatic in some cases is the large degree of soft tissue atrophy that can occur. Enophthalmos, caused by disappearance of orbital fat combined with atrophy of the temporalis and facial muscles, can give the patients a dramatically emaciated appearance (8).

Hypoperfusion of the retinal arteriolar circulation can be quantitatively documented by ophthalmodynamometry. In advanced cases of carotid insufficiency, light pressure on the globe or postural change may be enough to precipitate total retinal artery occlusion. Not only can the diastolic and systolic pressures be markedly reduced, but the pulse pressure can also be low. Often there is a significant difference between the ophthalmodynamometric readings of the two eyes. Because postural changes are common, pressure readings should be made with the patient in both the supine and the sitting positions. It should be noted that ophthalmodynamometry does not yield absolute pressure values; variable findings are common when the ophthalmic perfusion pressure is very low and there are changes in the systemic blood pressure (1,7,17).

Uyama and Asayama observed an apparent correlation between the systolic retinal artery pressure and the appearance of retinal microaneurysms (16). Microaneurysms developed at 30 mm Hg but disappeared with both an associated drop in systolic pressure, as seen with progressive disease, and an elevation in pressure following successful surgical treatment. A critical diastolic pressure for the development of microaneurysms was not found, but the frequency of microaneurysms was inversely proportional to the diastolic pressure.

RETINAL VASCULAR CHANGES

Chronic reduction of the orbital and ocular blood flow produces hypoxic retinal vascular changes (Table 1). Initially, the retinal veins become distended, and segmental beading may be evident (Uyama and Asayama stage 1). Stage 2 is characterized by microaneurysm formation but, as noted earlier, may depend on the systolic retinal artery pressure. Peripheral vascular hypoperfusion in stage 3 causes the formation of mid-peripheral and peripheral arterial venous anastomoses. Ocular complications are broadly classified as stage 4 (16). These include anterior segment changes, e.g., cataract and rubeosis iridis, and posterior segment complications, e.g., retinal ischemia, neovascularization, proliferative retinopathy, and vitreous hemorrhage (Table 2).

TABLE 1. *Classification of Takayasu's retinopathy*

Stage	Finding
1	Venous dilatation
2	Microaneurysm formation
3	Arterial venous anastomoses
4	Ocular complications

After Uyama and Asayama (16).

TABLE 2. *Ocular complications*

Fundus
  Retinal neovascularization
  Fibrovascular proliferation
  Vitreous hemorrhage
  Tractional retinal detachment
External
  Conjunctival vessel dilatation
  Episcleral vessel dilatation
  Corneal opacification
  Enophthalmos
  Phthisis bulbi
Anterior segment
  Hypotony
  Cataract
  Stromal iris atrophy
  Rubeosis iridis
  Iritis
Optic nerve
  Ischemic optic neuropathy
  Optic atrophy
  Disc neovascularization

Fluorescein angiography is particularly useful in assessing the state of the retinal circulation in patients with Takayasu's disease. This technique allows the clinician to study dynamically retinal vascular blood flow, circulation times, and retinal vascular lesions. In Takayasu's retinopathy, arm to retina and intraretinal circulation times are often reduced (16). Although no abnormalities of the choroidal circulation have been reported, it is likely that the choroidal circulation is also impaired as is suggested by histologic evidence of outer retinal segment damage (4,5). In contrast to the copious fluorescein leakage associated with microaneurysms in the early stages of diabetic retinopathy, the saccular dilatations seen in Takayasu's disease show sparse leakage. This may be due to low perfusion pressures rather than to intrinsic differences in vascular morphology, although leakage is much more pronounced in later stages. Again, in contrast to diabetes, the arterial venous anastomoses of stage 3 disease are sequelae of peripheral vascular nonperfusion which can be documented by angiography. The rarity of proliferative fibrovascular changes and vitreous hemorrhage (only two of Uyama and Asayama's cases) in these

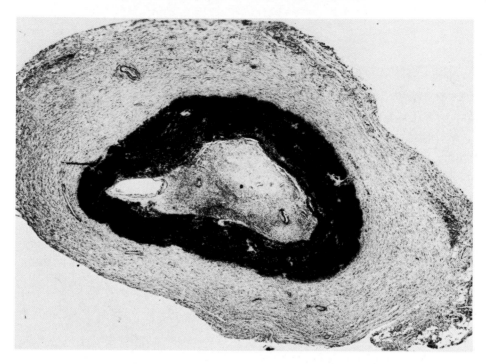

FIG. 1.   One of the large vessels from the aortic arch is almost occluded by subintimal fibrosis with eccentric displacement of the lumen. Focal scarring and destruction of elastic fibers are observed in the media. Marked sclerosis and thickening of adventitia are evident. (AFIP Neg.68-8176.) (Movat stain, × 15.) (From Font and Naumann, ref. 5, with permission.)

Takayasu's disease patients supports the distinction between Takayasu's retinopathy and diabetic retinopathy.

As is suggested by the correlation with the reduced retinal arterial perfusion pressures (16), microaneurysms do not form until extensive arterial disease has developed. Fluorescein angiography may detect early retinal neovascular changes which, as in the case of fibroproliferative changes seen in such diseases as sickle cell disease, may be amenable to photocoagulation which can reduce the risk of vitreous hemorrhage, proliferative retinopathy, and anterior segment neovascularization. When evaluating the degree of retinopathy by either direct observation or fluorescein angiography, the presence or absence of systemic hypertension must be considered.

Severe systemic hypertension can be seen in types II, III, and IV Takayasu's disease. Carotid vascular insufficiency (not present in type II disease) can minimize the retinal vascular changes, e.g., arteriolar narrowing, associated with hypertension. On the other hand, hypertension can exacerbate existing microvascular damage as commonly occurs in diabetic retinopathy (9).

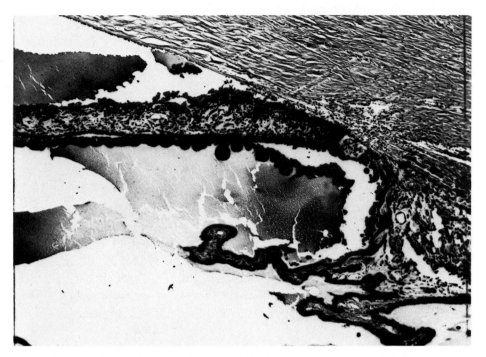

FIG. 2. Chamber angle is occluded by peripheral anterior synechiae. Proteinaceous exudate fills the anterior and posterior chambers. (AFIP Neg.69-3369.) (H&E, ×50.) (From Font and Naumann, ref. 5, with permission.)

INTRAOCULAR PRESSURE

Reduced intraocular pressure is a common manifestation of Takayasu's disease and is, in all probability, caused by suboptimal ciliary blood flow. Uyama and Asayama, in a clinical study of 80 cases, reported reduced intraocular pressure which became more prominent as the disease progressed (16). In a histopathologic study of a 35-year-old woman, Font and Naumann noted normal intraocular pressures in the face of extensive peripheral anterior synechiae (5). Severe, prolonged ocular hypotony can result in phthisis bulbi (11).

ANTERIOR SEGMENT COMPLICATIONS

Cataract formation is another manifestation of reduced ciliary blood flow. Cataracts do not become clinically apparent until several years after the onset of retinal vascular changes (7). In cases of ocular vascular insufficiency, cataractogenesis appears to be quite rapidly progressive (5). Cataract surgery in patients with Takayasu's disease can be complicated and often disappointing, for underlying retinal and optic nerve damage makes visual rehabilitation impossible (13).

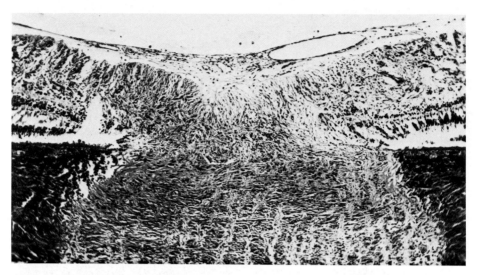

FIG. 3. Fibrovascular membrane extends from the optic disc along the inner surface of the juxtapapillary retina. (AFIP Neg.69-466.) (H&E, ×35.) (From Font and Naumann, ref. 5, with permission.)

Among the complicating factors to be considered are iris neovascularization and corneal opacification secondary to hypotony and anterior segment ischemia. When evaluating patients for cataract surgery, clinical estimation of retinal function by entoptic imagery and electrophysiological testing are indicated.

Abnormal pupillary light reflexes may be an indication of retinal or optic nerve ischemia and are sometimes accompanied by amaurosis. Persistent anisocoria may be a manifestation of stromal iris atrophy or iris neovascularization. The secondary glaucoma that can result from iris neovascularization is extremely difficult to treat and can result in blindness.

Iritis (inflammation of the anterior segment) can be a manifestation of rheumatoid arthritis, which is sometimes associated with Takayasu's disease (10), chronic orbital ischemia, or the mycobacterial infection frequently found in Takayasu's disease (12).

OCULAR HISTOPATHOLOGY

None of the histopathologic changes found in the eyes of Takayasu's cases is distinctive for this disease (5). All the changes resemble those found in ocular hypoxia.

In one reported case where there was complete thrombotic occlusion of the innominate (Fig. 1), left subclavian, and common carotid arteries, the eyes showed ischemic changes. The iris stroma was heavily pigmented and atrophic, and it was missing patches of the dilator muscle. The anterior chamber angle was occluded by peripheral anterior synechiae; proteinaceous exudate filled the anterior and poste-

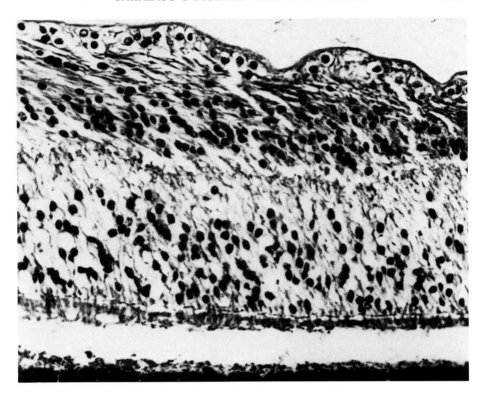

FIG. 4. The nuclei of the outer and inner nuclear and ganglion cell layers in macular area are moderately reduced in number, indicating impairment of retinal and choroidal circulation. (AFIP Neg.69-472.) (H&E, × 145.) (From Font and Naumann, ref. 5, with permission.)

rior chambers (Fig. 2). There was ectropion uveae with rubeosis iridis, and the iris pigment epithelium was partially attached to the anterior lens capsule. The ciliary muscle showed fibrosis with hyalinization of the processes. In the areas of posterior synechias, the nuclei of the lens epithelium were irregularly spaced and degenerated. The lens cortex and nucleus showed degeneration and clefts filled with Morgagnian globules. Pigment-laden macrophages were present in the posterior vitreous, and the optic disc showed a thin fibrovascular membrane extending into the juxtapapillary retina (Fig. 3).

The retinal periphery showed degeneration and thinning of all its layers; the macular retina showed degeneration of the outer nuclear layer (Fig. 4); the mid-peripheral and the macular retina showed an abnormal sparcity of ganglion and bipolar cells. Ganglion cells were best preserved adjacent to the retinal vessels.

Although the central retinal artery showed no abnormality on cross section, flat preparations of the capillaries showed the almost complete loss of endothelial cells but good preservation of the mural cells (Fig. 5).

These histopathologic changes appeared to result from a very slowly progressive, occlusive vascular disease affecting the entire blood supply to the eye (5). The

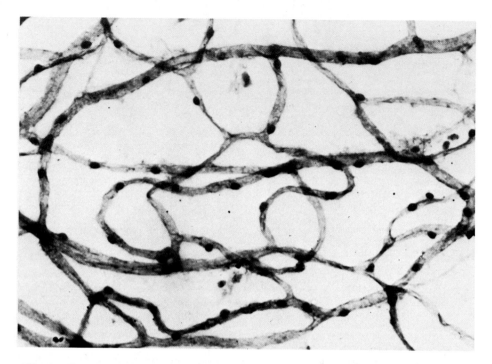

FIG. 5. Flat preparation of retinal vessels shows marked reduction of endothelial cells. Mural cells appear relatively preserved and slightly swollen. (AFIP Neg.69-3368.) (PAS, × 245.) (From Font and Naumann, ref. 5, with permission.)

similarity between the retinal changes of Takayasu's disease and the retinal changes following a central retinal artery occlusion is the relative sparing of the ganglion cells surrounding the retinal vessels. The damage to the outer retinal layers in Takayasu's disease cannot be explained by deficiency in only the retinal circulation; the outer retinal degeneration must result from impairment of the choroidal vascular supply. Although microaneurysms have been described, their histologic basis in Takayasu's disease is different from that of other types of ischemic retinopathy. Diabetic retinopathy is characterized by preferential loss of the intramural pericytes, but Takayasu's retinopathy is characterized by the selective loss of endothial cells of the capillaries. The anterior segment changes of Takayasu's disease can also be explained by inadequate circulation. The formation of extensive anterior synechias with occlusion of both the angle and the interior chamber would result in glaucoma were it not for the decreased production of aqueous humor caused by inadequate circulation to the ciliary body. Cataractogenesis is stimulated by the inadequate ciliary circulation and the secondary inadequacy of production of the aqueous humor which is necessary for the nutrition of the crystalline lens. Protcinaccous cxudatc within thc antcrior chamber results from increased vascular permeability secondary to endothelial cell disease.

BLINDNESS

Permanent monocular or binocular blindness is a grave prognostic sign in Takayasu's disease. Four of Ishikawa's 80 patients developed monocular or binocular blindness (10).

REFERENCES

1. Asayama, R., and Uyama, M. (1965): Ophthalmodynamometric study of pulseless disease. *Jpn. J. Clin. Ophthalmol.*, 19:397–413.
2. Ask-Upmark, E. (1954): On the "pulseless disease" outside of Japan. *Acta Med. Scand.*, 149:161–178.
3. Currier, R. D., DeJong, R. N., and Bole, G. G. (1954): Pulseless disease: Central nervous system manifestations. *Neurology* (NY), 4:818–830.
4. Dowling, J. L., and Smith, T. A. (1960): An ocular study of pulseless disease. *Arch. Ophthalmol.*, 64:236–243.
5. Font, R. L., and Naumann, G. (1969): Ocular histopathology in pulseless disease. *Arch. Ophthalmol.*, 82:784–788.
6. Frovig, A. G. (1946): Bilateral obliteration of the common carotid artery. *Acta Psychiatr. Neurol. Scand. [Suppl.]*, 39.
7. Hedges, T. R. (1964): The aortic arch syndromes. *Arch. Ophthalmol.*, 71:62–68.
8. Heydenreich, A. (1957): Die Durchblutungestorungen an Auge bei der "pulseless disease." *Z. Aertztl. Fortbild (Berl.)*, 51:199–204.
9. Hollenhorst, R. W. (1962): Carotid and vertebral-basilar arterial stenosis and occlusion: Neuro-ophthalmologic considerations. *Ophthalmol.*, 66:166–180.
10. Ishikawa, K. (1981): Survival and morbidity after diagnosis of occlusive thromboaortopathy (Takayasu's disease). *Am. J. Cardiol.*, 47:1026–1032.
11. Leo, M. (1955): Augenveranderungen bei Verscluss der grossen Gefasse am Aortenbogen. *Klin. Monatsbl. Augenheilkd.*, 217:284–294.
12. Lupi-Herrera, E., Sanchez-Torres, G., Marcushamer, J., Mispireta, J., Horwitz, S., and Vela, J. E. (1977): Takayasu's arteritis: Clinical study of 107 cases. *Am. Heart J.*, 93:94–103.
13. Mouillon, M., Bonnet, J-L., Ravault, M., and Maugery, J. (1974): Une observation de syndrome de Takayasu. *Bull. Soc. Ophthalmol.*, 74:765–769.
14. Shimizu, K., and Sano, K. (1954): Pulseless disease (thromboarteritis obliterans subclaviocarotica). *J. Neuropathol. Clin. Neurol.*, 1:37–47.
15. Takayasu, M. (1908): Case report of a peculiar abnormality of the retinal central vessels. *Acta Soc. Ophthalmol. Jpn.*, 12:554.
16. Uyama, M., and Asayama, K. (1976): Retinal vascular changes in Takayasu's disease (pulseless disease), occurrence and evolution of the lesion. *Doc. Ophthalmol. Proc. Series*, 9:549–554.
17. Walsh, F. B., and Hoyt, W. F. (1969): *Clinical Neuro-ophthalmology*. Williams & Wilkins, Baltimore.

Aortitis: Clinical, Pathologic, and Radiographic
Aspects, edited by A. Lande, Y. M. Berkmen, and
H. A. McAllister. Raven Press, New York © 1986.

Surgical Considerations in Aortitis

J. Michael Duncan and Denton A. Cooley

Division of Surgery, University of Texas Medical School of Houston, and Texas Heart Institute, St. Luke's Episcopal and Texas Children's Hospitals, Houston, Texas 77025

Atherosclerosis is the most common etiology for vascular disease in the United States, yet various forms of arteritis causing symptomatic occlusive or aneurysmal vascular lesions affect a significant number of patients each year. Although the incidence of some diseases known to cause arteritis has declined over the years as a result of antibiotic usage, most notably syphilis and rheumatic fever, other systemic diseases not initially thought to have vascular involvement as part of the clinical manifestations have, in some cases, been found to be associated with widespread arteritis.

Regardless of etiology, aortitis may result in an injury to the aorta or its branches. The inflammatory process which occurs in response to the injury may ultimately result in one of two morphological changes in the affected vessels: stenosis or occlusion from fibrosis, and dilatation or aneurysm formation from destruction and weakening of the arterial wall. All forms of arteritis of either known or unknown etiology are capable of producing dilatation or aneurysm formation, but only Takayasu's arteritis can produce narrowing or occlusion of the aorta or its branches, with the rare exception of stenosing arteritis, which sometimes follows radiation therapy in children.

Clinical symptoms occur depending on the extent and location of the vascular disease. Stenotic or occlusive lesions may result in ischemia to limbs or organs distal to the site of obstruction. Treatment of this stenosing type of arteritis is aimed at attempting to restore an adequate blood supply to the ischemic tissue before irreparable damage or infarction occurs. Aneurysms may result from any of the various types of arteritis. Perhaps the most important characteristic of any aneurysm is that once formed, from whatever etiology, it gradually enlarges until it either produces symptoms from compression on surrounding structures or death from rupture. The first and only manifestation of an aneurysm may be catastrophic rupture and death. Therefore the mere presence of an aneurysm is life-threatening, and surgical resection should be recommended in most patients.

Although similarities exist between the various forms of arteritis, differences in the clinical presentation, indications for surgery, surgical technique, and prognosis vary to some extent. Each of the more common types of arteritis is discussed with particular emphasis on the surgical treatment.

TAKAYASU'S ARTERITIS

Takayasu's arteritis is a disease of unknown etiology which can affect the aorta, its major branches, and the pulmonary arteries. It may cause stenosis, occlusion, or aneurysmal dilatation of the affected vessels.

Nonspecific arteritis was first reported by Savory in 1856 (60). In 1908 Takayasu (68) noted the peculiar ocular manifestations of the disease which consisted of a capillary flush in the ocular fundus, arteriovenous anastomosis, and cataracts which could lead to blindness. Onishi (50) noted the absence of pulses in the upper extremities in two additional patients with similar ocular findings. In 1951 Shimizu and Sano (63) detailed the clinical findings of the disease, and in 1954 the name Takayasu's arteritis was given to the disorder. Other names given to this disease in the past have been aortic arch syndrome (58), pulseless disease (2), Martorell's syndrome (45), atypical coarctation (26), brachiocephalic arteritis, and idiopathic aortitis (27). Although it was initially thought that Takayasu's disease was rare and confined to the Orient, subsequent reports (39,40,55) have shown that the disease is indeed worldwide in distribution and much more common than previously recognized.

The vascular abnormalities of the disease were initially thought to be confined to the aortic arch and its branches, but subsequent clinical and pathological studies have demonstrated that any segment of the aorta as well as the pulmonary arteries may be affected. The arteritis in the involved vessels may progress to narrowing, occlusion, coarctation, or aneurysmal dilatation. The clinical syndromes which result may be extremely varied and depend on the type, severity, and location of the vascular lesions (28).

In 1967 Ueno classified Takayasu's disease into four types depending on the location and extent of the arteritis (Fig. 1). In type I, originally described by Shimizu and Sano (63), the involvement is limited to the aortic arch and its branches. In type II, also referred to as "atypical coarctation of the aorta" or Kimoto type, the vascular lesions are confined to the descending thoracic and abdominal aorta without involvement of the aortic arch. Type III, also referred to as mixed or Inada type, contains features of types I and II. Type IV disease is characterized by dilatation and aneurysm formation in the affected vessels. In 1977 Lupi-Herrera et al. (44) described an additional variant, also called type IV, which has pulmonary artery involvement in addition to any of the features of types I, II, or III. This classification is useful in that it provides a convenient way to compare results of treatment, progression of disease, and prognosis in patients with occlusive lesions in similar anatomical locations.

Clinical Manifestations and Diagnosis

The clinical manifestations of Takayasu's arteritis are divided into two phases: an early systemic phase followed by a late occlusive phase. Symptoms present during the early phase are nonspecific and varied and include fever, myalgias, malaise, arthralgias, chest and abdominal pain, night sweats, vomiting, pleuritis,

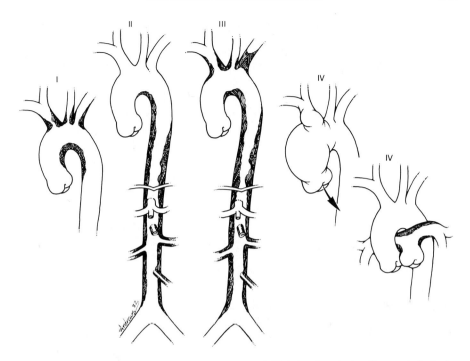

FIG. 1. Classification of Takayasu's disease. Type I (Shimizu-Sano): the disease is limited to the aortic arch and its branches. Type II (Kimoto): stenosis and occlusion are confined to the descending thoracic and abdominal aorta. Type III (Inada): contains features of types I and II. Type IV: dilatation or aneurysm formation in affected vessels or pulmonary artery involvement.

and skin rashes. The incidence of these symptoms varies. Lande and Bard (41) reported that a definite history of significant illness could be recorded in only 5 of 35 patients, whereas Nakao et al. (48) elicited a history of systemic illness in 53 of 84 patients. Apparently, many patients do manifest systemic symptoms at some time during the early phase of the disease, but in a significant number of patients these symptoms are absent or pass unrecognized (38).

The age of onset of the disease also varies, but in general most patients are young and there is a definite predilection for females. In the series of 107 cases reported by Lupi-Herrera et al. (44), the age of onset of the disease was between 10 and 20 years in 77% of the patients. Of the 84 patients reported by Nakao et al. (48), 67% had the onset between 10 and 29 years of age. In both of these large series, 85% of the patients were females.

The late occlusive phase of the disease results from marked fibrosis and thickening of the vessels affected by the arteritis. Occasionally, saccular aneurysms also result. The time elapsed from the onset of the systemic symptoms to the occurrence of symptoms from arterial occlusive disease may vary from months to years. During this period, patients may experience intermittent exacerbations of systemic symptoms, or they may be completely asymptomatic until localized signs and symptoms appear from regional ischemia secondary to arterial occlusive disease. Once symptoms appear, the clinical course is generally one of gradual deterioration.

The clinical manifestations and symptoms during the late phase are related to the location and severity of the occlusive disease. Stenosis or occlusion of one or more of the arch vessels (type I) may produce a wide range of neurological and ocular symptoms including headache, syncope, hemiplegia, paraplegia, visual disturbances, and cataract formation. In most patients the cardiovascular and neurological symptoms appear at the same time. The cardiovascular symptoms which predominate include hypertension, dyspnea, vascular bruits, and decreased amplitude of the peripheral pulses. Congestive heart failure and chest pain may be the presenting clinical manifestations in some patients.

Hypertension is common, except in type I disease, occurring in 72% of the patients reported by Lupi-Herrera et al. (44) and in 52% of those reported by Nakao et al. (48). It may occur as a result of stenosis of one or both of the renal arteries, or it may result from suprarenal aortic stenosis or coarctation. In many cases the hypertension is severe and refractory to drug management. Hypertensive congestive heart failure is the presenting complaint in some patients, particulary in those under 15 yeras of age (29).

Claudication and pain in the lower extremities can result from stenosis at the aortic bifurcation or the iliac or femoral arteries, or may be caused by stenosis in the thoracic or abdominal aorta. Chest pain, angina pectoris, and myocardial infarction have been reported as a result of coronary artery ostial stenosis (8,57,71). Pulmonary arteritis occurs in a significant number of patients and can be responsible for pulmonary hypertension (25,43,44).

Once symptoms occur, arteriography should be performed to define the extent and severity of the disease. Although aortodilatation and aneurysm formation may occur with any form of aortitis, stenosis and occlusion are specific for Takayasu's disease. Stenosis can occur at any level of the aorta and may affect any of the major branches. The lesions may be short and segmental or long and diffuse. Total arteriography is of extreme diagnostic importance because it gives a complete picture of both symptomatic and asymptomatic arterial lesions. Lande and co-workers (39,40) and others (21,22,59) have stressed the importance of aortography in the diagnostic evaluation of patients with Takayasu's disease.

Surgical Treatment

The surgical treatment of stenotic and occlusive lesions resulting from Takayasu's disease is based on the principle of restoring adequate circulation to ischemic tissue before irreversible damage occurs. Arterial dilation that causes a functional abnormality, such as dilatation of the ascending aorta with resultant aortic regurgitation, should be surgically corrected. Aneurysms, regardless of their size or location, should be resected, as it is known that these lesions progressively enlarge until they either produce symptoms from compression on surrounding structures or rupture, often with exsanguinating hemorrhage.

Surgical techniques used for treating stenotic and occlusive lesions in Takayasu's disease include endarterectomy, resection of the diseased arterial segment, and replacement with either a fabric or autogenous vein graft, bypassing the obstructed segment with a graft, and patch angioplasty (Fig. 2). Each of these techniques has its proponents; however, we have utilized resection and graft replacement or bypass in the majority of the patients we have treated with good results.

In order to clarify the therapeutic options of the surgeon in treating this disease, we discuss each type separately and indicate the methods of surgical treatment available.

Type I

Occlusive or stenotic lesions of the type I variety can produce a multiplicity of symptoms related to brachiocephalic ischemia. Neurological symptoms and ocular disturbances usually dominate the clinical manifestations. Cerebral symptoms may be absent, however, even in the presence of severe carotid stenosis or occlusion if sufficient time has elapsed for adequate collateral circulation to develop.

A variety of surgical techniques have been used to treat stenotic lesions in the brachiocephalic vessels. Inada et al. (25) and Kusaba et al. (36) have used thromboendarterectomy with good results. Both groups believe that this technique is superior to others because it avoids the use of prosthetic graft material. They also found that in patients undergoing bypass procedures the incidence of false aneurysms occurring at either anastomosis was significant and that the grafts had a high incidence of early thrombosis. Kusaba et al. stressed the importance of performing the endarterectomy through a long incision in the vessel under direct vision, using an onlay patch of saphenous vein to close the arteriotomy. In a series of 17 patients who had thromboendarterectomy of brachiocephalic lesions reported by Kusaba et al. in 1973, 16 had excellent immediate and long-term results, and there was only one death (5.9%) during the perioperative period.

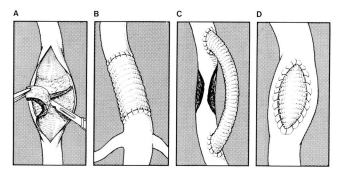

FIG. 2. Surgical techniques used in Takayasu's diease. **A**: Endarterectomy. **B**: Resection of diseased segment with graft replacement. **C**: Bypass of the stenosis or occlusion. **D**: Patch angioplasty.

Our own experience with endarterectomy, as well as that of others (35,41), has not been as good, and we believe that it is not the technique of choice in most patients. Unlike atherosclerotic stenotic lesions, which are often short and segmental, obstructions from Takayasu's arteritis are frequently more diffuse and affect longer segments of the involved vessel. More importantly, there is no plane of cleavage between the thick fibrous obstruction and the media of the vessel wall, making a satisfactory endarterectomy difficult to perform. The luminal surface that results following endarterectomy is often ragged and rough, leading to turbulence in blood flow over the repair and probably contributing to the high incidence of early thrombosis reported in several series (35,41).

We now believe that the most satisfactory method of treating brachiocephalic obstructions is with the bypass technique (6), or, on occasion, resection of the diseased segment and graft interposition. These two techniques offer several advantages over others. Arterial segments free of disease and at times quite distant from the obstructions can be used for the graft anastomoses. Choosing healthy tissue for the site of the graft anastomosis decreases the incidence of suture dehiscence and subsequent false aneurysm formation. Satisfactory nonturbulent flow in the vessel distal to the obstruction can be achieved by using a graft of adequate diameter, avoiding the possibility that flow through an endarterectomized vessel might be only marginal. The diseased segment of artery is often surrounded by dense perivascular fibrosis and inflammation. By working with normal tissue distant to the disease, the often tedious dissection and chance of injury to the vessel and surrounding structures is avoided.

Figure 3 illustrates a few of the possible combinations of brachiocephalic obstructions and some of the bypass techniques which can be utilized. Because there are six brachiocephalic vessels that may be diseased, there can be a variety of obstructions requiring bypass surgery. It is of paramount importance, however, that the anastomosis of each graft be to a segment of artery that is not involved with active arteritis because the incidence of graft failure and false aneurysm formation is high if diseased or unhealthy tissue is used. Figures 4 through 7 illustrate the arteriographic findings in three of our patients with severe forms of type I occlusive disease and the operative techniques used to bypass the lesions.

Type II

The pattern of lesions in patients with type II disease is characterized by stenosis or coarctation of the descending thoracic and abdominal aorta and often stenosis of the visceral branches as well. The renal arteries are frequently affected with stenotic lesions at their origins.

Hypertension dominates the clinical presentation in these patients and may result either from direct renal artery involvement or from decreased renal blood flow secondary to a suprarenal aortic stenosis or obstruction. Pulses may be strong in the upper extremities and severely diminished or absent in the lower extremities, and lower limb claudication may be present.

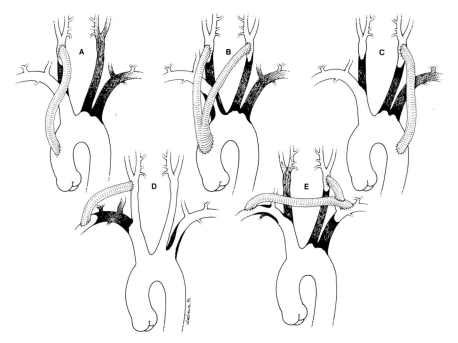

FIG. 3. Bypass techniques which can be used to treat brachiocephalic lesions in Takayasu's disease. Procedures **A** through **C** require a sternotomy incision in additiion to cervical incisions to create the bypass; procedures **D** and **E** can be done through cervical incisions only.

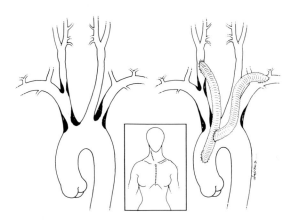

FIG. 4. A 29-year-old female had Takayasu's disease with symptoms of chronic headache and hypertension. Arteriography demonstrated stenosis of the innominate, right common carotid, and left subclavian arteries. Surgical treatment involved the creation of a bypass graft from the ascending aorta to the right carotid and left subclavian arteries.

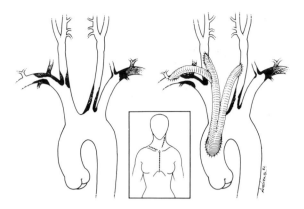

FIG. 5. A 46-year-old female had Takayasu's disease with symptoms of dizziness and decreased strength in both arms. Arteriography demonstrated stenosis or occlusion of all the brachiocephalic vessels. Adequate cerebral circulation was restored utilizing a bypass graft from the ascending aorta to both common carotid arteries; perfusion of the right subclavian artery was achieved using a bypass from the right carotid graft.

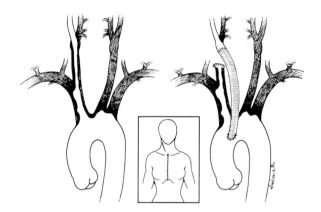

FIG. 6. A 35-year-old female had Takayasu's disease and symptoms of transient ischemic episodes. Arteriography revealed occlusion of all of the brachiocephalic vessels except the innominate artery, which was severely stenotic. A bypass graft from the ascending aorta to the distal innominate artery was performed to improve cerebral perfusion.

The stenotic areas may be located at any point in the descending thoracic or abdominal aorta (Figs. 8 and 9). The stenosis may be discrete and localized to a short aortic segment, or it may be diffuse, involving a long segment of descending or abdominal aorta. The discrete, localized areas of obstruction often appear angiographically to be similar to congenital coarctations found at the aortic isthmus. Many of these lesions were at one time considered to be atypical congenital coarctations, but studies by Lande (37), Nakao et al. (49), and others (12,46) have shown convincingly that almost all of these lesions represent variable localizations of Takayasu's arteritis, and that true isolated congenital coarctations in atypical

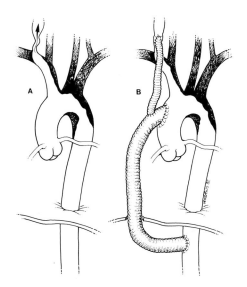

FIG. 7. A 19-year-old male had Takayasu's disease and symptoms of dizziness and chest pain. Arteriography demonstrated total occlusion of both common carotid arteries at their origins and a large right vertebral artery with 60% proximal stenosis. The aorta was stenotic in the distal arch. Surgical treatment involved creating a bypass from the ascending aorta to the supraceliac abdominal aorta; the vertebral artery stenosis was bypassed using a second graft from the aortic prosthesis.

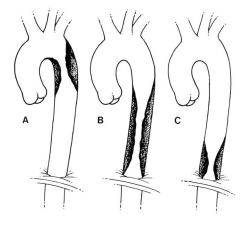

FIG. 8. Patterns of stenosis in the descending thoracic aorta in Takayasu's disease. **A,C**: Segmental stenosis in the proximal or distal thoracic aorta. **B**: Diffuse stenosis involving a long segment of descending thoracic aorta.

sites are extremely rare unless they exist as a part of well-known syndromes such as rubella (64) or neurofibromatosis (20).

Most cases of thoracic and abdominal coarctations and stenosis from Takayasu's arteritis develop during the chronic phase when systemic symptoms are absent. Many patients present with undiagnosed hypertension, and the lesions are suspected from the physical findings and confirmed with aortography. The disease in these patients is usually in an inactive form, and surgical treatment is often effective in relieving symptoms. However, in some patients, particularly the very young, the disease can pursue a fulminant course that is rapidly fatal (18).

Surgical techniques used in treating lesions of the type II variety primarily include the use of bypass grafts for diffuse disease or multiple obstructions and patch angioplasty if there is a single, discrete area of stenosis.

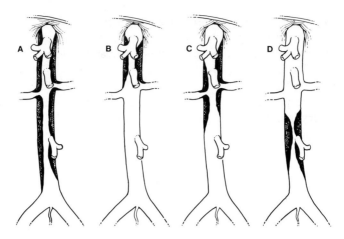

FIG. 9. Patterns of stenosis in the abdominal aorta in Takayasu's disease.   **A**: Diffuse narrowing of the entire abdominal aorta with bilateral renal artery stenosis.   **B**: Proximal stenosis (coarctation) of the abdominal aorta.   **C**: Mid-abdominal aorta stenosis (coarctation) with bilateral renal artery stenosis.   **D**: Distal abdominal aorta stenosis (coarctation).

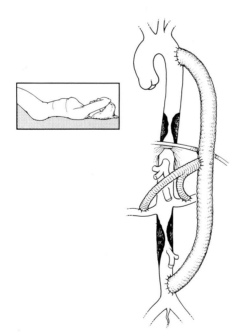

FIG. 10. Techniques for surgical repair of combined stenosis (coarctation) of the descending thoracic and abdominal aorta. The descending aorta is exposed through a left anterolateral thoracotomy, and the abdominal aorta is exposed through a separate flank incision. Visceral branch obstructions can also be bypassed with this exposure.

Patients with diffuse stenosis involving the thoracoabdominal aorta often require a bypass graft extending from the proximal descending thoracic aorta to the distal abdominal aorta (Fig. 10). The preferred surgical technique involves using a left thoracotomy incision for the proximal anastomosis and a left flank incision to expose the distal abdominal aorta in its retroperitoneal position. If mesenteric and/

or renal artery reconstruction is also necessary, separate grafts from the aortic prosthesis can be used to bypass the visceral branch obstructions.

An alternate technique which can be used in treating patients with complex thoracoabdominal obstructions involves the use of a bypass from the ascending aorta to the abdominal aorta. The advantage of this approach is that the entire procedure may be performed through a midline incision extended as a median sternotomy. Entry into the pleural spaces is thus avoided, and the midline approach gives the surgeon a greater degree of flexibility in treating multiple areas of obstruction (Fig. 11).

Short segmental lesions in the descending thoracic or supraceliac abdominal aorta can often be treated by patch aortoplasty or by resection of the diseased segment and replacement with an interposition graft (Fig. 12). It is, however, of paramount importance in utilizing either of these techniques that there must not be active aortitis present at the site of the suture line. The risk of suture dehiscence and subsequent false aneurysm formation is significant if sutures are placed in an area with active inflammation present.

Renovascular hypertension is common in these patients, and a significant number require some type of renal artery reconstruction or bypass procedure. In Kimoto's series (35), 22 of 27 patients with renovascular hypertension had aortitis as the etiology. Figure 13 illustrates the surgical techniques which can be used in reconstructing or bypassing occlusive lesions in the renal arteries. These techniques are similar to those used in treating renovascular hypertension from other etiologies, such as fibromuscular hyperplasia or arteriosclerosis. Nephrectomy should be per-

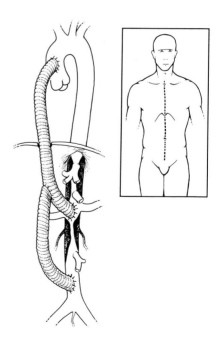

FIG. 11. Alternate technique for surgical repair of combined stenosis (coarctation) of the descending thoracic and abdominal aorta. The entire procedure is performed through a midline incision extended as a median sternotomy. This approach avoids entering the pleural spaces and provides a desirable degree of flexibility when dealing with complex situations.

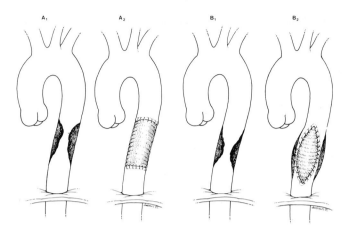

FIG. 12. Short segmental lesions in the descending thoracic aorta may be treated by segmental resection (**A**₁ and **A**₂) or by patch aortoplasty (**B**₁ and **B**₂).

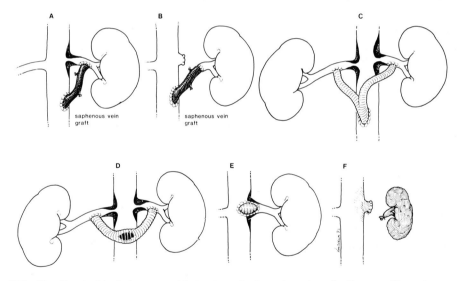

FIG. 13. Surgical techniques used to treat renal artery stenosis. **A**: Bypass with saphenous vein. **B**: Saphenous vein interposition graft. **C,D**: Bypass with prosthetic graft. **E**: Patch aortoplasty. **F**: Nephrectomy for nonfunctioning kidney.

formed when the affected kidney has been demonstrated to be atrophic and functionally diseased, and it is believed to be instrumental in producing hypertension.

The use of prosthetic grafts for bypassing obstructive lesions in the renal arteries secondary to arteriosclerosis is common, and results using this technqiue have generally been good. However, Sunamori et al. (67) and Kimoto (35) have noted that saphenous vein should be used for the bypass conduit whenever possible in treating renovascular obstructive disease caused by arteritis, as they have found a much higher incidence of bypass thrombosis with prosthetic grafts than with saphenous veins.

Type III

Patients with type III lesions have the most severe form of the disease with stenosis and obstructions involving the thoracic and abdominal aorta in addition to the brachiocephalic vessels. Cardiovascular and cerebral ischemic symptoms predominate, and almost all patients with this pattern of disease have hypertension. Visceral artery occlusive disease is also common, leading to symptoms of abdominal angina. Severe stenosis of the abdominal aorta or direct involvement of the iliac or femoral arteries can produce claudication in the lower extremities.

Patients with this form of disease offer an immense challenge to the vascular surgeon. The objective in treating these patients is to restore adequate circulation to ischemic tissue before loss of organ function occurs. Because of the extensive nature of this pattern of disease, the surgical treatment must often be staged with two or more operative procedures being necessary to treat all the involved areas. Symptomatic lesions in the brachiocephalic vessels generally should be treated first, as the threat of stroke is always present prior to surgical treatment. After restoring adequate cerebral circulation, lesions in the thoracoabdominal aorta and those involving the visceral branch vessels can be approached surgically.

Surgical techniques used in treating type III lesions are similar to those described and illustrated for treating types I and II. Bypass grafts are used almost exclusively to treat brachiocephalic disease and are also used occasionally, with resection and graft interposition, for treating thoracoabdominal and visceral branch lesions. Multiple grafts to the iliac, mesenteric, and renal vessels are sometimes needed to preserve organ function (Fig. 14).

Type IV

Dilatation and aneurysm formation of the aorta and its branches characterize type IV Takayasu's disease. It is the least common type encountered and is often found in association with stenotic and occlusive lesions as seen in types I, II, and III.

Aneurysms result from destruction of the supporting structure of the arterial wall by the inflammatory process. The weakening of the arterial wall results in gradual and progressive dilatation until a true aneurysm is formed. Dissecting aneurysm in this disease is uncommon.

Many aneurysms, especially those involving the visceral branches, are asymptomatic and are often discovered during total arteriographic evaluation of patients with coexisting symptomatic occlusive lesions or with undiagnosed hypertension. Aneurysmal dilatation of the ascending aorta can produce aortic regurgitation, and patients may present with symptoms of congestive heart failure. Aneurysms involving the brachiocephalic vessels may cause compression on surrounding structures such as the trachea, esophagus, or recurrent laryngeal nerve resulting in

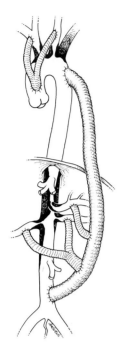

FIG. 14. Surgical approach to treating complex (type III) lesions. Brachiocephalic lesions are treated first utilizing a bypass graft from the ascending aorta to both carotid arteries. At a second operation, stenoses of the abdominal aorta and visceral arteries are bypassed.

dyspnea, dysphagia, or hoarseness. On occasion, aneurysms in this location reach a size sufficient to be palpated in the neck. Although most uncomplicated aneurysms from Takayasu's arteritis are clinically asymptomatic, sudden rupture resulting in death can occur at any time once a true aneurysm is established. Pokrovsky and Tsyneshkin reported two patients with ruptured aneurysms from Takayasu's arteritis, one involving the left subclavian artery that was successfully repaired and another in a patient who died following rupture of an abdominal aortic aneurysm (53).

Aneurysms involving the aorta and its major branches are all amenable to surgical resection. Although surgical techniques for treating aneurysms resulting from Takayasu's disease are similar to those used in treating atherosclerotic aneurysms, certain peculiarities of postarteritis aneurysms require special surgical considerations. There is a higher incidence of false aneurysm formation following surgical resection and graft replacement in Takayasu's disease. This occurs because suture lines are placed in areas where active arteritis is present. Although the aorta or branch artery adjacent to the aneurysm may appear normal grossly, there often is microscopic evidence of active arteritis present. As the disease slowly progresses over months or years, the strength of the arterial wall is gradually compromised and the sutures may pull through the wall, leading to dehiscence of the anastomosis and subsequent false aneurysm formation. A surgical technique which we have found beneficial in supplying additional strength to any arterial–prosthetic graft anastomosis is illustrated in Fig. 15. A tubular Dacron graft 8 to 10 mm in diameter

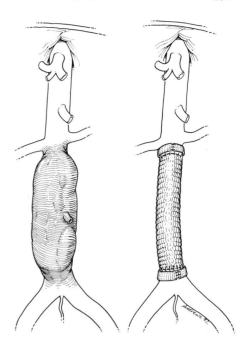

FIG. 15. A: Aneurysm of the infrarenal abdominal aorta from Takayasu's disease. **B**: Aneurysm resected and replaced with prosthetic graft. The proximal and distal suture lines are wrapped with a Dacron graft to prevent dehiscence at each anastomosis.

is used to wrap the proximal and distal anastomoses. We have found that the development of false aneurysms using this "collar" to support the suture line is rare.

As mentioned earlier, it is not uncommon to have stenotic or occlusive lesions of the brachiocephalic or visceral branches occurring along with aneurysms of the aorta. Occlusive lesions that are severe or symptomatic should be bypassed at the same time the aneurysm is repaired. When possible, bypass grafts to aortic branches should be anastomosed to the aortic graft to decrease the number of artery–graft anastomoses and thereby lessen the incidence of false aneurysm formation. Figure 16 illustrates the treatment of an ascending aneurysm causing aortic insufficiency and concomitant innominate artery occlusive disease. The aneurysm and aortic valve are replaced utilizing temporary cardiopulmonary bypass, and the innominate artery obstruction is bypassed with a second graft from the aortic prosthesis. Figure 17 illustrates the treatment of a patient with a distal abdominal aortic aneurysm and unilateral renal artery stenosis.

Coronary Artery Stenosis

Coronary artery involvement in Takayasu's disease is uncommon. Since Frovig and Loken (19) first described coronary artery narrowing in this disease, several reports have documented the clinical and pathological features that occur (8,57,71).

Almost all of the reported cases have documented that the narrowing involves the coronary ostia on the first few millimeters of the main coronary arteries. The

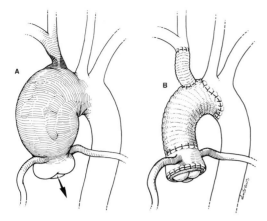

FIG. 16. Aneurysmal form of Takayasu's disease may also coexist with stenotic lesions. **A**: Large aneursym of the ascending aorta with aortic insufficiency and coexisting severe stenosis of the innominate artery. **B**: The ascending aortic aneurysm and aortic valve are replaced utilizing temporary cardiopulmonary bypass. The innominate artery obstruction is bypassed with a second graft from the aortic prosthesis.

FIG. 17. **A**: Aneurysm of the infrarenal abdominal aorta with right renal artery stenosis. **B**: Aneurysm is resected and replaced with a prosthetic graft; the renal artery lesion is bypassed with a second graft from the aortic prosthesis.

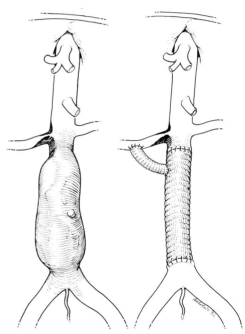

narrowing results from an extension into the coronary arteries of the processes of intimal proliferation, contraction, and fibrosis of the media and adventitia that affects the ascending aorta. The coronary arteries distal to this proximal obstruction are almost always of normal caliber and do not manifest arteritis.

Clinically, patients with coronary artery involvement may show symptoms of classical angina pectoris; however, a significant number of patients present initially with symptoms related to brachiocephalic, renal artery, or aortic obstructions. In a review of 16 patients with coronary artery narrowing from Takayasu's disease reported by Cipriano et al. (8), only 25% had chest pain as the presenting symptom.

The first indication that the coronary arteries are diseased might be a myocardial infarction, congestive heart failure, or sudden death.

The fact that the distal coronary arteries are normal makes these patients ideal candidates for coronary bypass surgery. The operation is effective in relieving myocardial ischemia and should be performed as soon as possible once the diagnosis of significant occlusive coronary disease is documented. Delay in surgical treatment of these patients, particularly those with ostial narrowing of the left coronary artery, can result in sudden death from myocardial infarction or arrhythmia (7).

MYCOTIC ANEURYSM

In 1885 William Osler first used the term "mycotic aneurysm" to describe aneurysms that resulted from nonsyphilitic bacterial infection of the arterial wall (51). These aneurysms were much more common prior to the era of antibiotics and often were caused by septic emboli from bacterial endocarditis (66). Although the incidence of mycotic aneurysms has decreased significantly over the past few decades, they are not rare. They may occur in patients of all ages and can affect any systemic artery, giving rise to a wide spectrum of clinical manifestations.

Finseth and Abbot (17) have classified mycotic aneurysms according to their etiology. Primary mycotic aneurysms arise from direct extension from a surrounding area of suppuration, trauma, or infection or may result indirectly from lymphatic spread from an area of cellulitis or abscess. Secondary mycotic aneurysms occur from septic embolization of infected vegetations that lodge intraluminally in peripheral arteries. Cryptic mycotic aneurysms are those that arise without a known cause but are believed to occur following a prior episode of bacteremia or septicemia, with the infecting organisms entering the arterial wall either through an atherosclerotic defect in the endothelial lining or through the vasa vasorum. Once formed, mycotic aneurysms are associated with morbidity from continued sepsis or distal embolization and a high mortality from rupture. Emergency surgical intervention therefore should be instituted once the diagnosis is confirmed.

In many instances systemic illness or anatomical abnormalities predispose patients to the development of mycotic aneurysms. Patients with diabetes mellitus or those who are receiving chronic steroid treatment for various systemic diseases are particularly susceptible to developing infections which might give rise to mycotic aneurysms. Bacterial endocarditis occurring on abnormal valves and bacterial infection on cardiac valve prostheses are likely to cause septic emboli and mycotic aneurysm formation. Coarctation of the aorta is associated with mycotic aneurysm formation (1,15,62), the aneurysm occurring most often just distal to the coarcted segment. Arteries with severe atherosclerosis are also susceptible to the development of cryptic mycotic aneurysms (13,17).

Although a wide variety of pathogens have been associated with mycotic aneurysms, the organisms most commonly cultured are *Staphylococcus aureus*, *Escherichia coli*, *Streptococcus viridans*, *Pseudomonas*, and *Salmonella* (4,17,47,54). Failure to identify a causative organism is not uncommon, however, and in one series blood cultures were negative in almost half the cases reported (47).

Clinical Manifestations and Diagnosis

Although mycotic aneurysms may arise in any artery, the aorta is most often affected (3,47,52). Other vessels commonly involved are the mesenteric, intracranial, and popliteal arteries (14).

The clinical manifestations of mycotic aneurysms are related to the symptoms and signs of systemic infection and to the local effects produced by the aneurysm. Fever and leukocytosis are almost always present unless specific antibiotic therapy has been successful in eliminating the causative organisms. A high index of suspicion for the presence of a mycotic aneurysm should exist in patients known to have conditions which predispose to aneurysm formation or who have a general increased susceptibility to infection. Patients with coarctation of the aorta who develop signs of sepsis should be evaluated for the presence of a mycotic aneurysm. Patients with congenital or acquired valvular heart disease who develop endocarditis or those who develop prosthetic valve endocarditis should be suspected of having a mycotic aneurysm if appropriate localizing signs appear.

The diagnosis of a mycotic aneurysm arising in a peripheral artery can usually be made clinically. The presence of a tender, pulsatile mass in the popliteal or antecubital space in a patient with signs of sepsis is strong evidence for a popliteal or brachial artery mycotic aneurysm. The diagnosis of mycotic aneurysms involving the thoracic aorta or brachiocephalic vessels can be more difficult to make, and other studies are often necessary to confirm the diagnosis. Chest or back pain is common in patients with intrathoracic aneurysms (33). The chest x-ray film may show mediastinal widening or even a discrete, localized mass with an aneurysm of the ascending or descending aorta. Tracheal deviation on the chest radiograph is common with larger aneurysms. An aneurysm of the abdominal aorta may be palpated as a pulsatile mass. Involvement of the splenic, hepatic, mesenteric, or renal arteries may present as nonspecific abdominal pain without a palpable abdominal mass. Hemoperitoneum can occur with rupture of visceral artery aneurysms (33). Hepatic artery involvement may cause jaundice and hematobilia (65). Renal artery aneurysms may cause hematuria (9) and hypertension (33), and splenic artery aneurysms may present as splenic or subphrenic abscesses (30).

Angiography should be performed in all patients suspected of having a mycotic aneurysm to confirm the diagnosis, establish the status of the circulation distal to the aneurysm, and aid in the design of the operation. These aneurysms usually appear as saccular projections arising eccentrically from one wall of the vessel. Arteriography occasionally reveals the presence of multiple aneurysms that were not previously suspected.

Treatment

Once the diagnosis of a mycotic aneurysm is confirmed, all patients should be placed on high doses of antibiotics appropriate for the offending pathogen. If positive blood cultures cannot be obtained prior to surgery, an antibiotic with a wide spectrum of activity should be chosen to decrease the risk of distal embolization of viable vegetations.

The goal of surgical treatment is complete removal of the infected aneurysm and preservation of the distal circulation. Aneurysms involving small peripheral vessels, e.g., the posterior tibial artery, can be resected and the artery ligated without compromise to the distal circulation. Aneurysms of visceral or medium-sized arteries should be completely resected and vascular continuity restored with either an autogenous saphenous vein graft or a Dacron graft.

Mycotic Aneurysms of the Aorta

Mycotic aneurysms of the aorta are severe, life-threatening lesions that require urgent surgical treatment once the diagnosis is made. These aneurysms have a propensity for early rupture, particularly when the causative organism is virulent. When rupture occurs prior to surgical intervention, the mortality approaches 100% (33,47).

Mycotic aneurysms involving the thoracic aorta present a major challenge to thoracic surgeons. The two problems which must be overcome with these lesions are complete removal of the aneurysm along with any infected segment of aortic wall and restoration of blood flow in the aorta distal to the aneurysm.

Surgical techniques used to treat mycotic aneurysms in the thoracic aorta include patch angioplasty, segmental resection with prosthetic graft interposition, and resection with creation of a bypass graft. Small saccular mycotic aneurysms of the ascending aorta can often be managed by patch aortoplasty or by segmental resection with the use of temporary cardiopulmonary bypass support. Although placement of a prosthetic patch or graft into a potentially contaminated area should be avoided whenever possible, lesions in the ascending aorta or transverse arch are not amenable to alternative forms of surgical treatment. The basic surgical principle of excising all infected tissue and attempting to make the wound as "clean" as possible prior to restoring aortic continuity must be paramount at the time of operation. When cultures obtained at the time of surgery reveal the causative pathogen, high doses of an appropriate antibiotic should be started and continued well into the recovery period.

Mycotic aneurysms occurring at the site of a coarctation or in other segments of the descending thoracic aorta can be treated using several surgical techniques. If appropriate antibiotic therapy is effective in alleviating active infection, elective aneurysm resection and repair of the coarctation with a prosthetic graft is often possible. It is important to note, however, that there is a 75% incidence of aneurysmal rupture during the period of active infection and that the mortality of emergency surgery in this setting is 62% (62). Waiting for bacteriological sterilization imparts a high risk of aneurysmal rupture; therefore once the diagnosis is established, operative treatment should usually be instituted.

When active infection is present in or around the aneurysm, the risk of an interposition graft becoming infected is significant. Under these circumstances, some type of extra-anatomical conduit should be utilized to bypass the infected aneurysmal segment. A technique favored by some (5,11,13,42) is the creation of an axillofemoral bypass using a prosthetic graft. After establishing flow through the graft, the chest is opened and the aneurysm resected. The proximal and distal ends of the aorta are debrided to healthy tissue and then oversewn. When the patient recovers following successful antibiotic therapy, usually weeks to months later, elective anatomical aortic reconstruction can be performed.

An alternate technique which we have utilized with success is the creation of a bypass from the ascending aorta to the supraceliac abdominal aorta (70). This technique also allows for placement of the graft in a noninfected site. A large-caliber prosthetic graft can be used for the bypass, obviating the need for further aortic reconstruction, as is usually the case with axillofemoral grafts. The incidence of graft thrombosis is also much less than with an axillofemoral bypass. After the ascending aorto-abdominal-aorta bypass is created, the mycotic aneurysm in the descending aorta is resected and the ends of the aorta closed.

Mycotic aneurysm of the abdominal aorta is a serious disorder. Because this lesion usually results in rapid destruction of the aortic wall, rupture of the aneurysm with fatal hemorrhage often occurs before the diagnosis can be made. In a review of 34 mycotic aneurysms reported by Bennett and Cherry, rupture of the aneurysm occurred in 79% of the cases prior to surgical intervention and was uniformly fatal (4).

Prior to widespread use of antibiotics, most mycotic abdominal aneurysms were believed to result from septic emboli from bacterial endocarditis. More recently, the etiology in the majority of these aneurysms is believed to result from secondary blood-borne infection of a preexisting aneurysm or vessel diseased from atherosclerosis. Of the 13 cases of mycotic abdominal aneurysms reported by Mundth et al. in 1969, none were associated with bacterial endocarditis (47); and among the 34 patients reported by Bennett and Cherry in 1967, only 9% resulted from bacterial endocarditis (4). Thus a transient bacteremia from any cause may result in secondary bacterial invasion of a preexisting diseased vessel, leading to the formation of a mycotic aneurysm.

Whereas peripheral mycotic aneurysms are associated with bacterial organisms frequently seen with bacterial endocarditis, the bacteriology of abdominal mycotic aneurysms is different. *Salmonella* was found to be the causative pathogen in 35% of the cases reported by Bennett and Cherry (4) and in 44% of the aortic mycotic aneurysms reported by Mundth et al. (47). Apparently, the *Salmonella* organism has a distinct predilection for diseased arteries (4,61,69). Other pathogens which have been reported include *Staphylococcus, E. coli, Bacillus proteus, Streptococcus, Enterococcus*, and *Pneumococcus*. Once the infection is established, destruction of the arterial wall is rapid, leading to early aneurysm rupture (47).

Clinical manifestations of mycotic aortic aneurysms are often vague or obscure. Fever and leukocytosis are always present, but positive blood cultures can be obtained in only about 50% of the cases. Early rupture is common and is associated with a high mortality rate (13,47). In over half of the reported cases, the aneurysm could not be palpated prior to rupture. Therefore abdominal pain in the presence of fever and palpable mass should immediately suggest a mycotic aneurysm, and angiography should be performed as soon as possible to confirm the diagnosis.

Successful therapy is contingent on a prompt diagnosis and early surgery before the aneurysm ruptures. When rupture occurs prior to surgical treatment, the mortality approaches 100%. The importance of giving massive doses of antibiotics prior to surgery has been stressed (13,47). When the causative pathogen has been identified preoperatively, high doses of an antibiotic specific for the bacteria cultured should be given. When no organisms have been cultured, massive doses of a broad-spectrum antibiotic should be started.

The goal of surgery should be complete excision of the aneurysm and all infected tissue surrounding the aneurysm while preserving or restoring blood flow distally with the use of either an anatomical or extra-anatomical bypass. The extra-anatomical axillofemoral bypass, as initially described by Blaisdell and Hall (5) and Louw (42) in 1962, is probably the surgical technique most widely used to treat mycotic aneurysms of the infrarenal abdominal aorta. It was initially devised as an alternative means of aortofemoral reconstruction in debilitated patients thought to be too sick for major abdominal vascular surgery. The technique was subsequently used to treat patients who developed prosthetic aortic graft infections and in those with mycotic aortic aneurysms. The operation is simple and can be performed under local anesthesia. The bypass can be constructed through clean tissue prior to aneurysm resection. Successful treatment using this technique has been reported in a number of series (5,11,42).

Although enthusiasm for the axillofemoral bypass remains high, there are problems and complications associated with the procedure. Richardson and McDowell (56) reported a 50% incidence of graft thrombosis after 24 months. Late graft infection is another complication. However well planned the procedure might be, emergency circumstances and changing clinical situations can lead to cross-contamination and subsequent graft infection.

Alternate methods of treating these lesions include the use of bypass grafts from the suprarenal abdominal aorta or ascending aorta to the iliac arteries (Fig. 18). The aneurysm is resected and all infected tissues are debrided prior to insertion of the bypass graft. Every attempt is made to place the new graft in a clean, uncontaminated location to reduce the possibility of late graft infection. There have been some reported cases of mycotic aneurysms being successfully treated with prosthetic interposition grafts (47). James and Gillespie (31) reported a remarkable case in which a mycotic aneurysm involving the abdominal aorta and four visceral arteries was successfully resected and treated with an aortic interposition graft with side branches to the four visceral arteries. The patient was well and free from infection 1 year after surgery. It appears that in some patients placement of a prosthetic graft into a contaminated, but not grossly infected, site is successful and that late graft infections do not necessarily occur. The virulence of the offending pathogen and the sensitivity to antibiotic therapy must also play a significant role in the success of these procedures.

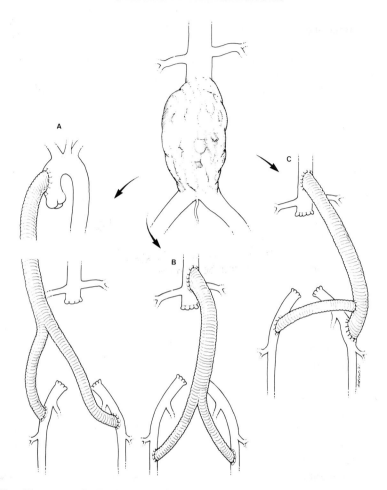

FIG. 18. Alternate methods of treating a mycotic aneurysm of the abdominal aorta. **A**: Bypass from the ascendiing aorta to both external iliac arteries. **B,C**: Bypass from the suprarenal abdominal aorta to both external iliac arteries.

SYPHILITIC AORTITIS

Although the incidence of syphilis has declined significantly since the discovery of penicillin, the disease is not uncommon and still accounts for a significant percentage of inflammatory lesions affecting the aorta. The fundamental lesion of cardiovascular syphilis is aortitis. The inflammatory response results from invasion of the aortic wall by *Treponema pallidum*. The spirochetes localize in the aortic wall early following the primary infection. They are found initially in the adventitia but eventually enter the media of the aortic wall via the lymphatics surrounding the vasa vasorum. Necrosis of the elastic fibers and connective tissue in the aortic media results from obliterative endarteritis of the vasa vasorum. The intima ultimately thickens over the areas of medial necrosis with intervening segments of wrinkling, giving the characteristic "tree-bark" appearance in the late stages of the disease.

Cardiovascular manifestations of syphilis can be grouped into five categories: uncomplicated syphilitic aortitis, syphilitic aortic aneurysm, syphilitic aortic valvulitis with aortic insufficiency, syphilitic coronary ostial stenosis, and syphilitic myocarditis.

Uncomplicated Syphilitic Aortitis

Uncomplicated syphilitic aortitis usually appears early following the primary infection and reportedly occurs in 70 to 80% of untreated cases. It is important because it is the precursor of the lethal and symptomatic complications of cardiovascular syphilis. If the disease is adequately treated during this stage, progression does not occur and the later development of severe cardiovascular complications is avoided. If the disease is unrecognized or if treatment is inadequate, the aortitis remains active, forming the basis for the later development of complications. Approximately 10% of patients with untreated syphilitic aortitis develop significant cardiovascular complications (10).

The ascending aorta and transverse aortic arch are the two areas most commonly affected by syphilitic aortitis. It is thought that the predilection for the two sites results from the rich lymphatic networks found in these two aortic segments (32). The descending thoracic aorta is less commonly affected, and involvement of the abdominal aorta, especially the infrarenal segments, is rare. The affinity for aortitis to affect the proximal aorta often leads to secondary involvement of the coronary ostia and aortic valve leaflets.

Syphilitic aortitis is a disease which can be treated successfully if an accurate diagnosis is made early and appropriate antibiotic therapy is instituted. With adequate medical therapy, the disease can be arrested and progression does not occur. When patients go untreated or are treated inadequately, late cardiovascular complications can occur, i.e., aortic aneurysm, aortic valvular insufficiency, and coronary ostial stenosis. Surgical treatment should be considered when any of these late complications becomes manifest.

Syphilitic Aortic Aneurysm

The development of an aortic aneurysm following syphilitic aortitis is a serious disorder. The time from onset of the primary infection to the formation of an aneurysm may vary from 15 to 30 years. These aneurysms can occur anywhere in the aorta but most commonly are found in the ascending aorta or transverse aortic arch. In an autopsy series of 40 patients with 51 syphilitic aortic aneurysms reported by Heggtveit (23), over half of the aneurysms were located in the ascending aorta or transverse arch. Most syphilitic aneurysms are saccular; less commonly, fusiform aneurysms result from generalized dilatation in the involved aortic segment.

Clinical Manifestations and Diagnosis of Syphilitic Aortic Aneurysms

Clinical symptoms result from compression by the aneurysm on surrounding structures. A large aneurysm of the ascending aorta may compress the pulmonary artery, superior vena cava, or right bronchus with symptoms referable to the obstructed structure. If the aneurysm expands laterally, it may extend into the right hemithorax and reach an enormous size before dyspnea occurs from compression of surrounding lung parenchyma. Ascending aneurysms can also expand anteriorly, eventually eroding into the sternum or deforming the chest wall. Aneurysms of the transverse arch may impinge on the trachea, esophagus, or recurrent laryngeal nerve resulting in stridor, dyspnea, dysphagia, hoarseness, and pain. Aneurysms in the descending aorta may cause compression and atelectasis of surrounding lung parenchyma, or they may cause pain from impingement on nerve roots or erosion of vertebrae.

The diagnosis of a thoracic aneurysm can be suspected from the plain chest radiograph and confirmed with arteriography or computed tomography. The chest roentgenogram reveals a widened mediastinum. Most ascending aneurysms are seen as a mass projecting to the right side of the mediastinal silhouette (Fig. 19); descending aneurysms more commonly project to the left. Linear calcifications in the aneurysm wall are common but are not diagnostic for syphilitic aneurysms (24).

Computed tomography reveals the aneurysm, but aortography should be performed to confirm the diagnosis, define the extent of the aneurysm, and aid in the design of the operation. In addition, the presence of concomitant aortic insufficiency

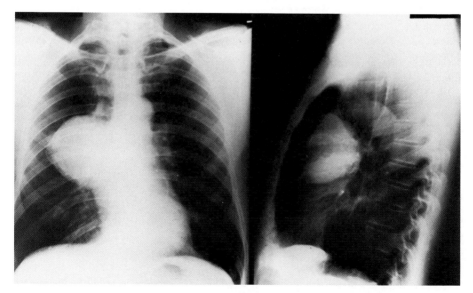

FIG. 19. Posteroanterior and lateral chest radiographs revealing a large syphilic aneurysm of the ascending aorta. Fine linear calcifications can be seen in the wall of the aneurysm.

or obstructive coronary artery disease should be assessed in all patients undergoing aortography.

Once a syphilitic aneurysm is formed, its course is one of progressive enlargement until it either produces symptoms from compression on surrounding structures or death from rupture. As the aneurysm gradually enlarges, the thin fibrous wall becomes weaker, increasing the risk of rupture. Of the 40 patients with syphilitic aneurysms reported by Heggtveit (23), aneurysmal rupture with fatal hemorrhage occurred in 35% (14 patients). Once the diagnosis is confirmed, surgery should be recommended for most patients.

Operative treatment for aneurysm of the ascending aorta involves resecting the aneurysmal segment and restoring continuity with a fabric tube graft. The operation is performed with the use of temporary cardiopulmonary bypass (Fig. 20). If significant aortic valvular insufficiency is also present, valvuloplasty or replacement of the diseased valve with a prosthetic valve should be performed at the same time. If the aortitis has resulted in coronary ostial stenosis or if atherosclerotic coronary artery occlusive disease is present, coronary bypass grafting should also be considered.

Results following surgery are generally good. In a series from our institution, 83 patients underwent surgery for ascending aneurysms of various etiologies with a hospital mortality of 9% (34).

Aneurysm of the transverse aortic arch presents a formidable surgical challenge. Our present technique for arch resection involves the use of cardiopulmonary bypass, moderate systemic hypothermia (26° to 24°C) and temporary circulatory arrest. We have used this technique in 40 patients with an operative mortality of 10%.

Syphilitic Aortic Valvular Insufficiency

Gradual enlargement of the aortic root following syphilitic aortitis can result in dilatation of the aortic valve annulus. As the annulus dilates, the commissures widen. With sufficient dilatation, the leaflets no longer coapt, leading to regurgitation through the valve. Other pathological changes that can occur are thickening and rolling of the edges of the leaflets. Calcification in the leaflets usually does not occur unless there is also underlying rheumatic disease present. Coronary ostial stenosis and aortic aneurysm can also coexist.

A mild to moderate degree of aortic insufficiency can usually be tolerated for years, and medical treatment is generally successful. Prosthetic valve replacement should be reserved for patients with more significant aortic insufficiency, but surgery should be performed prior to the development of heart failure.

Coronary Ostial Stenosis

Extension of the syphilitic process in the ascending aorta can lead to encroachment on the coronary ostia and can result in ostial stenosis. Coronary ostial stenosis occurred in 29% of the cases of syphilitic aortitis reported by Heggtveit (23). This

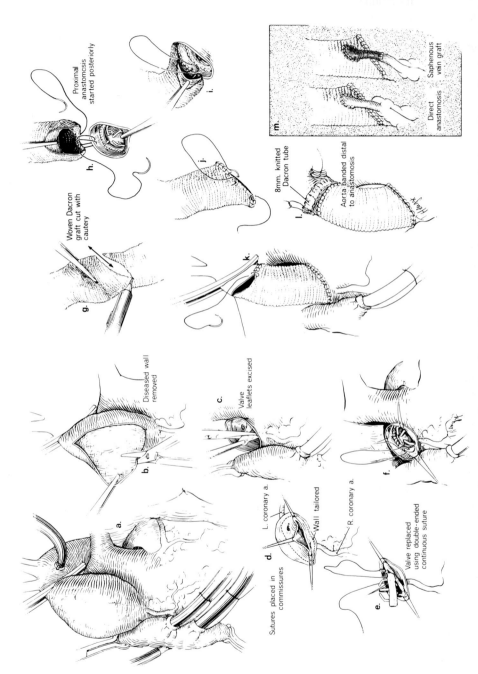

FIG. 20. Technique for resection and replacement of an ascending aortic aneurysm and aortic valve using temporary cardiopulmonary bypass.

process occurs gradually and is often associated with aortic insufficiency. Angina pectoris occurs when the stenosis is severe enough to result in myocardial ischemia.

Surgical treatment should focus on bypassing the obstructed coronary arteries with saphenous vein grafts, often in conjunction with aortic valve replacement.

OTHER FORMS OF AORTITIS

Although the majority of cases with clinically significant aortitis result from Takayasu's disease, syphilis, and mycotic aneurysms, aortitis may occur as a part of the clinical manifestations in other diseases of known and unknown etiology. In most instances the vascular involvement is usually incidental to other major clinical manifestations of the disease, and severe vascular complications are rare. At times, however, these lesions assume clinical importance and may require surgical treatment.

Aortitis can occur with rheumatic fever. Pathologically, the vascular lesion is a true panaortitis involving the adventitia, media, and intima. Patients with rheumatic aortitis are usually less than 30 years of age, and there is no sex predominance. Any segment of the aorta may be involved, but there is a predilection for severe lesions to occur in the abdominal aorta (16). Large saccular or fusiform aneurysms may develop. Valvular heart disease following rheumatic fever may be severe. Surgery is indicated in patients with significant valvular heart disease or in the rare patient in whom an aortic aneurysm develops.

Aortitis occasionally occurs with rheumatoid arthritis. Histologically, there is distinct intimitis and involvement of the media, but adventitial inflammation is minimal. The aortitis occurs in about 5% of the cases and is associated with rheumatoid spondylitis in men. The aortitis almost always affects the ascending aorta just above the aortic valve, resulting in dilatation of the ascending aorta. With progressive aortic enlargement, a discrete aneurysm may result and aortic insufficiency may occur as the aortic annulus dilates. Surgery is indicated when a true aneurysm is formed or when aortic insufficiency becomes hemodynamically significant.

Giant cell arteritis is a disease that can affect large, medium, or small arteries. The aortitis which develops usually occurs in patients over 50 years of age, and there is a female predominance. The entire aorta may be affected. It is the only form of aortitis commonly associated with dissecting aneurysm of the aorta. Corticosteroids are effective in treating the active form of the disease and can usually prevent the development of later severe complications. Surgery is indicated when a dissecting aneurysm develops.

REFERENCES

1. Abbott, M. (1928): Coarctation of the aorta. II. Statistical study and historical retrospective of 200 recorded cases, with autopsy, of stenosis or obliteration of the descending arch. *Am. Heart J.*, 3:392–400.
2. Ask-Upmark, E. (1954): On the "pulseless disease" outside of Japan. *Acta Med. Scand.*, 149:161–178.

3. Bennett, D. (1967): Primary mycotic aneurysms of the aorta. *Arch. Surg.*, 94:758–765.
4. Bennett, D., and Cherry, J. (1967): Bacterial infections of aortic aneurysms: A clinicopathologic study. *Am. J. Surg.*, 113:32–37.
5. Blaisdell, F., and Hall, A. (1963): Axillary femoral bypass for lower extremity ischemia. *Surgery*, 54:563–568.
6. Bloss, R., Duncan, M., Cooley, D., Leatherman, L., and Schnee, M. (1979): Takayasu's arteritis: Surgical considerations. *Ann. Thorac. Surg.*, 27:574–579.
7. Chun, P., Jones, R., Robinowitz, M., David, J., and Lawrence, P. (1980): Coronary ostial stenosis in Takayasu's arteritis. *Chest*, 78:330–331.
8. Cipriano, P., Silverman, J., Perbroth, M., Griepp, R., and Wexler, L. (1977): Coronary arterial narrowing in Takayasu's arteritis. *Am. J. Cardiol.*, 39:744–750.
9. Clark, R., Jacobson, A., and Petty, W. (1975): Intrarenal mycotic (false) aneurysm secondary to staphylococcal septicemia. *Radiology*, 115:421–422.
10. Cole, H. (1937): Cooperative clinical studies in the treatment of syphilis. *JAMA*, 108:1861–1866.
11. Cooke, P., and Efnenfeld, W. (1974): Successful management of mycotic aortic aneurysm: Report of a case. *Surgery*, 75:132–136.
12. Cooley, D., and DeBakey, M. (1955): Resection of the thoracic aorta with replacement by homograft for aneurysms and constrictive lesions. *J. Thorac. Surg.*, 19:66–104.
13. Davies, O., Thorburn, J., and Powell, P. (1978): Cryptic mycotic abdominal aortic aneurysms: Diagnosis and management. *Am. J. Surg.*, 136:96–101.
14. Dickman, F., and Moore, I. (1968): Mycotic aneurysm: A case report of a popliteal mycotic aneurysm. *Ann. Surg.*, 167:590–594.
15. Dotter, C. (1961): Impending aortic rupture: pathogenesis of x-ray signs. *N. Engl. J. Med.*, 265:214–221.
16. Fassbender, H. (1975): *Pathology of Rheumatic Diseases*, pp. 57–62. Springer-Verlag, Berlin.
17. Finseth, F., and Abbot, W. (1974): One stage operative therapy of Salmonella mycotic abdominal aneurysm. *Ann. Surg.*, 179:8–11.
18. Fisher, R., and Corcoran, C. (1952): Congenital coarctation of the abdominal aorta with resultant renal hypertension. *Arch. Intern. Med.*, 89:943–950.
19. Frovig, A., and Loken, A. (1951): Syndrome of obliteration of the arterial branches of the aortic arch due to arteritis. *Acta Psychiatr. Neurol. Scand.*, 26:313–337.
20. Glenn, F., Keefer, C., Speer, S., and Dotter, T. (1952): Coarctation of the lower thoracic and abdominal aorta immediately proximal to celiac axis. *Surg. Gynecol. Obstet.*, 94:561–569.
21. Gotsman, M., Beck, W., and Schrine, V. (1967): Selective angiography in arteritis of the aorta and its major branches. *Radiology*, 88:232–248.
22. Hachiya, J. (1970): Current concepts of Takayasu's arteritis. *Semin. Roentgenol.*, 5:245–259.
23. Heggtveit, H. (1964): Syphilitic aortitis: A clinico-pathologic autopsy study of 100 cases, 1950 to 1960. *Circulation*, 24:346–355.
24. Higgins, C., and Reinke, R. (1974): Nonsyphilitic etiology of linear calcification of the ascending aorta. *Radiology*, 113:609–613.
25. Inada, K., Katsumura, T., Hirai, J., and Sunada, T. (1970): Surgical treatment in the aortitis syndrome. *Arch. Surg.*, 100:220–224.
26. Inada, K., Shimiyu, H., and Yokoyama, T. (1962): Pulseless disease and atypical coarctation of the aorta with special reference to their genesis. *Surgery*, 52:433–443.
27. Isaacson, C. (1961): An idiopathic aortitis in young Africans. *J. Pathol. Bacteriol.*, 81:69–79.
28. Ishikawa, K. (1978): Natural history and classification of occlusive thromboaortopathy (Takayasu's disease). *Circulation*, 57:27–35.
29. Ishikawa, K. (1981): Survival and morbidity after diagnosis of occlusive thromboaortopathy (Takayasu's disease). *Am. J. Cardiol.*, 47:1026–1032.
30. Jacobs, R., Shanser, J., Lawson, D., and Palubinskas, A. (1974): Angiography of splenic abscesses. *AJR*, 12:419–424.
31. James, E., and Gillespie, J. (1977): Aortic mycotic abdominal aneurysm involving all visceral branches: Excision and Dacron graft replacement. *J. Cardiovasc. Surg.*, 18:353–356.
32. Kampmeier, R., and Morgan, H. (1952): The specific treatment of syphilitic aortitis. *Circulation*, 5:771–778.
33. Kaufman, S., White, R., Harrington, D., Bartts, K., and Siegelman, S. (1978): Protean manifestations of mycotic aneurysms. *AJR*, 131:1019–1025.

34. Kidd, J., Reul, G., Cooley, D., Sandiford, F., Kyger, E., and Wukash, D. (1976): Surgical treatment of aneurysms of the ascending aorta. *Circulation [Suppl. 3]*, 54:188–195.
35. Kimoto, S. (1979): The history and present status of aortic surgery in Japan particularly for aortitis syndrome. *J. Cardiovasc. Surg.*, 20:107–126.
36. Kusaba, A., Inokuchi, K., Kiyose, T., and Oka, N. (1973): Carotid reconstruction for Takayasu's (pulseless) disease using open thromboendarterectomy at aortocarotid junction. *Jpn. J. Surg.*, 3:91–97.
37. Lande, A. (1976): Takayasu's arteritis and congenital coarctations of the descending thoracic and abdominal aorta: a critical review. *AJR*, 127:227–233.
38. Lande, A., and Berkmen, U. (1976): Aortitis: pathologic, clinical and arteriographic review. *Radiol. Clin. North Am.*, 14:219–240.
39. Lande, A., and Gross, A. (1972): Total aortography in the diagnosis of Takayasu's arteritis. *AJR*, 116:165–178.
40. Lande, A., and Rossi, P. (1975): The value of total aortography in the diagnosis of Takayasu's arteritis. *Radiology*, 114:297.
41. Lande, A., Bard, R., Bold, P., and Guarnaccia, M. (1978): Aortic arch syndrome (Takayasu's arteritis): Arteriographic and surgical considerations. *J. Cardiovasc. Surg.*, 19:507–593.
42. Louw, J. (1963): Splenic-to-femoral and axillary-to-femoral bypass grafts in diffuse atherosclerotic disease. *Lancet*, 1:140–142.
43. Lupi-Herrera, E., Sanchey, G., Horwitz, S., and Gutierrey, E. (1975): Pulmonary artery involvement in Takayasu's arteritis. *Chest*, 67:69–74.
44. Lupi-Herrera, E., Sanchez-Torres, G., Marcushamer, J., et al. (1977): Takayasu's arteritis: Clinical study of 107 cases. *Am. Heart J.*, 93:94–103.
45. Martorell, F., and Fabre, J. (1944): El sindrome de obliteracion de los troncos supraaorticos. *Med. Clin. (Barc.)*, 2:26–35.
46. Morris, G., DeBakey, M., Cooley, D., and Crawford, E. (1960): Subisthmic aortic stenosis and occlusive disease. *Arch. Surg.*, 80:87–104.
47. Mundth, E., Darling, R., Alvarado, R., Buckley, M., Linton, R., and Austen, W. (1969): Surgical management of mycotic aneurysms and the complications of infection in vascular reconstructive surgery. *Am. J. Surg.*, 117:460.
48. Nakao, K., Ikida, M., Kimata, S., et al. (1967): Takayasu's arteritis: Clinical report of eighty-four cases and immunologic studies of seven cases. *Circulation*, 35:1141–1155.
49. Nako, K., Ikeda, M., Kimata, S., Nutani, H., Miyahara, M., Ishimi, Z., Hashiba, K., Takeda, Y., Ozawa, T., Mitsushita, S., and Kuramochi, M. (1967): Takayasu's arteritis. *Circulation*, 35:1141–1155.
50. Onishi (1908): Quoted by Takayasu, M., ref. 68.
51. Osler, W. (1885): The Gulstonian lectures on malignant endocarditis. *Br. Med. J.*, 1:467–470.
52. Parkhurst, G., and Decker, J. (1955): Bacterial aortitis and mycotic aneurysm of the aorta: A report of twelve cases. *Am. J. Pathol.*, 31:831–835.
53. Pokrovsky, A., and Tsyneshkin, D. (1975): Nonspecific aorto-arteritis. *J. Cardiovasc. Surg.*, 16:181–191.
54. Reichle, R., Tyson, R., Soloff, L., Lautch, E., and Rosmond, G. (1970): Salmonellosis and aneurysm of the distal abdominal aorta. *Ann. Surg.*, 171:219–228.
55. Restrepo, C., Tejeda, C., and Correa, P. (1969): Nonsyphilitic aortitis. *Arch. Pathol.*, 87:1–12.
56. Richardson, J., and McDowell, H. (1977): Extra-anatomic bypass grafting in aortoiliac occlusive disease: Seven-year experience. *South. Med. J.*, 70:1287–1291.
57. Rosen, N., and Gaton, E. (1972): Takayasu's arteritis of coronary arteries. *Arch. Pathol.*, 94:225–229.
58. Sanding, H., and Welin, G. (1961): Aortic arch syndrome with special reference to rheumatoid arteritis. *Acta Med. Scand.*, 170:1–19.
59. Sano, K., Aiba, T., and Saito, I. (1970): Angiography in pulseless disease. *Radiology*, 94:69–74.
60. Savory, W. S. (1856): Case of a young woman in whom the main arteries of both upper extremities and of the left side of the neck were throughout completely obliterated. *Med. Chir. Trans. Lond.*, 39:205–211.
61. Sawer, N., and Whelan, J. (1962): Suppurative arteritis due to Salmonella. *Surgery*, 52:851–859.
62. Schneider, J., Rheuban, K., and Crossby, I. (1979): Rupture of post coarctation mycotic aneurysm of the aorta. *Ann. Thorac. Surg.*, 27:185–190.
63. Shimizu, K., and Sano, K. (1951): Pulseless disease. *J. Neuropathol. Exp. Neurol.*, 1:37–47.

64. Siassi, B., Klyman, G., and Emmanouilides, C. (1970): Hypoplasia of the abdominal aorta associated with the rubella syndrome. *Am. J. Dis. Child.*, 120:476–479.
65. Stack, B., Runkin, J., and Bentley, R. (1968): Hepatic artery aneurysm after staphylococcal endocarditis. *Br. Med. J.*, 2:659–660.
66. Stengel, A., and Wolferth, C. (1923): Mycotic (bacterial) aneurysms of intravascular origin. *Arch. Intern. Med.*, 31:527–554.
67. Sunamori, M., Hatano, R., Yamada, T., Tsukuura, T., Sakamoto, T., Suzuki, T., Murakami, T., Yokokawa, M., and Numano, R. (1976): Aortitis syndrome due to Takayasu's disease: A guideline to the surgical indication. *J. Cardiovasc. Surg.*, 17:443–456.
68. Takayasu, M. (1908): Case with unusual changes of the vessels in the retina. *Acta Soc. Ophthalmol. Jpn.*, 12:554–563.
69. Tillotson, J., and Lerner, M. (1966): Mycotic aneurysm and endocarditis: Two uncommon complications of Salmonella infections. *Am. J. Cardiol.*, 18:267–274.
70. Wukasch, D., Cooley, D., Sandiford, F., Nappi, G., and Reul, G. (1977): Ascending aorta-abdominal aorta bypass: Indications, techniques and report of 12 patients. *Ann. Thorac. Surg.*, 23:442–448.
71. Young, J., Sengupta, A., and Khaja, F. (1973): Coronary arterial stenosis, angina pectoris and atypical coarctation of the aorta due to nonspecific arteritis. *Am. J. Cardiol.*, 32:356–360.

Subject Index